Atlas of Endocrine Diseases

The preparation and publication of this study was supported through the Special Foreign Currency Program of the National Library of Medicine, National Institutes of Health, Public Health Service, U.S. Department of Health, Education and Welfare, Bethesda, Maryland, under an agreement with the Coordinating Commission for Polish–American Scientific Collaboration, Scientific Council to the Minister of Health and Social Welfare, Warsaw, Poland.

The study was published pursuant to an agreement with the National Science Foundation, Washington, D.C., by the Foreign Scientific Publications Department of the National Center for Scientific, Technical and Economic Information

and Economic Information

Warsaw, Poland, 1978

Jerzy Kosowicz

Atlas of Endocrine Diseases

The Charles Press Publishers, Inc.
Bowie, Maryland

Copyright © 1978 by The Charles Press Publishers, Inc., Bowie, Maryland 20715
Library of Congress Cataloging in Publication Data

Kosowicz, Jerzy.
    Atlas of endocrine diseases.

    1. Endocrine glands–Diseases–Atlases. I. Title.
[DNLM: 1. Endocrine diseases–Diagnosis–Atlases
WK17 K86a]
RC649.K67   616.4′07′2   77-21493
ISBN 0-913486-86-8

INTRODUCTION

Most endocrine diseases present characteristic alterations in facial features and general appearance of the patient. In acromegaly, hypopituitarism, thyrotoxicosis, hypothyroidism, adrenogenital syndrome, Cushing's syndrome, eunuchoidism or Turner's syndrome, the patients afflicted with these diseases lose their individual features and gradually assume those characteristic of the disease. Each endocrine disorder produces a striking physical similarity among its sufferers; these changes are so obvious and so characteristic that experienced endocrinologists can make a diagnosis at first glance. Thus, seeing one patient with a given endocrine syndrome greatly facilitates recognition of this syndrome in others.

On the other hand, diagnosis of endocrine diseases is more difficult for general practitioners or medical students who have not previously had the chance to examine patients with these diseases. This is especially true with some of the lesser known endocrine diseases, and there is little probability of seeing every variant. Hence, the first intention of this Atlas is to present variations of endocrine disorders to facilitate rapid recognition of their typical signs and characteristic features.

Due to inhibited perception, deficient intellect and impaired memory, the case history as given by the patients is often vague and incomplete, and many symptoms are ignored. The family does not immediately notice the insidious onset of the disease and the gradual changes in the appearance of the patients, and so, consequently, is of little help in assisting the doctor in his diagnosis. For these reasons hormonal disturbances may remain undiagnosed for several years. Patients with acromegaly are treated for arthritis; an erroneous diagnosis of neurosis or heart disease is frequent in patients suffering from thyrotoxicosis. Patients with hypopituitarism occasionally undergo treatment from anemia because of their striking pallor; and hypothyroid subjects, because of edema, cyanosis, fatigability and electrocardiographic abnormalities, are treated for heart failure.

Thus, of primary importance in diagnosis of endocrine diseases is the awareness and perceptiveness of general practitioners in noticing the slightest signs of these diseases. Hence, dry, coarse skin, hoarseness, slow speech, pallor, lack of axillary hair, swelling of eyelids, stare, coarsening features, pigmentation of scars or a rounded plethoric face should arouse the doctor's suspicion and initiate a detailed interrogation of the patient and subsequent hormonal studies. The recently introduced technique of radioimmunoassay of most hormones permits rapid confirmation of the suspected disease, or its exclusion.

I would like to thank Professor H. L. Sheehan, Liverpool University, for his kindness in reviewing the chapter on hypopituitarism and for his invaluable comments. Dr. Jack Insley, Institute of Child Health, Birmingham University, was kind enough to read the chapter on gonadal dysgenesis and make many useful suggestions. Dr. A. D. Wright, Hammersmith Hospital, London, kindly reviewed the text of the Atlas and offered helpful advice.

Professor M. Gembicki, M.D., Head of the Department of Endocrinology, School of Medicine, Poznań, Poland, allowed me to take full advantage of the vast diagnostic facilities of the Department and kindly shared his knowledge gained from long experience in diagnosis and treatment of thyroid diseases with me.

My colleagues from the above mentioned Department, Dr. S. Sobieszczyk and Dr. W. Kozak, were of great assistance in the daily care of patients; Mrs. J. Porawska, M.A., offered help in radioimmunoassays; Dr. M. Białecki kindly performed chromosome analyses on our patients. I would like to express my sincere thanks to all of them.

I should also like to thank most sincerely those authors, mentioned in the text, by whose courtesy I was able to reproduce the excellent illustrations which were a great contribution to the Atlas.

I am grateful to all the patients who, realizing that their photographs will help in diagnosis and treatment of other patients, kindly consented to publication of these prints.

September 1975   *Jerzy Kosowicz, M.D.*

Chapter 1

THE PITUITARY

I. THE ADENOHYPOPHYSIS

ACROMEGALY

(HYPERSOMATOTROPISM)

Acromegaly is a disease characterized by an excess of growth hormone, causing progressive enlargement of the hands and feet and characteristic changes in the face. The disease affects men and women with equal frequency and usually occurs in the third or fourth decades of life. It is caused by an eosinophilic or chromophobe adenoma of the pituitary, and very rarely by hyperplasia of the eosinophilic cells. The onset is insidious, and the progression of the disease may appear to be intermittent, with periods of stabilization.

Complications such as hypertension with congestive heart failure or cerebral hemorrhages, diabetes, and local complications caused by an expanding pituitary tumor may shorten the life of some patients, while others, despite grotesque appearance and physical disability, survive for decades.

Endocrine Signs and Symptoms

1. Gradual, progressive enlargement of the hands and feet.
2. Change in the facial appearance.
3. Difficulty in mastication due to overbite of the teeth of the lower jaw.
4. Change in the voice to a deeper pitch; slurred speech; loud snoring at night.
5. Excessive perspiration, even in cold weather.
6. Pain in the joints; easy fatigability.
7. Paresthesia in the fingertips that may hinder precision work.
8. Diminished potency in males; menstrual disturbances, amenorrhea and sterility in females.
9. Impaired hearing.
10. Thyroid enlargement.

Fig. 1A. A male patient aged 43, with acromegaly of 12 years duration. Note heavy, stocky build, broad chest, large head, enlarged hands and feet. Serum HGH greatly increased (basal values from 130 to 240 ng/ml).

Fig. 1B. Increased dorsal kyphosis, barrel-like chest.

Fig. 2. Comparison of acromegalic hand with a normal one. The fingers are thick and broad; the hand is heavy.

PLATE 1

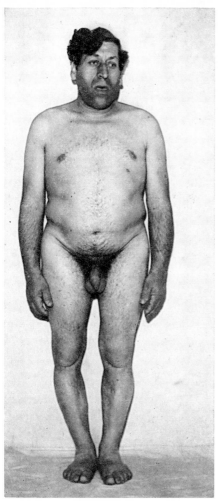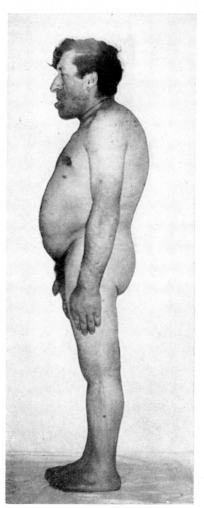

Fig. 1A   Fig. 1B

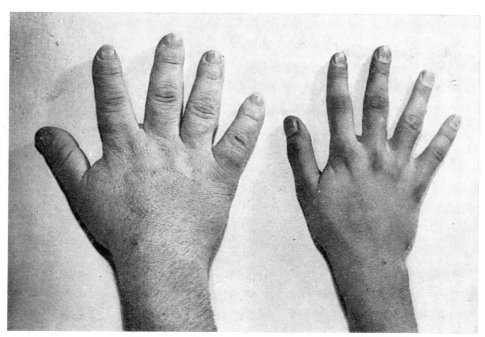

Fig. 2

Neurologic (Local) Manifestations

1. Severe headaches.
2. Impairment of vision, limited visual fields, optic atrophy.

Complications

1. Diabetes mellitus.
2. Hypertension; congestive heart failure.
3. Cerebral hemorrhages.
4. Hypopituitarism in the later stages of acromegaly.
5. Diabetes insipidus.
6. Carpal-tunnel syndrome.

General Appearance

The body becomes heavy, stocky. Attending symptoms include definite muscle hypertrophy, weight increase and chest cavity enlargement with protruding sternum due to the continued growth of the rib cartilages. Male patients experience an excessive growth of hair on the trunk and extremities. The large head, typical acromegalic changes of the face, thick and broad hands and enlarged feet are pathognomonic clinical manifestations.

In some patients kyphosis occurs, resulting in a shortening of the trunk. This gives an illusion of an elongation of the upper extremities, since the hands reach almost to the knees.

Fig. 1. Face of an acromegalic patient with long standing disease. The nose is long and enlarged; the jaw is of huge dimensions.

Fig. 2. A 38-year-old patient with acromegaly. Facial features are coarse, the nose enlarged, the lips swollen, the jaw elongated.

Fig. 3. A 35-year-old acromegalic patient showing hypertrophy of the nose, deep frontal folds, swollen upper eyelids.

Fig. 4. Coarse features of the face, enlarged nose, thick lips, deep skin folds and swollen eyelids in a 60-year-old patient with acromegaly.

PLATE 2

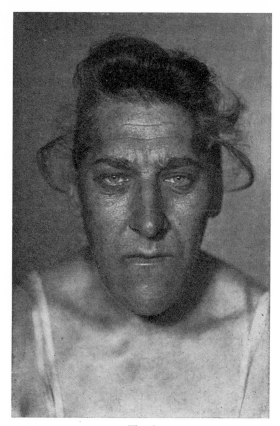

Fig. 1

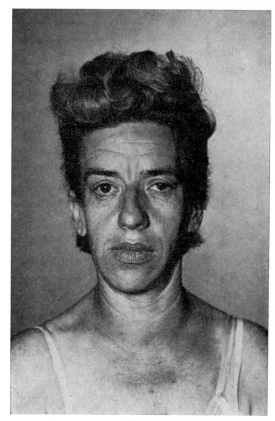

Fig. 2

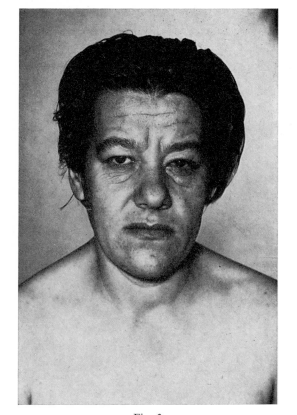

Fig. 3

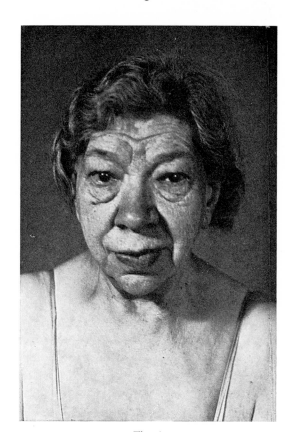

Fig. 4

The Face

The head is very large; the face especially is prominent owing to overgrowth of the facial bones, thickening of the skin and further growth of nose and ear cartilage. Conspicuous acromegalic changes of the face include a protruding, large, thick nose, thick lips, accentuation of the nasolabial folds, marked elongation of the mandible and prominent chin. The contour of the face becomes more oval. In male patients the supraorbital ridges protrude owing to excessive pneumatization of the frontal sinuses. The forehead is furrowed; vertical folds sometimes appear resembling those of a bulldog, hence the term "bulldog scalp." The ears become enlarged.

Following all these changes the face of the male subject assumes a coarse and "villainous" appearance. In female patients the face loses its delicate, feminine features, becomes heavy and assumes a grim, determined expression.

Photographs of the face taken at intervals of several years are helpful in evaluating the progression of the disease.

Fig. 1. Coarsened features, huge nose, thick lips and deep nasolabial and frontal folds in a 58-year-old acromegalic patient.

Fig. 2. Face of an acromegalic patient, aged 49. There is striking coarsening of features, large nose, deep skin folds, thick lips.

Fig. 3. Face of a 30-year-old acromegalic patient shows marked elongation and hypertrophy of the jaw, with folds appearing on the cheeks.

Fig. 4. Acromegalic patient, aged 58. Many deep skin folds on the forehead and cheeks. The nose is bulbous and markedly enlarged.

PLATE 3

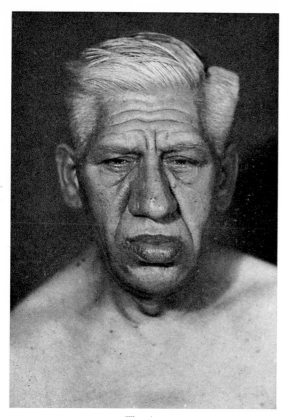

Fig. 1

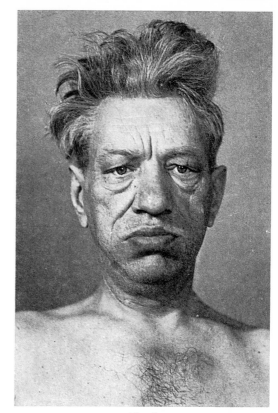

Fig. 2

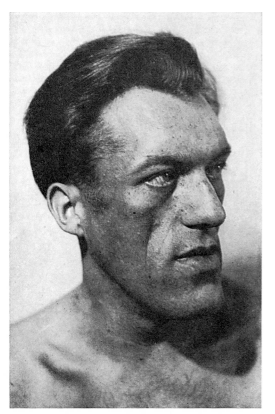

Fig. 3

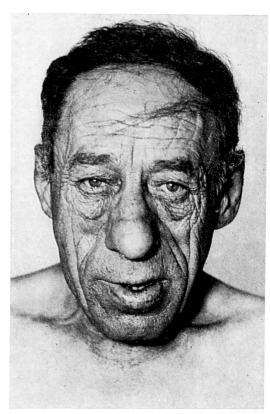

Fig. 4

The Tongue and Teeth

The tongue very frequently becomes enlarged and thickens because of hypertrophy of its muscles. Speech becomes unintelligible, slurred and of a nasal quality; further growth of laryngeal cartilage gives the voice a lower pitch. During sleep the enlarged tongue fills the mouth and hinders respiration causing patients to snore loudly.

The teeth, especially those in the mandible, become widely spaced as the jaw undergoes further growth. The widened interdental spaces and the pressure of the hypertrophied tongue cause the teeth to slope outwards and impair the bite. The elongation of the mandible causes the teeth to protrude beyond those of the upper jaw. This also hinders mastication.

Fig. 1. Note wide interdental spaces, malocclusion. Lower teeth protrude beyond the upper teeth and are obliquely pushed to the front by a thick, large tongue.

Fig. 2. Thickened lips and widely spaced teeth of an acromegalic patient.

Fig. 3. Comparison of an acromegalic mandible to a normal one (artist's rendering). The acromegalic jaw is grossly enlarged, elongated. The neck is long, and there is a heavy articular condyle. The teeth are markedly decayed, widely spaced and slanted obliquely to the front.

Fig. 4. Greatly enlarged, elongated and broadened tongue of an acromegalic patient.

PLATE 4

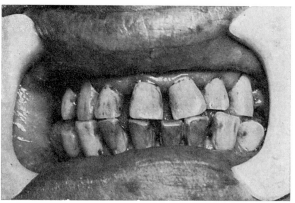

Fig. 1

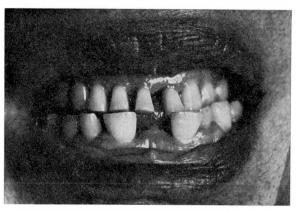

Fig. 2

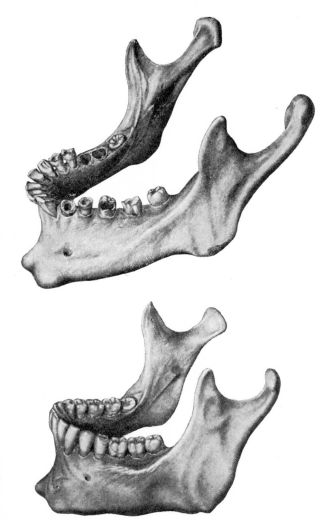

Fig. 3

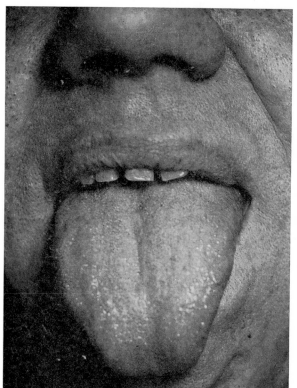

Fig. 4

The Hands

A classic manifestation in acromegaly is the progressive enlargement of the hands and feet. Some patients complain of pains in joints and stiffness in the fingers, especially in the morning hours; other patients experience paresthesia of the fingertips that hinders precision work. On physical examination the hands are enlarged, broad and thick. The spade-like hands of acromegalic patients have thickened, sausage-like fingers. There is usually no impairment of flexion and ability to extend the fingers.

In advanced stages, fingerprints show disruption of the ridges into small fragments. At the onset of the disease this fragmentation is seen only in alternating ridges, but later they are all affected, forming a mosaic pattern.

The Feet

Gradual enlargement of the feet is frequently the first symptom noted by patients, as they require frequent refitting for larger shoes. Women with acromegaly cannot wear ladies' shoes and are often obliged to buy men's shoes. On examination the feet appear broad and enlarged; the big toe especially may reach enormous dimensions.

Fig. 1. Heavy, enlarged hand of an acromegalic patient with long standing disease (*left*) compared to a normal hand. The fingers have markedly thickened and broadened, but their length remains normal.

Fig. 2. A typical acromegalic foot with a huge toe compared to the foot of a normal subject.

Fig. 3. Athletic appearance of a 40-year-old acromegalic patient. Hypertrichosis, hypertrophied muscles, large hands and coarse facial features are seen.

Fig. 4A. Skin on the back of the hand of an acromegalic patient shows accentuation of pores.

Fig. 4B. Same area of the hand, greatly magnified, shows thickening of the skin and deepening of the pores.

PLATE 5

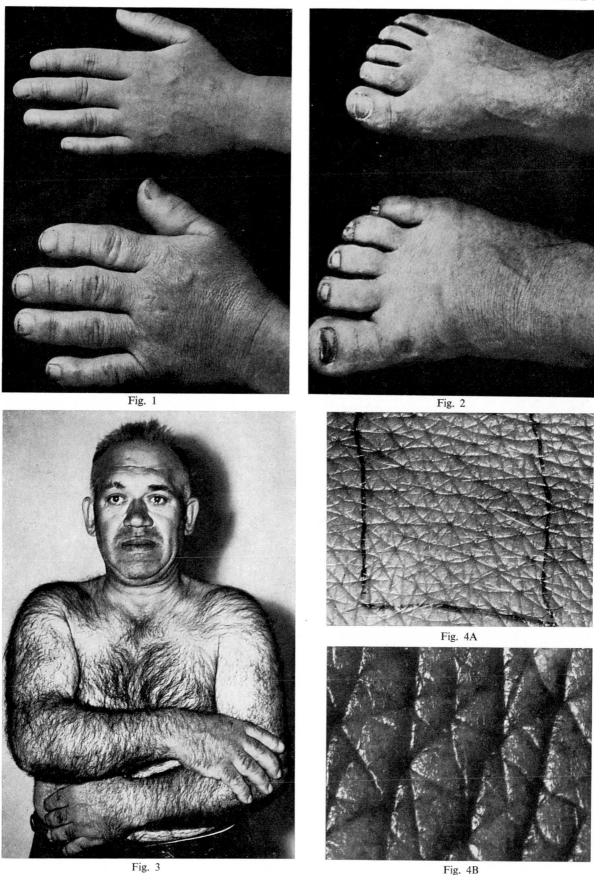

Fig. 1

Fig. 2

Fig. 3

Fig. 4A

Fig. 4B

Roentgen Findings

1. Skull: enlargement of the sella turcica; thinning of the dorsum sellae; flattening of the sphenoid sinuses; enlargement and excessive pneumatization of the frontal sinuses; thickening of the cranial vault; elongation of the mandible.
2. Spine: increased anteroposterior diameter of the vertebral bodies; increased intervertebral spaces.

Figs. 1A and 1B. Skull roentgenograms of male acromegalic patients. The bones of the vault are markedly thickened, the frontal sinuses excessively enlarged and protruding, the sella deepened and enlarged, the mandible elongated with marked progenia. Figs. 2A to 2D. Roentgenograms of the sella turcica in 4 patients with acromegaly. *A*. Enlarged fossa with double floor, thinning of the dorsum, elongated anterior clinoid processes. *B*. Enlarged sella with uneven floor, the dorsum displaced posteriorly, the sphenoidal sinuses flattened. *C*. Deepening of the fossa, the anterior clinoid processes markedly pseudoelongated due to erosion of bone beneath them. *D*. Gross enlargement and ballooning of the sella, disappearance of the sphenoidal sinuses, thinning and posterior displacement of the dorsum.

PLATE 6

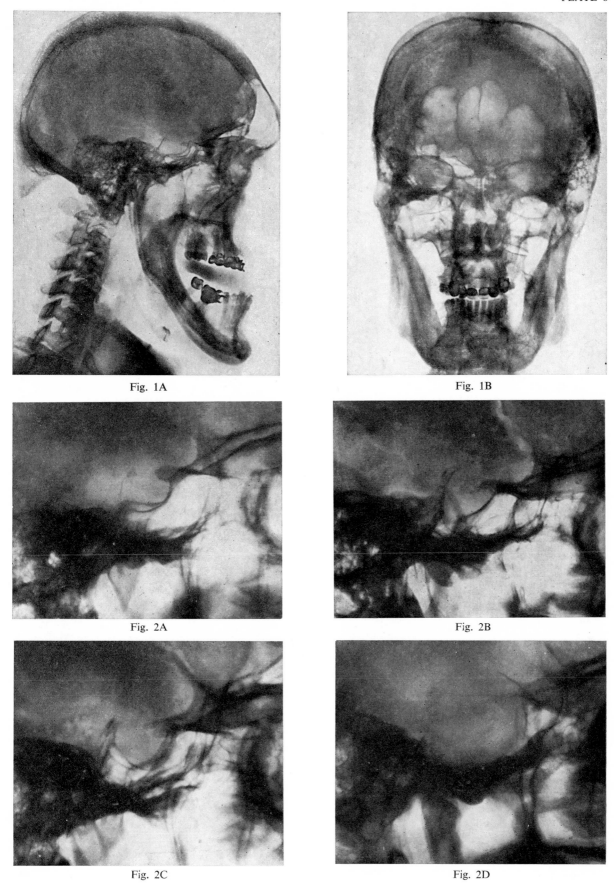

Fig. 1A

Fig. 1B

Fig. 2A

Fig. 2B

Fig. 2C

Fig. 2D

3. Hands: enlargement of the tufts and broadening of the bases of the distal phalanges with formation of exostoses distally; squared metacarpal heads; widening of the joint spaces; increased distance between the metacarpals; thickening of the soft tissues; enlargement of the sesamoid bones of the thumb.
4. Joints: enlargement of the epiphyses; widening of the joint space; accentuation of the muscular insertions. Arthritic changes with pronounced exostoses limiting the joint movements in advanced stages.
5. Calves: increased muscle thickness; decreased thickness of subcutaneous fat.
6. Feet: increased heelpad thickness.

Fig. 1. Roentgenogram of the hand and wrist of a 50-year-old acromegalic patient shows typical changes: mushroom enlargement of the tufts; broadening of the base of the distal phalanges with exostoses; squared metacarpal heads; widening of the articular fissures; widely spaced metacarpals; thickened, soft tissue around the fingers and large sesamoid bones of the thumb; minute cysts in the carpal bones.

PLATE 7

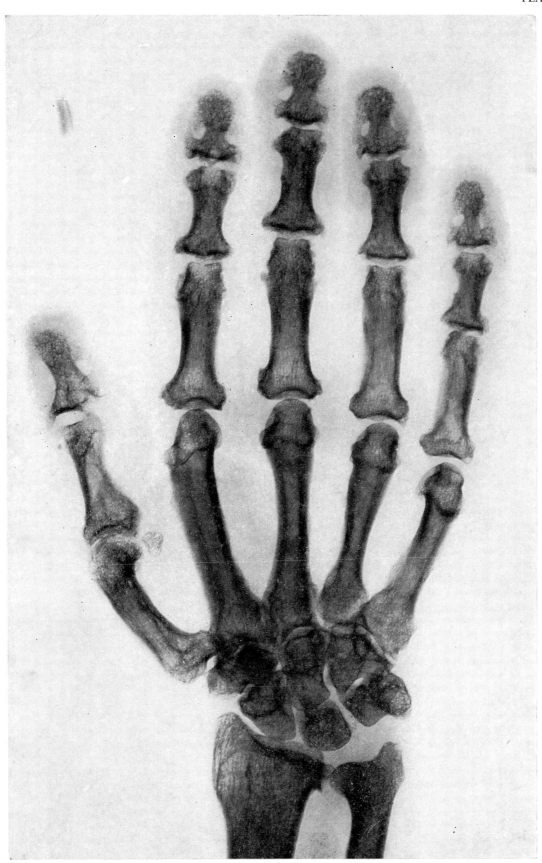

Fig. 1

Laboratory Findings

1. Increased basal serum growth hormone (HGH, GH) concentration.
2. No suppression of elevated serum GH level by glucose administration. In normal subjects, in the first and second hours following ingestion of 100 g glucose, there is an abrupt drop in serum GH concentration to very low levels, while in acromegalic patients the serum GH remains high.
3. Increased serum somatomedin (serum sulfation factor). The serum of acromegalic patients stimulates the incorporation of radiosulfate into cartilages.
4. Increased serum inorganic phosphorus in one third of the cases.
5. Impaired glucose tolerance despite a high serum insulin concentration.
6. Decreased sensitivity to insulin. Larger doses of insulin than normal are required to obtain a hypoglycemic response.
7. Increased urinary hydroxyproline.
8. Increased basal metabolic rate.
9. L-dopa administration leads to a paradoxical drop in serum HGH concentration.
10. TRH stimulation test: increase in serum HGH not observed in control subjects.

Fig. 1. Serum HGH in 43 patients with acromegaly. In the majority of cases serum HGH concentration ranges from 10 to 160 ng/ml, while in normal subjects it is usually between 0 to 7 ng/ml.

Fig. 2. Effects of glucose loading on serum HGH concentration in acromegaly and in control subjects. There is a rapid fall in serum HGH after glucose load in normal subjects, whereas in acromegaly serum HGH remains elevated.

Fig. 3. Serum HGH concentration in response to L-dopa administration (0.5 g orally) in acromegaly and in normal subjects. In normal subjects L-dopa evokes a rise in serum HGH, whereas in acromegaly elevated serum HGH remains unaltered, or there is a paradoxical drop in serum HGH after L-dopa.

PLATE 8

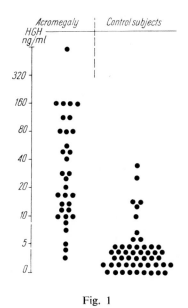

Fig. 1

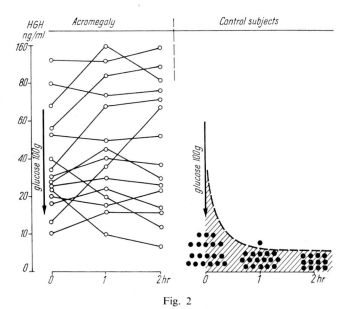

Fig. 2

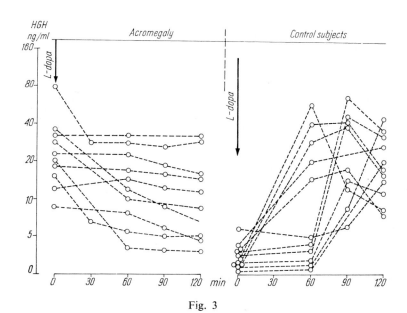

Fig. 3

PITUITARY GIGANTISM

(HYPERSOMATOTROPIC GIGANTISM; ACROMEGALOGIGANTISM)

Gigantism is a rare disease characterized by growth exceeding the average height by more than three standard deviations, i.e., height above 203 cm in males and above 195 cm in females. Two different forms may be distinguished: pituitary gigantism, due to growth hormone excess, and primordial gigantism, dependent on genetic factors.

Pituitary gigantism, a rare disease whose onset occurs in childhood or adolescence at a time when the epiphyses have not yet fused, is caused by excessive growth hormone secretion from a pituitary adenoma, or from hyperplasia of eosinophilic cells. An abnormally rapid spurt in growth is usually noted at about ages 10 to 12 years, and after several years the patients attain gigantic stature. In some patients gonadotropic deficiency may delay puberty and eunuchoid body proportions develop. Despite their huge size and excellent muscle development the patients are weak, easily fatigued and ungainly.

Acromegalic features appear, usually by the third decade. The head is heavy and large; the mandible greatly elongated. There is progressive enlargement of the hands and feet, muscle hypertrophy, hypertrichosis, increased body weight, expansion of the chest and sometimes kyphosis and genu valgum.

The serum growth hormone is greatly increased and even after glucose administration, 100 g per os, there is no drop in growth hormone as is seen in normal subjects. Other laboratory findings typical of acromegaly are also present.

Frontal roentgenograms of the skull show an abnormally large vault and face, huge dimensions of the mandible and excessive development of the frontal sinuses. Lateral roentgenograms reveal an enlargement of the sella turcica with thinning of the dorsum (in cases with pituitary adenoma), pronounced development of the paranasal sinuses, protruding supraorbital ridges, increased thickness of the vault bones. Roentgenograms of the hand show the bones to be greatly elongated and thick, the metacarpals widely spaced, the joint spaces of increased width, the tufts and bases of the distal phalanges broadened, the metacarpal heads squared and the soft tissues of the fingers thickened.

Fig. 1A. General appearance of a 36-year-old pituitary giant. Height 205 cm (81 in.); weight 102 kg. Large head, strong build, hypertrichosis, pronounced varicose veins on the legs. Basal serum HGH 22 ng/ml; no suppression of serum HGH (21, 24 ng/ml) after oral glucose administration.

Fig. 1B. Face of the same pituitary giant showing marked bulging of the forehead, especially at supraorbital ridges, large nose, elongated jaw and deepened labionasal folds.

Fig. 2. Silhouettes of the hands of a healthy man (*left*) and a pituitary giant (*right*). The hand of the giant is much bigger, broader and heavier.

Figs. 3A and 3B. Roentgenograms of the knee joints of a healthy, tall man (height 198 cm) and the pituitary giant (Fig. 1). The knee roentgenogram of the giant (*B*) reveals squared enlarged epiphyses with exostoses at the sites of tendon attachments and definite increase in width of the joint space.

PLATE 9

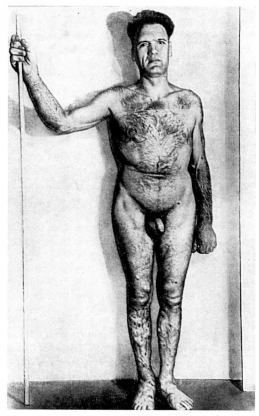

Fig. 1A

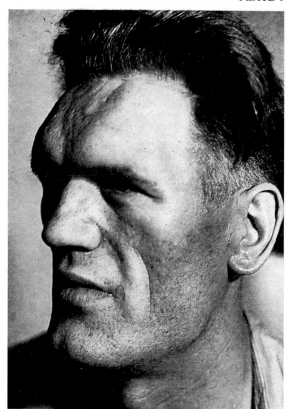

Fig. 1B

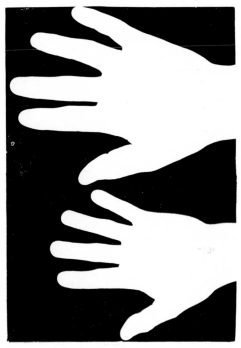

Fig. 2

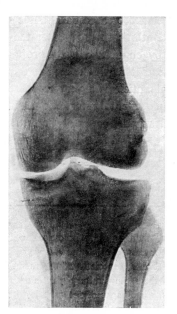

Fig. 3A

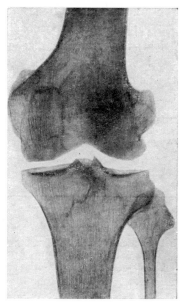

Fig. 3B

CONSTITUTIONAL TALL STATURE

(FAMILIAL TALLNESS; PRIMORDIAL GIGANTISM)

In some races and in some families there is a tendency to excessive height. The growth rate is accelerated from early childhood, but otherwise the subjects do not differ in any way from other people. By puberty some of these subjects have attained excessive height (over 205 cm in males, over 197 cm in females) and may be termed primordial giants. After puberty further growth ceases and sexual development is normal. These tall subjects are of proportional build, physically fit and mentally normal.

Serum growth hormone concentration is normal and decreases rapidly to very low levels following glucose administration.

Roentgenograms of the skull show an increased size (but normal proportions) of the bones; no changes in sella turcica are seen. Roentgenograms of the hand show the bones to be of proportionally increased dimensions, but acromegalic changes such as increased joint spaces, enlargement and squaring of the epiphyses, increased thickness of soft tissues are never present. Normal suppression of serum growth hormone after glucose administration and the absence of roentgen abnormalities permit a clear differentiation from pituitary gigantism in which serum growth hormone level is elevated, both in basal conditions and after glucose load.

Some patients with extra Y chromosomes attain a height of 200 cm or more; their karyotype shows 47,XYY or 48,XYYY constitution. In buccal smears two or three fluorescent Y-bodies are seen in the cell nucleus. The patients frequently have a decreased basal angle and other roentgen abnormalities of the skull.

Patients with hypogonadism continue to grow after the age of puberty and may reach an excessive height; they are easily diagnosed by eunuchoid body proportions and sexual infantilism.

Marfan's syndrome is also associated with excessive growth, but it is easily recognizable by characteristic clinical features. Cerebral gigantism is a very rare entity characterized by excessive growth rate in the first five years of life, macrocrania, mental retardation, neuromuscular disturbances, seizures, frequently also dilatation of cerebral ventricles and abnormal electroencephalograms.

Fig. 1A. General appearance of a pituitary giant, age 19, who experienced excessive growth since age 9. Height 204 cm (81 in.); heavy muscular build. Skull roentgenogram showed moderate enlargement of the sella turcica and greatly increased dimensions of the vault and facial bones, especially of the mandible. Basal serum HGH 120 ng/ml.

Fig. 1B. Roentgenogram of the hand of the same pituitary giant shows increased dimensions of all bones, and acromegalic changes: mushroom enlargement of tufts, widely spaced metacarpals with squared heads and increased width of joint fissures.

Figs. 2A and 2B. Comparison of the hands of a healthy male (*left*) and a pituitary giant (*right*) illustrates the greatly incraesed dimensions of the latter's hand.

PLATE 10

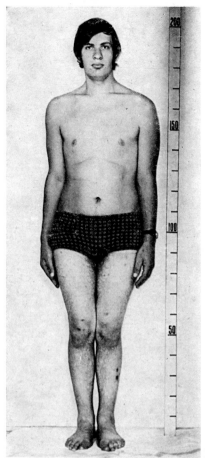

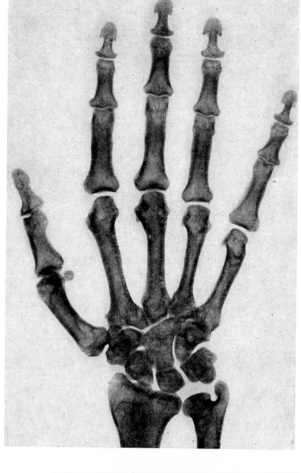

Fig. 1A   Fig. 1B

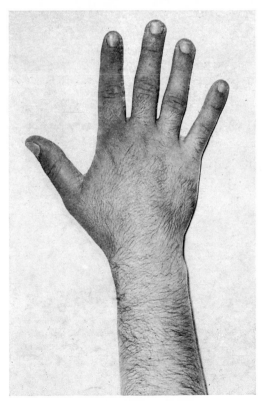

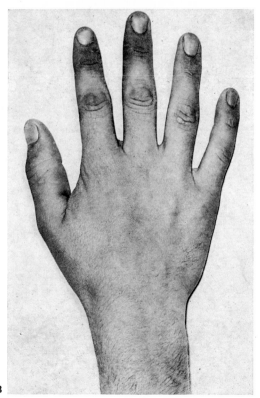

Fig. 2A   Fig. 2B

HYPOPITUITARISM

(PANHYPOPITUITARISM; ANTERIOR PITUITARY INSUFFICIENCY; SHEEHAN'S SYNDROME; SIMMONDS' DISEASE)

Hypopituitarism is a chronic disease resulting from gross destruction of the anterior pituitary with subsequent loss of pituitary hormones: the gonadotropins, growth hormone, ACTH and TSH. The clinical features depend on signs and symptoms of secondary gonadal and adrenocortical insufficiency and varied degrees of thyroid insufficiency.

A prominent description of the pathology and clinical findings was given by Sheehan in 1937 (and in subsequent works). He stated that the most common cause of the disease is pituitary necrosis in obstetric patients from circulatory collapse during delivery. Some earlier reports by Simmonds and other authors erroneously emphasized loss of weight as a cardinal and characteristic feature. This led to publication of cases involving anorexia nervosa or other debilitating diseases under a false diagnosis of hypopituitarism.

Fig. 1. A 26-year-old patient with postpartum hypopituitarism showing skin pallor, expressionless face, complete lack of sexual hair.

Fig. 2. A 30-year-old patient with hypopituitarism which commenced 6 years before showing swollen face with typical myxedematous appearance, loss of axillary and pubic hair, bloated body, dry skin.

Fig. 3. Face of a 48-year-old patient with hypopituitarism. No graying of hair, nose delicate, slight puffiness of the eyelids and base of the nose, narrow lips, numerous fine wrinkles are seen.

Fig. 4. Face of a 34-year-old patient with hypopituitarism. Many fine wrinkles around the eyes and the mouth and on the cheeks; deepened tarsal folds are present.

PLATE 11

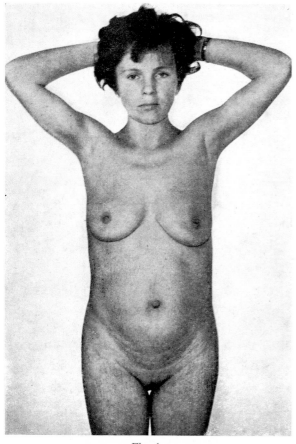

Fig. 1

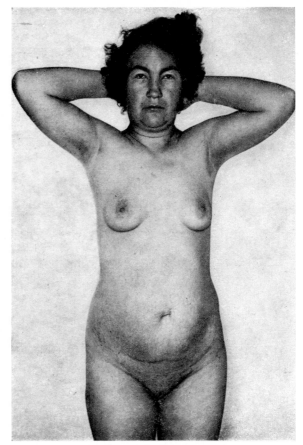

Fig. 2

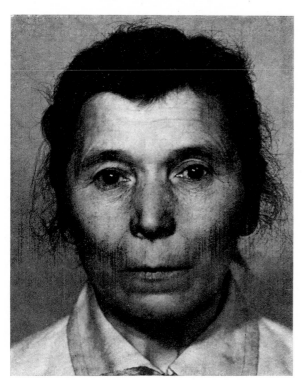

Fig. 3

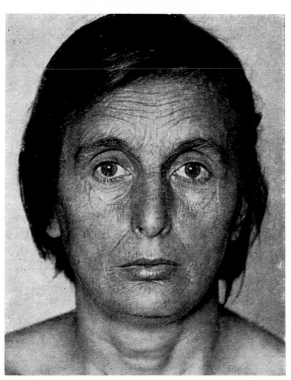

Fig. 4

Symptoms

1. Asthenia and fatigue (usually progressive), mild in some cases where the patients are able to do light work; severe in other cases where patients spend much of their time in a chair or bed.
2. Loss of sexual function; loss of potency in males; amenorrhea in females. Complete loss of libido.
3. Apathy, lassitude, loss of sense of wellbeing. The patient neglects his health, finds no interest in his work and appearance, avoids company; decrease in physical and mental activity.
4. Somnolence, the patient sleeps 8 to 10 hr at night, often falls asleep during the day.
5. Constant feeling of cold. Increased sensitivity to cold even in hot weather.
6. Loss of appetite. The intake of food is reduced; despite this there is no considerable weight loss because of greatly diminished activity and lowered metabolic rate.
7. Gradual onset of all symptoms after puerperal shock in female patients with postpartum hypopituitarism; in the puerperium there is lack of breast engorgement and activity, amenorrhea and no regrowth of the shaved pubic hair.
8. Headaches and impairment of vision may occur in patients with sellar or parasellar tumors.

Fig. 1. A 26-year-old patient who developed hypopituitarism after a skull fracture. Note apathetic facial expression, squint, complete loss of axillary and pubic hair, pale and dry skin, atrophy of the genitals.

Fig. 2. A 54-year-old patient with pituitary tumor and hypopituitarism exhibiting bloated body, loss of axillary and pubic hair, marked atrophy of the genitals, reduced nipples.

Fig. 3A. A 34-year-old man before the onset of the disease.

Fig. 3B. Face of the same subject at age 50, with a pituitary tumor and manifestations of hypopituitarism. Note puffiness of the upper lids and cheeks, typical bloated myxedematous appearance.

PLATE 12

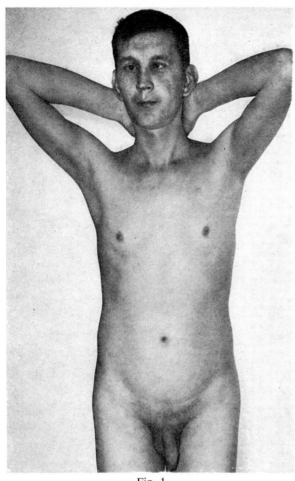

Fig. 1

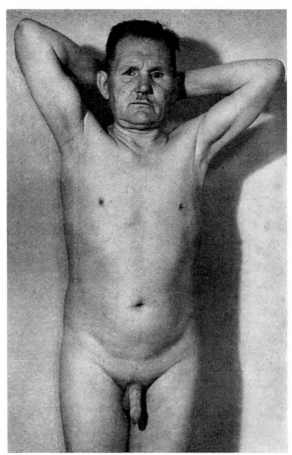

Fig. 2

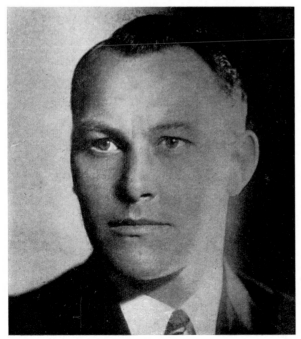

Fig. 3A

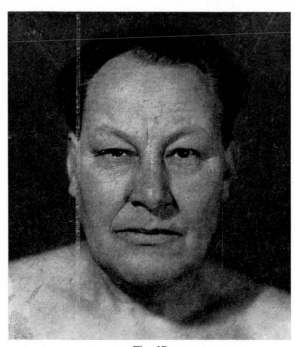

Fig. 3B

Signs

1. Striking pallor due to lack of both skin pigmentation and capillary flush.
2. The face has a vacant or weary expression; in some cases it has a bloated appearance.
3. Poor muscle development; fat deposits on the abdomen and above the hips obscure the waist.
4. Disappearance of axillary and pubic hair in females. In males the pubic hair is reduced to a female escutcheon, is sparse or lost completely. There is always loss of body hair on the chest and extremities.
5. Atrophy of the genitals; lack of pigmentation in the pubic and scrotal areas. In females the areola and nipples are poorly pigmented.

Fig. 1. Face of a 29-year-old patient with a pituitary tumor and pituitary insufficiency of 6 years duration shows many fine wrinkles about the eyes and nose, on the forehead and cheeks. Note progeroid appearance, deep set eyes (enophthalmos), lack of beard growth.

Fig. 2. A 40-year-old patient following removal of a chromophobe adenoma. Sunken cheeks; many wrinkles; progeroid features can be seen.

Fig. 3. A closeup view of the cheeks of a 42-year-old female with hypopituitarism showing abundant fine wrinkles on the cheeks and about the mouth.

Fig. 4. Numerous fine wrinkles on the face and ear of a 59-year-old patient with long standing hypopituitarism.

32

PLATE 13

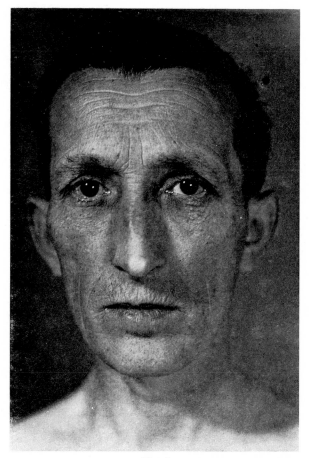

Fig. 1

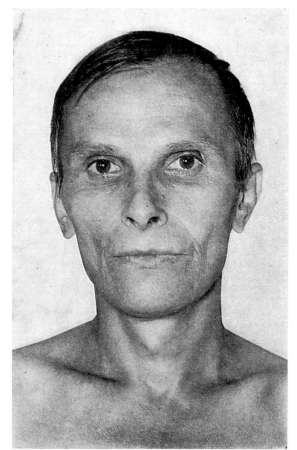

Fig. 2

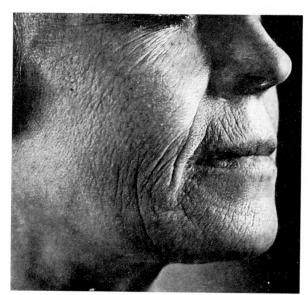

Fig. 3

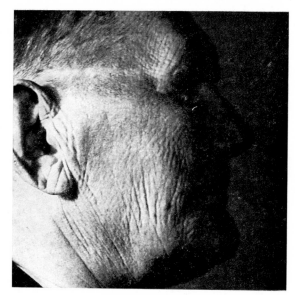

Fig. 4

The Face

The face is usually characteristic in that it is uniformly pale without capillary flush on the cheeks, ears and nose; there is complete lack of animation, giving an impression of fatigue, dullness or somnolence. In long standing cases, especially in females, the face is slightly puffed from edema of the eyelids and narrowing of the palpebral fissures — an appearance suggestive of myxedema. Cyanosis of the lips and cheeks, typical of the latter disease, is not seen in hypopituitarism.

The lips are narrower than before the onset of the disease. In patients with hypopituitarism, predominantly in males with pituitary tumors, numerous fine wrinkles appear as a result of prolonged androgen deficiency. The wrinkles form around the mouth, the base of the nose, the corners of the eye and on the cheeks, so the skin looks like parchment. These fine wrinkles in hypopituitarism differ from those in aged persons in whom they are deeper but not so numerous.

The general appearance of the face is a mixture of premature senility and myxedema, characteristics that occur in various degrees and with varying predominance in individual patients.

With the inception of the disease in childhood or adolescence, as in some cases of craniopharyngioma or pituitary tumors, the face retains some juvenile characteristics such as small nose, underdeveloped chin and lack of facial hair. Pale, wrinkled skin gives the face a progeroid look, so that curiously enough it has at the same time both a juvenile and progeroid appearance.

The hair on the scalp is fine and soft and retains its color, even in patients over the age of 60. In male patients the beard and mustache is either sparse or is lost.

Fig. 1. A 32-year-old female patient with hypopituitarism. Look of fatigue and apathy, narrowed lips; deepened tarsal folds can be seen.

Fig. 2. Pale and bloated myxedematous face of a 34-year-old patient with hypopituitarism has swollen upper lids; narrowed palpebral fissures.

Fig. 3. A 33-year-old patient with postpartum hypopituitarism. Sunken cheeks; wrinkles; aged appearance are seen.

Fig. 4. Pale and swollen face of a 38-year-old patient with hypopituitarism. Marked edema of the lids, narrow palpebral fissures, give a sleepy and oriental appearance.

PLATE 14

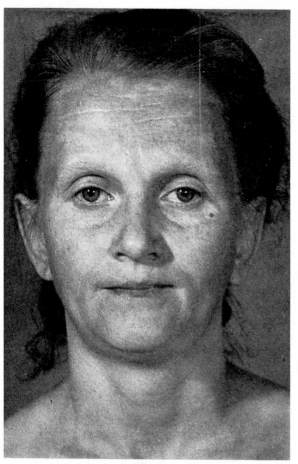

Fig. 1

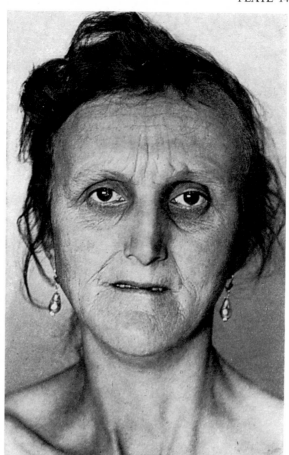

Fig. 2

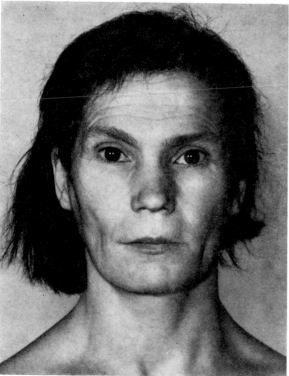

Fig. 3

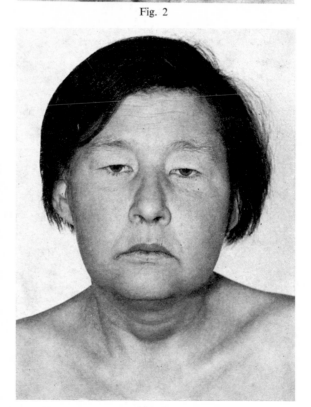

Fig. 4

The Eyes

In the majority of patients with long standing hypopituitarism, especially in females with Sheehan's syndrome, the upper and lower eyelids are puffed and the eyebrows are thinned at the periphery. In some patients the edema diminishes with cortisone treatment alone, while most need both cortisone and thyroxine before the edema disappears.

In other patients, especially in males with pituitary tumors, the eyes are more deeply set than before the onset of the disease. There is sometimes a real enophthalmos; keratometric examinations show values below normal. Simultaneously the tarsal folds, i.e., folds in the skin of the upper eyelids, are markedly deepened, and the skin of the supraorbital ridges together with that of the eyebrows is drawn into these folds. The deep set of the eyes and deepening of the tarsal folds are probably due to atrophy of retrobulbar tissues and reduced tonicity of the orbital muscles. Multiple, delicate wrinkles develop around and especially below the eyes that, together with the deepened tarsal folds, give the eyes a tired look.

Fig. 1. Puffiness of the upper lids and periorbital area, drooping eyelids; narrowed palpebral fissures give the eyes a myxedematous appearance in a 35-year-old patient with postpartum hypopituitarism.

Fig. 2. Deeply sunk tarsal folds, deep set eyes, numerous fine wrinkles in a 36-year-old patient with hypopituitarism.

PLATE 15

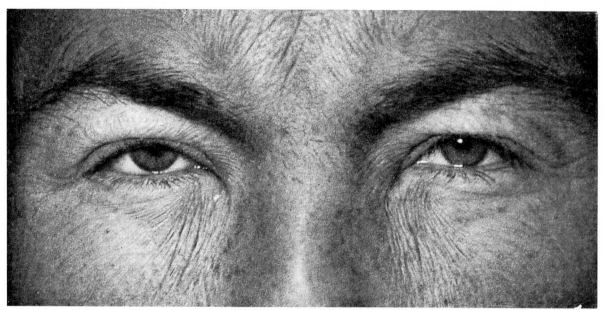

Fig. 1

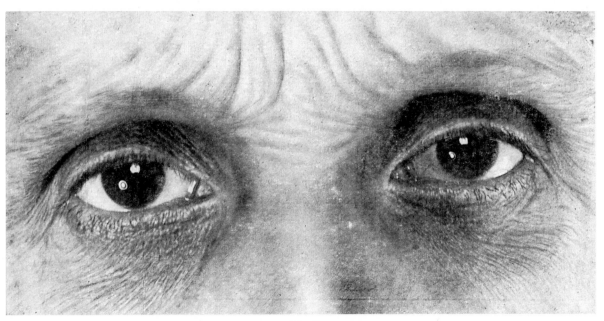

Fig. 2

The Skin and Subcutaneous Fat

The skin lacks pigmentation, is sometimes sallow and does not tan on exposure to sun. Furthermore, the skin on the extremities is dry owing to diminished sweating; it remains dry even in the axillae where, in normal subjects, there is always a slight dampness. Even in patients as young as age 30 the skin has atrophied and thinned, forming numerous extremely fine wrinkles on the face and on the dorsa of the hands. Owing to the thinned skin of some patients, veins are more easily seen on the chest, especially in the subclavicular region.

In some patients edema that does not pit on pressure appears on the face and hands. In these patients the skin on the fingers may be shiny. The hair on the extremities, like sexual hair and chest hair, disappears completely. The pH of the axillary vault is acid instead of alkaline.

Well developed fat deposits in subcutaneous tissues of the trunk, atrophy of the muscles, hairlessness and lack of pigmentation lead to an immature appearance.

Fig. 1. Hand of a 32-year-old man with a pituitary adenoma and pituitary insufficiency shows loss of downy hair. The skin, inelastic with atropic epidermis, exhibits numerous fine wrinkles — unusual at that age.

Fig. 2. Hand of a 35-year-old female with hypopituitarism. The back of the hand and fingers appears puffy; the skin is dry and shiny.

Fig. 3. Dry and scaly skin about the knee of a 23-year-old male with hypopituitarism.

Fig. 4. Skin of the back of the hand, greatly magnified, shows excessive wrinkling in a patient with hypopituitarism.

PLATE 16

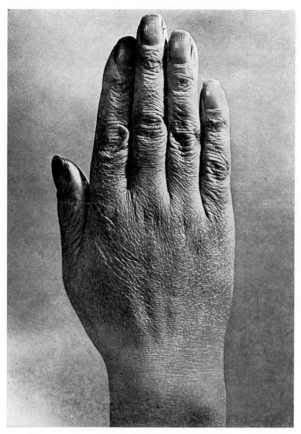

Fig. 1

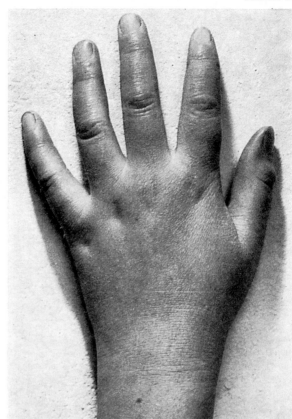

Fig. 2

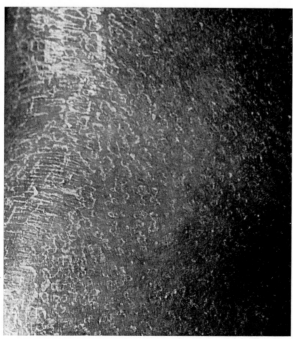

Fig. 3

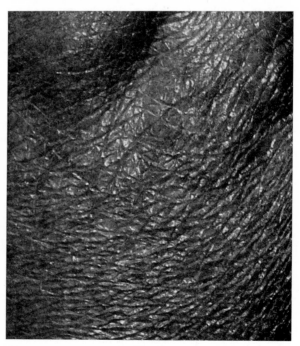

Fig. 4

The Male Genitals

Lack of the pituitary gonadotropins results in atrophy of the testes and a failure to produce androgens. Impotency and lack of libido are early and constant symptoms. Furthermore hair loss, weakness, skin and muscle atrophy, increased deposition of fat on the abdomen and above the hips result from androgen deficiency. On physical examination progressive atrophy of the genitals is always found. The testes are small and soft; the penis and scrotum undersized. There is lack of pigmentation of the scrotal area and lack of pubic hair or only sparse hair of female escutcheon. The prostate is very small.

Histology of testicular biopsy specimens shows widely spaced seminiferous tubules, decreased in size, and with narrowed lumen. The tubules are usually composed of a single layer of Sertoli cells, but no germinal cells. In a few cases in their early stages, remnants of the degenerating germinal cells displaced into the lumen may be seen. The Leydig cells disappear completely or are greatly reduced in number, while the interstitial tissue increases.

Smears taken from the distal part of the urethra show a striking predominance of parabasal cells and anucleated squamous cells which together constitute from 88% to 100% of the cell population. The number of the intermediate and superficial cells is reduced, by from 2% to 12%. In urethral smears taken from control subjects, the number of intermediate and superficial cells vary from 20% to 68%.

Fig. 1. Genitals of a 29-year-old patient with hypopituitarism show marked atrophy and loss of pubic hair.
Fig. 2. Atrophic genitals of a 42-year-old patient with hypopituitarism. The testes are small and soft; there is complete absence of sexual hair and loss of pigmentation.
Fig. 3. Testicular biopsy specimen in a case of hypopituitarism shows advanced tubular atrophy and interstitial fibrosis.
Figs. 4A and 4B. *A*. Urethral smears of a patient with hypopituitarism showing only parabasal cells. *B*. Urethral smears of a control male reveal the presence of intermediate and superficial cells.

PLATE 17

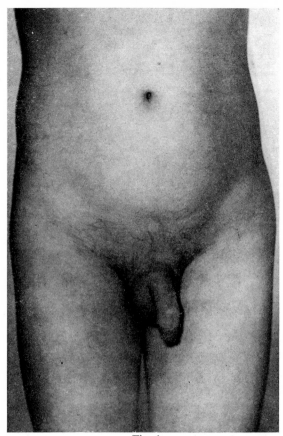

Fig. 1

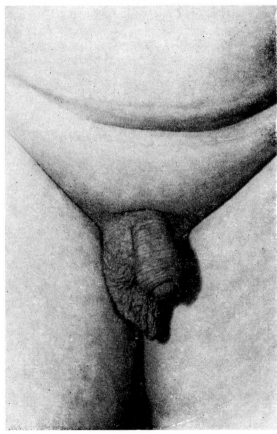

Fig. 2

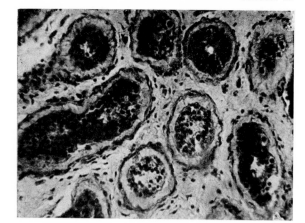

Fig. 3

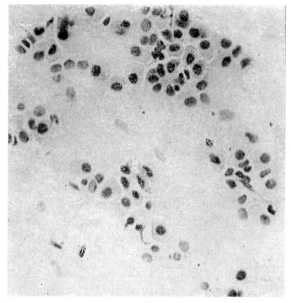

Fig. 4A

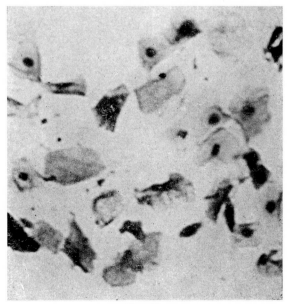

Fig. 4B

The Female Genitals

All female patients with hypopituitarism experience a cessation of menstruation as a result of lack of pituitary gonadotropins. Amenorrhea may be preceded by a period of scanty, irregular menses. In patients with Sheehan's syndrome there is a complete absence of breast activity following childbirth. The areolae are small and depigmented. Loss of libido occurs; atrophic changes of the vagina and its dryness may cause difficulties in sexual relations. On gynecologic examination extreme atrophy of the genitalia is found. The uterus and cervix are very small and difficult to palpate, the labia majora and minora are paper thin and lack the normal pigmentation, the sexual hair is completely absent. The vagina is greatly shrunken with smooth atrophic epithelium. Absence of glycogen in the vaginal epithelium is determined by painting the vaginal mucosa with iodine solutions which produce a slight yellow stain. In sexually mature, healthy women, a deep mahogany color is obtained due to the presence of glycogen. On curettage no endometrium is obtained and the atrophied uterus is easy to perforate.

Pelvic pneumography (roentgenograms of the pelvis after gas insufflation into the peritoneum) reveals a marked involution of the uterus as well as ovaries greatly reduced in size.

In the majority of cases, vaginal smears stained by Shorr's method are profoundly atrophic, showing only parabasal cells; small, intermediate cells may also be seen, indicating a moderate estrogen deficiency.

Fig. 1A. Genitals of a 35-year-old female with hypopituitarism show marked atrophy of the labia majora and minora; loss of pigmentation and pubic hair.

Fig. 1B. Roentgen pelvic pneumography in the same patient shows a very small, flattened uterus, and flat, oyster-shaped ovaries.

Fig. 2. Vaginal smears of a patient with hypopituitarism showing lack of estrogen effect. Only parabasal and intermediate cells are seen.

42

PLATE 18

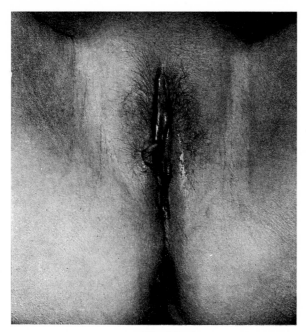

Fig. 1A

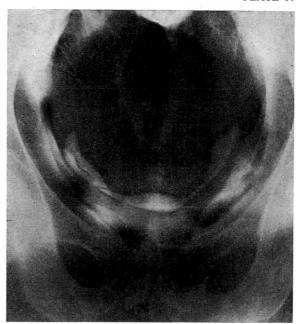

Fig. 1B

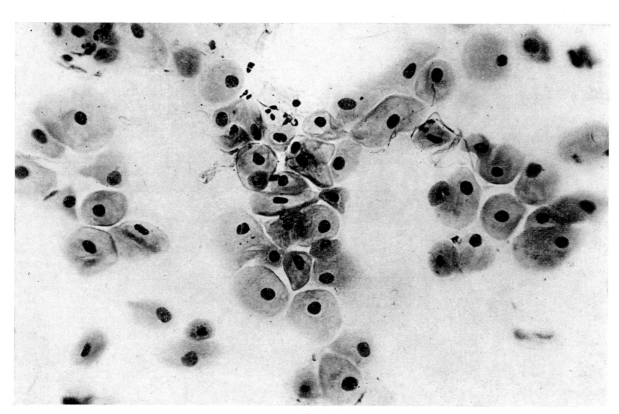

Fig. 2

Monitoring the Disease

Electrocardiogram. In nearly all patients the electrocardiogram (ECG) shows definite abnormalities. The most frequent is inversion or flattening of the T waves in all standard and left precordial leads. In half the cases a low voltage of QRS complexes in standard leads, the ST depression in left precordial leads and QT prolongation are found.

In patients with secondary gonadal and adrenocortical insufficiency, but without secondary hypothyroidism, all the electrocardiographic changes disappear on administration of cortisone or other glucocorticoids. In cases where secondary hypothyroidism has also developed, the electrocardiographic abnormalities do not regress with cortisone treatment alone. In these patients the ECG reverts to normal only when adequate doses of thyroxine are given.

Reflexogram. The Achilles tendon reflex in patients with hypopituitarism differs from that found in normal subjects. The recordings of the reflex, called reflexograms, are made with the use of a photoelectric device (photomotograph), or with a simple displacement ballistocardiographic device attached to the electrocardiograph. In 90% of the patients the reflexogram is abnormal; there is a plateau, i.e., the initial part of the relaxation phase flattens. In half the patients the reflex time, and especially the relaxation phase, is prolonged above normal values. The mean reflex time in hypopituitarism is 0.40 ± 0.06 sec (where N = 0.28 ± 0.06), and relaxation time is 0.32 ± 0.05 sec (N = 0.17 ± 0.04). These values are above the normal but usually below those in primary hypothyroidism.

Fig. 1A. ECG of a patient with hypopituitarism: negative or flattened T waves in all standard and precordial leads.
Fig. 1B. ECG of same patient on replacement therapy shows regression of the abnormalities. T waves are now positive and of normal voltage.
Figs. 2A to 2C. Recordings of the Achilles tendon reflexes in patients with hypopituitarism reveal flattening in the initial part of the relaxation phase (*A*). *B*. Marked prolongation of the reflex time, and especially of the relaxation phase. *C*. Comparable reflexograms of normal subjects.

PLATE 19

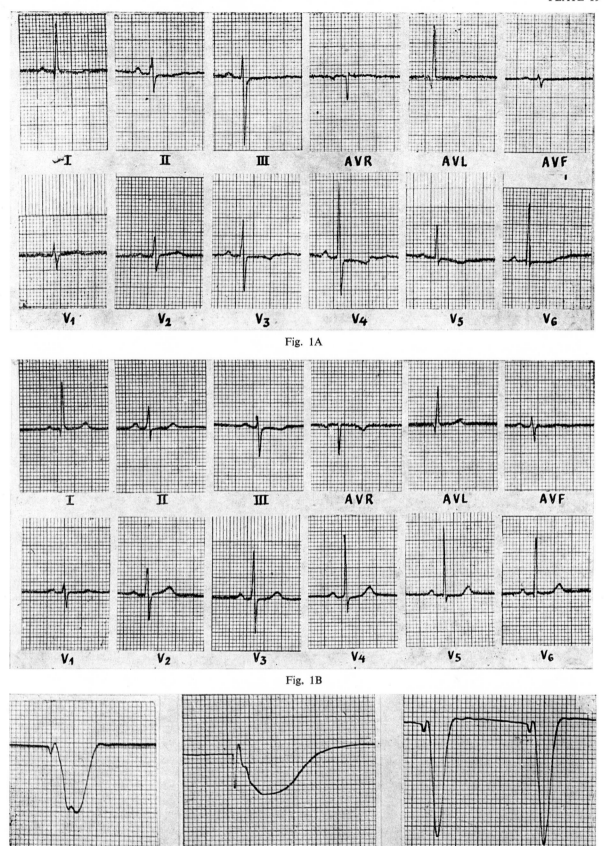

Fig. 1A

Fig. 1B

Fig. 2A   Fig. 2B   Fig. 2C

Laboratory Findings

Deficiency or excess of pituitary hormones

1. Low serum HGH; no rise in serum HGH during insulin hypoglycemia and after L-dopa administration.
2. Low serum and urinary LH and FSH; deficient or no response in the stimulation tests with LH-releasing hormone and clomiphene.
3. Low serum ACTH; no rise after metyrapone administration.
4. Low serum TSH.
5. Increased serum prolactin in some patients with pituitary tumors.

Deficiency of corticosteroids

1. Very low basal plasma cortisol even in the morning hours.
2. Urinary 17-hydroxycorticoids and 17-ketosteroids very low.
3. No response in urinary 17-hydroxycorticoids to metyrapone (Metopirone) administration.
4. Gradual increase in plasma cortisol and urinary 17-hydroxycorticoids after several day administration of ACTH.
5. Strikingly impaired diuresis in water loading test and inability to excrete diluted urine.
6. Prolonged hypoglycemia in insulin tolerance test.
7. Markedly increased taste and smell sensitivity.
8. Abnormal ECG with flat or inverted T waves in standard and left precordial leads.
9. Low glomerular filtration rate.
10. Occasional hyponatremia.
11. Abnormal encephalogram: θ and δ waves; slowing of the basic frequency.

Fig. 1. Plasma ACTH concentration in primary and secondary adrenocortical hypofunction. Markedly elevated ACTH concentration occurs in chronic adrenal insufficiency, but is undetectable or at a low level in hypopituitarism.

Fig. 2. Urinary 17-hydroxycorticoids in hypopituitarism and in control subjects. Urinary 17-hydroxycorticoids are definitely lowered in the former.

Fig. 3. Water loading test in hypopituitarism. There is marked impairment of diuresis in the first 4 hours following water ingestion (20 ml/kg of body weight) in all cases.

Fig. 4. Taste threshold for galvanic current in hypopituitarism. Patients with hypopituitarism are able to detect galvanic current at 1 to 10 μA, while taste threshold in normal subjects fluctuates, according to age, between 10 and 120 μA as shown by the shaded area.

PLATE 20

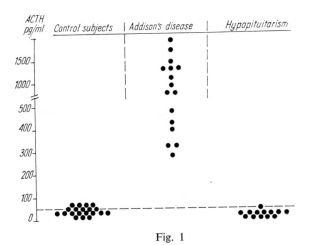

Fig. 1

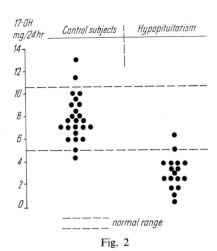

Fig. 2

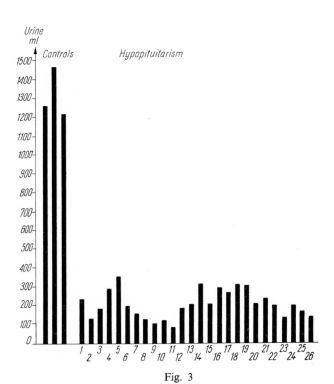

Fig. 3

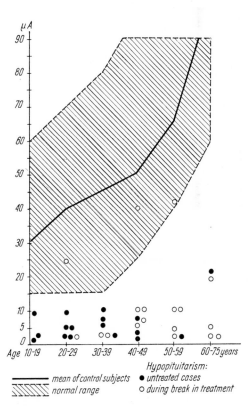

Fig. 4

Deficiency of sex hormones

1. Low plasma and urinary testosterone.
2. Low plasma and urinary estrogens.
3. Atrophic vaginal smears in female patients; atrophic urethral smears in male patients.
4. Acid pH reaction of the skin in the axillary area.

Deficiency of thyroid hormones

1. Lowered or low-normal serum thyroxine and triiodothyronine.
2. Decrease in basal metabolic rate.
3. Thyroidal ^{131}I uptake decreased in some cases.
4. Occasional increase in plasma cholesterol.
5. Abnormal reflexogram of the Achilles' tendon.

SECONDARY HYPOPITUITARISM

Damage to the hypothalamus by suprasellar tumors such as craniopharyngiomas, gliomas, trauma, hydrocephalus, granulomas may lead to cessation of hypophysiotropic hormone synthesis or impairment of their transport to the anterior pituitary resulting in secondary pituitary hypofunction. Clinical features do not differ from those of hypopituitarism. However, the results of stimulating tests with the use of TRH and LH-RH are different. In primary hypopituitarism there is usually no response to TRH or LH-RH administration. In contrast, in secondary hypopituitarism the patients respond to these neurohormones by increased secretion of TSH, or LH and FSH, respectively. In addition, serum prolactin concentration is frequently increased in secondary hypopituitarism.

Fig. 1. Serum HGH concentration following insulin administration (0.1 U/kg iv) in patients with hypopituitarism. Basal HGH concentration 0 to 4 ng/ml; no rise is observed during insulin hypoglycemia. In all control subjects a prompt rise in serum HGH occurs, after insulin administration, in the range of from 10 to above 100 ng/ml.

Fig. 2. Effects of L-dopa (0.5 g orally) on HGH concentration: no change in hypopituitarism; rise in serum HGH within 60, 90 or 120 minutes after oral L-dopa administration in control subjects.

Fig. 3. Basal serum LH and FSH concentrations in hypopituitarism; LH and FSH concentrations are undetectable or very low (0 to 3 mIU/ml).

Fig. 4. Pituitary stimulation test using LH-RH. No response or deficient response is seen in hypopituitarism after LH-RH administration. Normal subjects show a prompt rise in serum LH after LH-RH administration.

PLATE 21

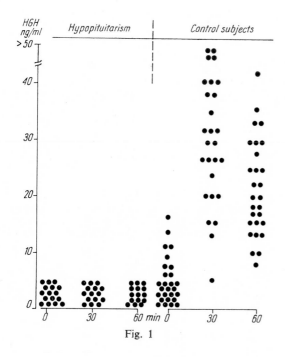

Fig. 1

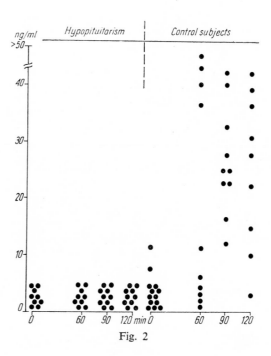

Fig. 2

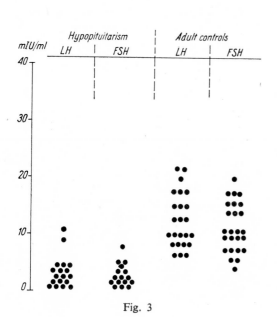

Fig. 3

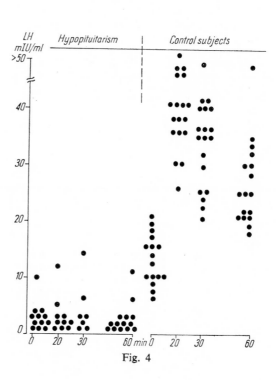

Fig. 4

PITUITARY TUMORS

Pituitary tumors may cause local manifestations, or they may lead to hormonal disturbances due to involvement of the hypothalamus, or to impaired function of anterior and posterior pituitary. The most frequent local manifestations are headaches and visual disturbances. Loss of visual acuity may be the first symptom. If the tumor exerts pressure upon the optic chiasm it gives rise to bitemporal defects of the visual field; these defects are sometimes asymmetric, involving a single quadrant. Involvement of the third, fourth and sixth nerves may result in diplopia. Seizures and signs of increased intracranial pressure may occur in cases involving large tumors.

Roentgen Manifestations

Intracranial tumors are characterized by enlargement of the sella turcica, deepening of the fossa toward the sphenoidal sinus, sometimes a double floor and thinning of the dorsum. In cases of craniopharyngioma, the sella may be of normal size, but the dorsum is shortened, with destruction of the posterior clinoid processes occurring. A characteristic feature of craniopharyngioma is the presence of intensive patchy shadows in the suprasellar area due to calcifications in the walls of the cyst. In some cases semicircular calcifications are seen. Cerebral angiography and pneumoencephalography are helpful in locating the tumor and evaluating its size.

Fig. 1. A 22-year-old female with an intrasellar tumor. Height 146 cm. Complete lack of sexual development; slender extremities; double chin; fat accumulation on abdomen obscuring the waistline; atrophic vaginal smears. Lowered serum LH and FSH (0 and 1 mIU/ml); no response to LH-RH stimulation. Serum HGH during insulin tolerance test: 1–1–1 ng/ml.

Fig. 2. An 18-year-old patient with pituitary chromophobe adenoma confirmed at craniotomy. There is no sexual development; the penis is infantile; the scrotum greatly shrunken; the testes small and soft; the nipples are small. The facies is immature. Poor muscle development; slender extremities. Plasma testosterone 0.2 ng/ml (N = 5 to 8 ng/ml), serum LH is 0 mIU/ml, serum FSH is 1 mIU/ml. No response of serum HGH to insulin hypoglycemia.

Fig. 3. A 26-year-old patient with Fröhlich's syndrome: craniopharyngioma, obesity, diabetes insipidus, stunted growth and sexual infantilism are present. First symptoms, polyuria and polydypsia, appeared at age 10. Growth gradually ceased and no sexual maturation occurred. Following massive doses of testosterone sparse pubic hair appeared. Serum LH and FSH are undetectable.

Figs. 4A to 4D. Roentgenograms of the sella turcica in 4 patients with pituitary insufficiency. *A*. A large, calcified tumor expands pituitary fossa. *B*. Ballooning of the sella from an intrasellar tumor. The floor is depressed toward the sphenoidal sinus; the anterior clinoid processes pseudoelongated due to erosion of the bone beneath them; the dorsum is thin and displaced posteriorly. *C*. Enlargement of sella, thinning of dorsum, pseudoelongation of anterior clinoid processes and double floor are seen. *D*. Extensive patchy densities in suprasellar area in calcified craniopharyngioma.

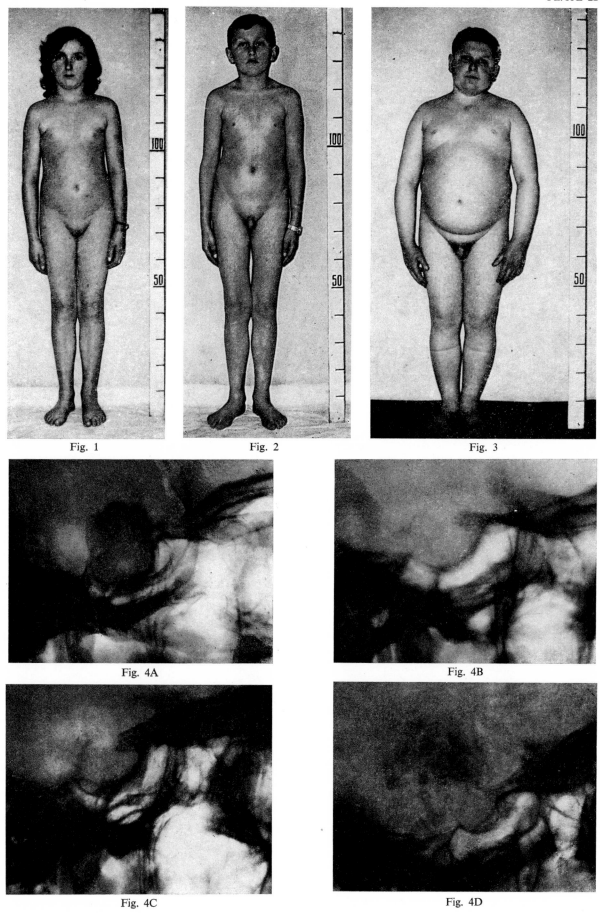

PLATE 22

Fig. 1   Fig. 2   Fig. 3

Fig. 4A   Fig. 4B

Fig. 4C   Fig. 4D

Hormonal Manifestations

Chromophobe and acidophilic adenomas secrete large quantities of growth hormone, causing gigantism in children and acromegaly in adults. Tumors secreting an excess of prolactin give rise to galactorrhea and amenorrhea. Corticotropin-secreting pituitary tumors, usually small, basophilic adenomas, are frequently found in Cushing's disease.

Other, non-secreting tumors, due to pressure on the anterior pituitary, may cause pituitary insufficiency. In the earliest stage of the disease there is a deficiency in pituitary gonadotropin and growth hormone secretion. Children with the disease do not achieve sexual maturation; in adult patients there is cessation of sexual functions and atrophy of the genitalia. The obesity, diabetes insipidus and sexual infantilism that sometimes appear are referred to as Froehlich's syndrome. In exceptional cases the pressure of suprasellar tumors on the hypothalamus causes sexual precocity.

Fig. 1. Face of a 25-year-old patient with craniopharyngioma and partial pituitary insufficiency, first symptoms of which were noted at age 16. Height 172 cm; no sexual development. The face shows lack of expression, infantile features, delicate nose, absence of facial hair and male characteristics, double chin. Serum HGH during insulin tolerance test was undetectable, serum LH and FSH from 0 to 2 mIU/ml.

Fig. 2. Genitals of the patients shown in Fig. 1 are extremely underdeveloped. The penis is tiny; the scrotum greatly shrunken, and the testes very small and soft. Lack of pubic hair and pigmentation.

Fig. 3. A 28-year-old patient with chromophobe pituitary adenoma resulting in progressive loss of vision and regression of sexual function. The face is pale, lacking expression; no beard growth; skin slightly wrinkled; edema of the upper lids. Serum LH and FSH are undetectable.

Fig. 4. Genitals of the patient shown in Fig. 3. There is complete loss of sexual hair; the testes are small and soft.

PLATE 23

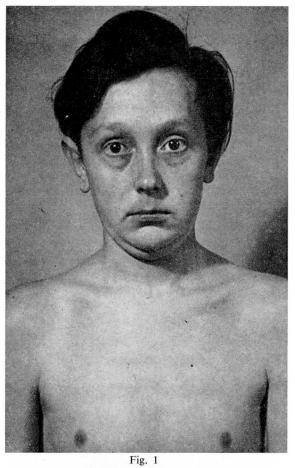

Fig. 1

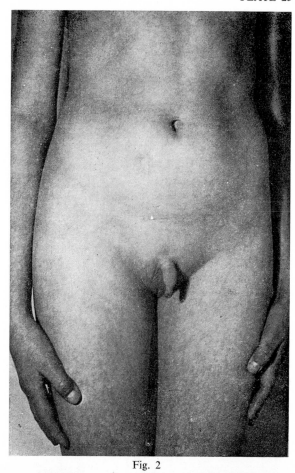

Fig. 2

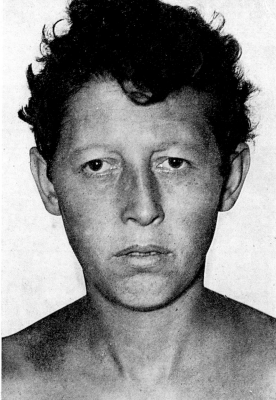

Fig. 3

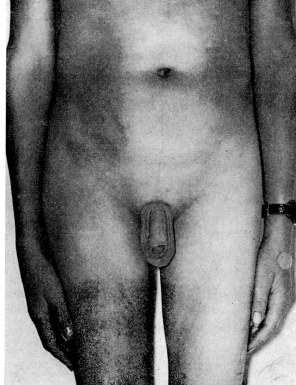

Fig. 4

PITUITARY DWARFISM

(HYPOPITUITARY DWARFISM; HYPOPITUITARISM IN CHILDHOOD)

Pituitary dwarfism is characterized by dwarfism and sexual infantilism, the result of a deficiency in pituitary growth hormone and gonadotropins. The mental development of dwarfs is normal. In some patients signs of secondary adrenocortical insufficiency and secondary thyroid insufficiency develop due to a deficiency in ACTH and TSH. There are two forms of pituitary dwarfism: 1) idiopathic of unknown etiology, and 2) organic, due to destruction of the pituitary.

The idiopathic form probably represents a congenital defect in the hypothalamus leading to a deficiency in GH-releasing hormone, or a defect in the eosinophilic cells of the pituitary that results in a growth hormone deficiency. This form is occasionally seen in siblings, indicating its congenital origin. Clinical manifestations, especially cessation of growth, begin in the first, second or third year. The growth does not completely cease but continues at a very slow rate of about 1 to 3 cm a year, even into the second and third decades. In the majority of patients aged 30 to 40 years, signs of precocious senility develop, but this progeria may be occasionally seen in younger patients. In untreated dwarfs the stature remains markedly stunted, finally reaching 105 to 140 cm (41 to 55 in.).

The organic form of pituitary dwarfism is usually caused by tumors of the pituitary area such as craniopharyngioma or glioma, and in other cases by inflammatory, traumatic or other types of lesions damaging the pituitary. In the organic form manifestations usually appear between the ages of 5 and 10 years, and the shortness of stature is not so pronounced, but sexual infantilism predominates the clinical picture. Neurologic symptoms such as headaches, vomiting and impaired vision are common.

Fig. 1. A 21-year-old pituitary dwarf. Height 118 cm (47 in.). Immature facial features; complete lack of sexual development; slender extremities can be seen.

Fig. 2. A 42-year-old pituitary dwarf. Height 122 cm (48 in.). Note round face; fat accumulation on the abdomen; atrophic genitals.

Fig. 3. A 28-year-old female with pituitary dwarfism. Height 114 cm (45 in.). Round face; fat deposits on the breasts and abdomen; complete lack of sexual development are observed.

Fig. 4. Comparison of an 8-year-old female with pituitary dwarfism with her healthy 6-year-old sister. The patient exhibits stunted growth (89 cm, 35 in.), round dollface, short neck and fat deposits on the abdomen.

PLATE 24

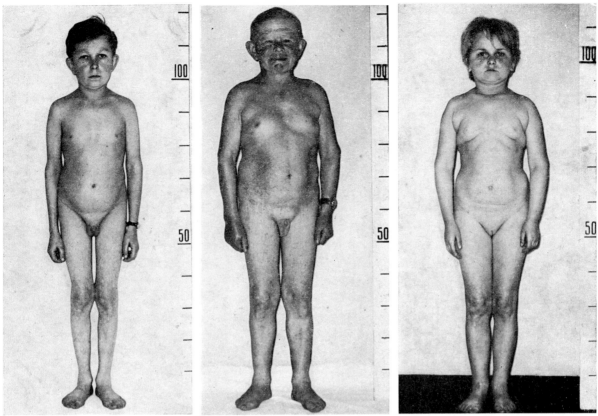

Fig. 1   Fig. 2   Fig. 3

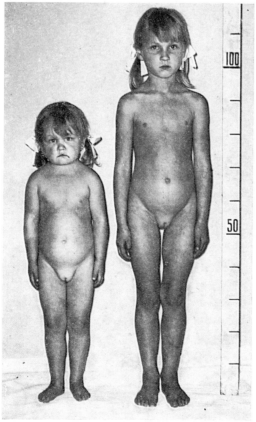

Fig. 4

Symptoms

1. Stunted, very slow rate of growth.
2. Poor appetite; pituitary dwarfs eat half the amount of normal children; their weight remains proportional to their height.
3. Lack of sexual development at and past the age of puberty; primary amenorrhea in females.
4. Fatigue of lesser degree.
5. Normal mental development, but not interest in sex; no libido.
6. Occasional headaches; increased thirst and polyuria; impairment of vision with tumors of the pituitary or the hypothalamus.

Signs

1. Short stature; growth deficiency becomes more pronounced with increasing age. At the age of 8 years or more the patients are 20 to 40 cm (8 to 16 in.) below the mean height standards.
2. Complete lack of sexual development at and past the age of puberty.
3. Truncal obesity; slender limbs.
4. Normal or slightly younger body proportions; small hands and feet.
5. Skin somewhat dry; occasionally has a yellowish tint.
6. Poor muscle development, especially evident in males.
7. Childlike, or childlike-progeroid, facial features.

Fig. 1. Comparison of faces of 2 pituitary dwarfs, ages 5 and 7 (*left*) with that of their healthy, 3-year-old sister (*right*). Note the round face, delicate nose and narrow lips of the dwarfs.

Fig. 2. Face of a 22-year-old pituitary dwarf displaying an infantile appearance; delicate nose, prominent cheeks, small chin, low hairline on the forehead.

Fig. 3. Face of a 54-year-old pituitary dwarf showing a mixture of childlike and progeroid traits: prominent cheeks, puffiness of the upper lids, delicate nose, many wrinkles, complete lack of beard growth and of male characteristics.

PLATE 25

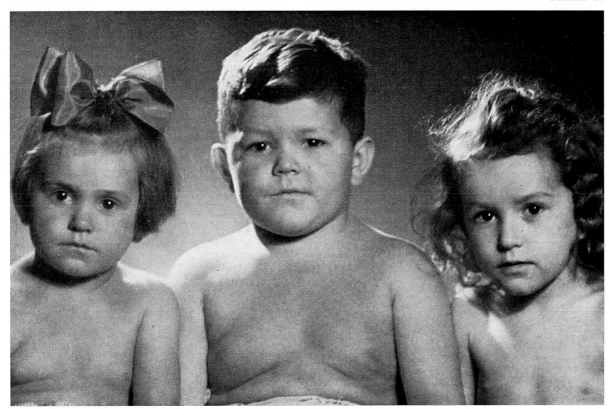

Fig. 1

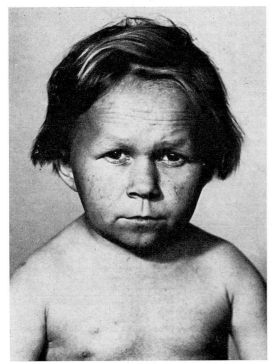

Fig. 2

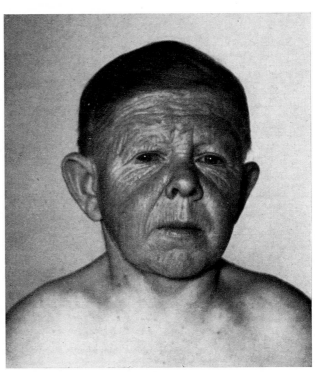

Fig. 3

The Head and Neck

A common finding is a poor facial development in contrast to normal dimensions of the vault. The face of pituitary dwarfs is childlike in appearance; the contours are soft and rounded, the cheeks prominent, the nose short and small. The chin is underdeveloped, sometimes recessed; the lips are narrow.

In patients over 30 years of age, but occasionally in younger patients, many fine wrinkles appear around the mouth, at the base of the nose and at the corners of the eyes. These features, as well as a yellowish tint to the cheeks, give patients a progeroid look. On the other hand, a round face, lack of facial hair (in males), a small mandible, recessed chin and shortened nose are reminiscent of the faces of young children. Thus, the features represent a peculiar mixture of childlike and progeroid characteristics. Slight puffiness of the upper lids is sometimes present.

The scalp hair is thin, fine and does not curl easily. In male patients the hairline extends low on the forehead with no recession at the temples.

The permanent teeth appear late, and due to small dimensions of the mandible and maxilla are sometimes displaced beyond the alveolar ridges.

The neck is short; the inelastic skin of the neck may form several folds.

Fig. 1. A 15-year-old patient, childlike in appearance, with a delicate nose, recessed chin, slight puffiness in cheeks and upper lids, narrow lips.

Fig. 2. A 21-year-old patient with doll-like face, narrow lips, short nose, puffed cheeks, swollen upper lids.

Fig. 3. A 17-year-old dwarf with pituitary tumor exhibiting stunted growth and infantile facial features.

Fig. 4. A 36-year-old patient with idiopathic pituitary dwarfism. Swollen cheeks and upper eyelids, no beard growth, short neck, double chin are seen.

PLATE 26

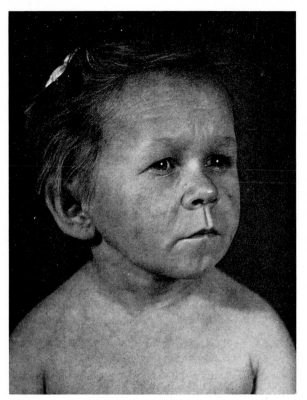

Fig. 1

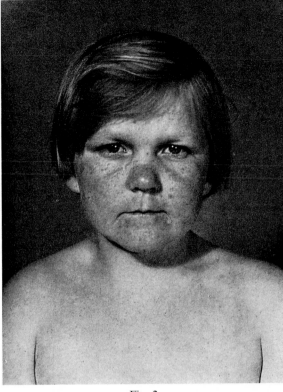

Fig. 2

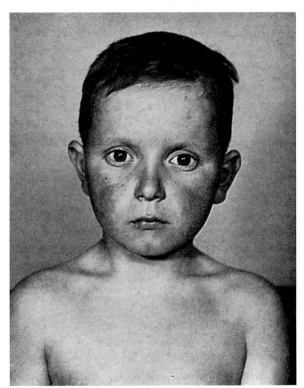

Fig. 3

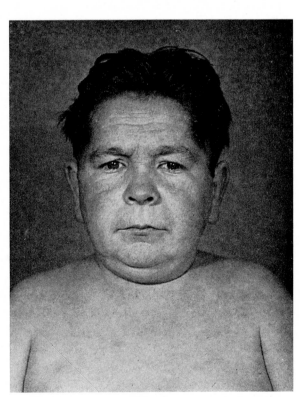

Fig. 4

The Hands

The hands are short and small with slender, tapering fingers. The dorsa of the hands are puffed, and the skin is somewhat dry. The dermatoglyphics do not reveal any abnormalities; the palmar creases are normal; the nails are normal. There is an increased sensitivity to cold and a tendency to frostbite.

Fig. 1. Face of a 46-year-old pituitary dwarf. Numerous wrinkles are seen on the forehead, at the base of the nose, around the eyes and mouth. Note short nose and narrowed lips.

Fig. 2. Trunk of a 19-year-old pituitary dwarf shows accumulation of fat on the abdomen, especially at the epigastric area, and on the lower chest; slender extremities; lack of sexual development are also seen.

Fig. 3. Hand of a 21-year-old pituitary dwarf is short but proportionate; fat pads are seen on the back of the hand.

Fig. 4. Veins are easily seen on the chest through thin, transparent skin in a 20-year-old pituitary dwarf.

PLATE 27

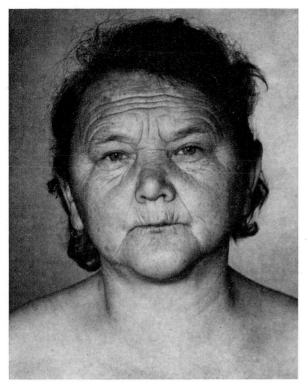

Fig. 1

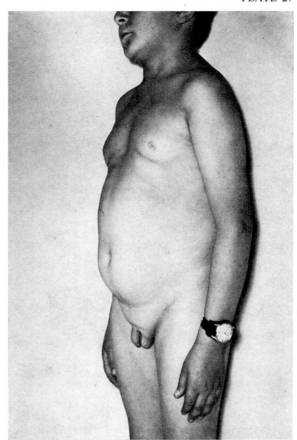

Fig. 2

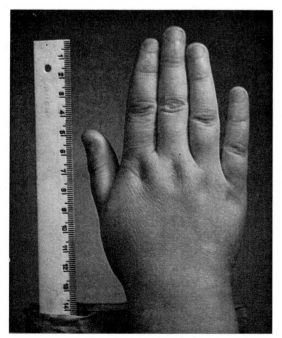

Fig. 3

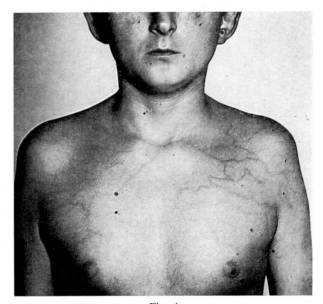

Fig. 4

Gonadal Function

Always present in pituitary dwarfs is a severe gonadal insufficiency caused by a complete absence of pituitary gonadotropins.

In males no sexual development occurs at or past the age of puberty. The voice remains high pitched, the genitals underdeveloped. There is no growth of sexual hair or facial hair. The patients have no interest in the opposite sex. The testes are very small and soft, measuring only a few millimeters; the penis is tiny, and the scrotum greatly shrunken, with no physiologic pigmentation. The prostate is also small. Histologic examination of testicular biopsy reveals an immature testis with small, densely packed tubules and no Leydig cells.

In females, menstruation never begins; there is no breast development and no sexual hair. The external genitals remain infantile; the labia majora and minora are pale and very small. The vaginal smears show a complete lack of estrogen effect, the pH of the vagina is alkaline, as in children. Roentgen pelvic pneumography shows the ovaries, uterus and tubes to be small. The ovaries have the shape of an elongated oval.

In all pituitary dwarfs the pH of the axiliary vault and fossa is always strongly acid in contrast to normal subjects in whom the pH is alkaline after puberty. Even after prolonged and careful sex hormone administration the patients remain sterile.

Fig. 1. The conspicuously undeveloped genitals of a 16-year-old pituitary dwarf. The penis is tiny; the scrotum greatly shrunken There is no sexual hair and no pigmentation. Fat deposits appear on the abdomen.

Fig. 2. Genitals of a 21-year-old patient showing complete lack of sexual development.

Fig. 3. Genitals of a 26-year-old female dwarf. The labia majora and minora are very small; no sexual hair is seen.

Fig. 4. On roentgen pelvic pneumography the uterus is small; the ovaries are of flattened oval shape similar to ovaries in early infancy.

Fig. 5. Vaginal smear shows complete lack of estrogen effects; only parabasal cells are seen.

PLATE 28

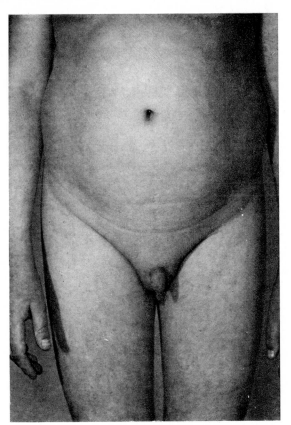

Fig. 1

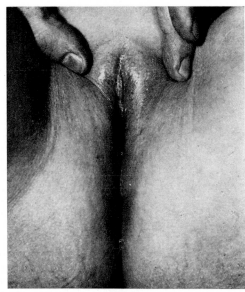

Fig. 3

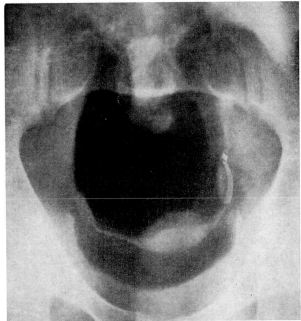

Fig. 4

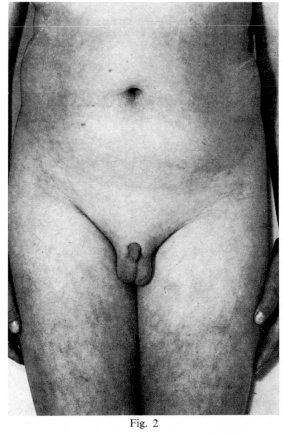

Fig. 2

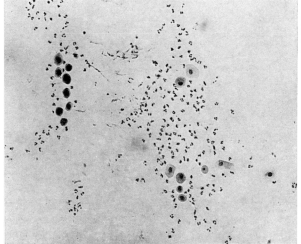

Fig. 5

Thyroid Function

The skin is usually dry; there is some puffiness of the dorsa of the hands and sometimes of the upper eyelids also. These findings suggest secondary hypothyroidism. Serum T_3 and T_4 are lowered or low-normal.

ECG findings are similar to the ECGs of children: negative deep T waves in leads V_1 to V_3 and rS pattern in left precordial leads. In most patients over age 20, and occasionally those a few years younger, additional changes appear depending on secondary hypothyroidism: negative or flat T waves and lowered ST segments in standard and left precordial leads. After administration of thyroxine the changes completely disappear; the T waves become positive and ST segments return to the isoelectric line.

Recordings of the Achilles tendon reflex frequently reveal a flattening of the initial part of the relaxation phase that is also common in adult patients with hypopituitarism. The relaxation time is at the upper limit of normal values, exceeding this limit only in some cases.

In contrast to congenital hypothyroidism, in pituitary dwarfs the mental development is normal. Radioimmunoassay of serum TSH is of decisive value in differentiating primary from secondary hypothyroidism, as TSH concentration is very low in pituitary dwarfs, ranging from 0 to 5 mU/liter. It is constantly elevated from 20 to 500 mU/liter in congenital or juvenile hypothyroidism.

Fig. 1. ECG of a 32-year-old pituitary dwarf. The T waves are deep and negative in leads V_1 to V_4 and are flattened in standard and other precordial leads.

Fig. 2. ECG of a 21-year-old pituitary dwarf shows negative deep T waves in precordial leads V_1 to V_4.

Fig. 3. Recordings of the Achilles tendon reflexes in 3 control subjects (*upper row*) and in 3 pituitary dwarfs (*lower row*). *A* and *B*. A flattening of the initial part of the relaxation phase. *C*. A marked prolongation of the relaxation time, indicating secondary hypothyroidism.

PLATE 29

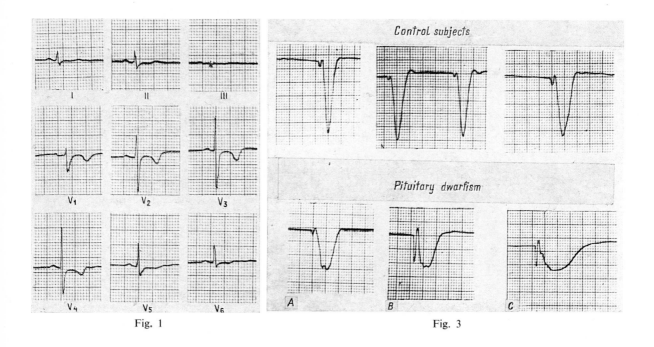

Fig. 1

Fig. 3

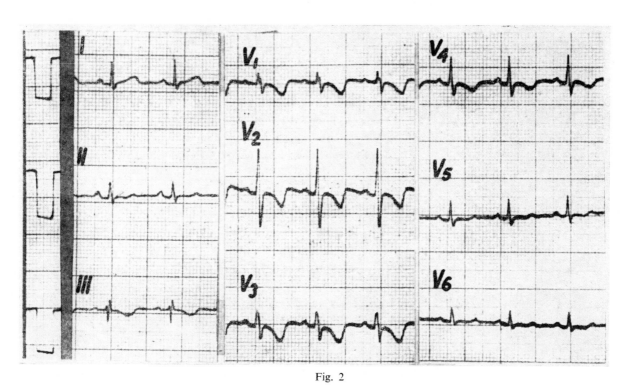

Fig. 2

Roentgen Findings

Roentgenograms of the bones are of significant value in the diagnosis of pituitary dwarfism, especially in the prepubertal period. A delay in bone age — 5 years or more in the second decade of life — and persistent lack of epiphyseal fusion in later years, are common findings. The delay in bone age is proportional to height age. A normal bone age, as is found in primordial dwarfism and gonadal dysgenesis, is never seen. The metacarpals and phalanges are short but relatively broad in older patients. The distal phalanges are pawn-shaped with broad base, straight sides, short triangular shaft and small tuft.

On frontal roentgenograms of the skull a disproportion between a normal sized vault and tiny facies is clearly evident. The vault has the appearance of a large sized helmet resting on the small facies, i.e., the so-called helmet sign. In control adults the distance from the lower margin of the mandible to the sphenoidal plane is equal to the distance from this plane to the vertex; whereas in pituitary dwarfs the mandible-sphenoidal plane distance is from 2 to 3 cm less than the sphenoidal-vertex distance.

The mandible is small and delicate; several permanent teeth are seen in its shaft. The mastoid processes are small, 2.5 to 3.5 cm in height (N = 4.0 to 6.0 cm). The frontal sinuses do not develop, while the sphenoidal sinuses are undersized.

Figs. 1A and 1B. Roentgenograms of the skull of a 22-year-old pituitary dwarf show striking underdevelopment of the facies. The mandible is small and delicate, with teeth overcrowding. The sphenoidal sinuses are very small; the frontal sinuses are completely undeveloped.

Fig. 2. Comparison in development of the skull in pituitary dwarfs and in healthy subjects. In healthy children the facial part is small but increases in size with the advance of age. In adult healthy subjects the height of the vault equals the height of the facies. In pituitary dwarfs the vault is of normal size, but the contour is usually more rounded than usual; the facial part of the skull is strikingly undeveloped even in the third decade of life. The childish proportions of the skull, large vault and small face, persist permanently in pituitary dwarfs.

Fig. 3. Roentgenogram of a hand and wrist of a 16-year-old pituitary dwarf showing a marked delay in bone maturation. The bone age is 8 years.

PLATE 30

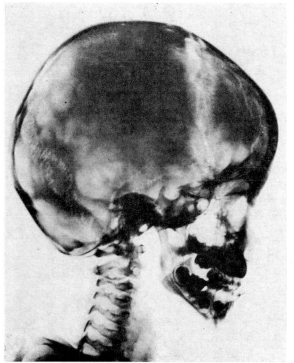

Fig. 1A

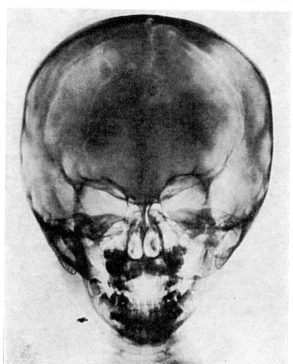

Fig. 1B

Pituitary dwarfism

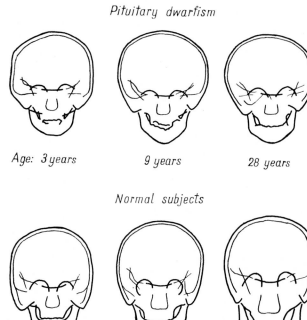

Age: *3 years*   *9 years*   *28 years*

Normal subjects

Age: *3 years*   *7 years*   *adult*

Fig. 2

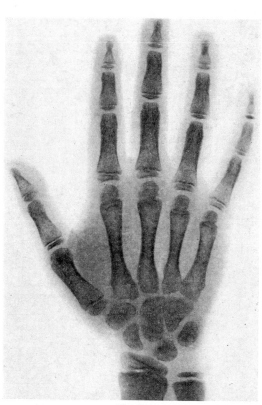

Fig. 3

67

Laboratory Findings

Classic findings

1. Serum HGH concentration is very low, 0 to 2 ng/ml. No rise in serum HGH during insulin-induced hypoglycemia and after administration of L-dopa.
2. Serum and urinary LH and FSH are undetectable or very low. No response to administration of LH-releasing hormone.
3. Lowered plasma testosterone.
4. Low plasma estrogens.
5. Atrophic vaginal smears; only parabasal cells are seen.
6. Low plasma TSH concentration.

Occasional findings

1. Low serum T_3 and T_4.
2. "Hypopituitary" reflexograms showing flattening in the initial part of the relaxation phase.
3. ECG abnormalities: deep, negative T waves in leads V_1, V_2, V_3 and sometimes in V_4.
4. Deficient diuresis in water loading test.
5. Occasional slight decrease in plasma cortisol.
6. Low urinary 17-ketosteroids, but usually in the range of that found in prepubertal children.
7. Increased taste sensitivity in some patients.
8. Slightly elevated plasma cholesterol.

Fig. 1. Results of HGH radioimmunoassays during insulin tolerance test. In all pituitary dwarfs serum HGH concentration is low (0 to 4 ng/ml) and does not increase after intravenous insulin administration. Normal subjects constantly show a definite increase in serum HGH above 10 ng/ml during insulin-induced hypoglycemia.

Fig. 2. LH radioimmunoassays before and after intravenous LH-RH administration. On the left, a normal response in patients with delayed puberty. In pituitary dwarfs the low basal LH does not increase after LH-RH stimulation.

PLATE 31

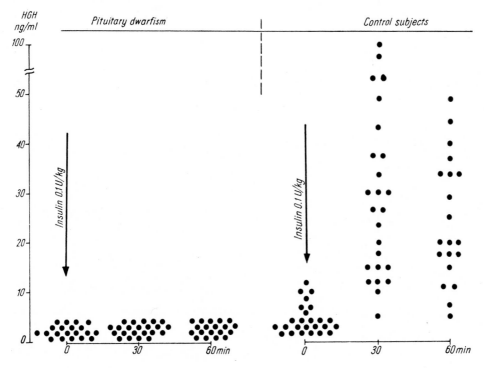

Fig. 1

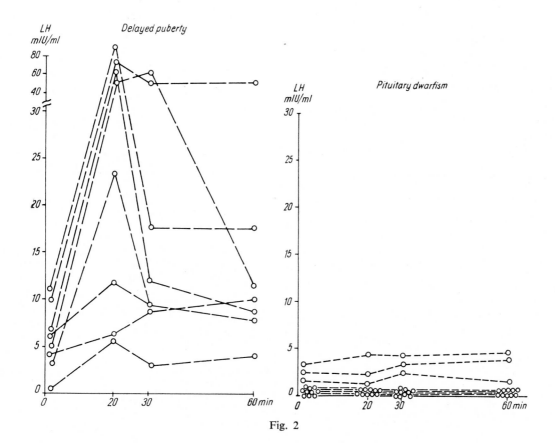

Fig. 2

Differential Diagnosis

Patients with congenital or juvenile hypothyroidism are of short stature and their serum growth hormone is low, both in basal conditions and during insulin-induced hypoglycemia. However, serum TSH is greatly elevated in these patients whereas it is low in pituitary dwarfism. Deformity of the lumbar vertebral body and epiphyseal dysgenesis are frequent in congenital hypothyroidism and do not occur in pituitary dwarfs. On proper replacement therapy patients with hypothyroidism attain a normal rise in serum growth hormone after insulin administration.

Patients with Turner's syndrome are sometimes confused with pituitary dwarfs due to their stunted growth but can be properly diagnosed on findings of congenital anomalies, sex chromosome aberrations, absence of the ovaries, and numerous roentgenographic changes which do not occur in pituitary dwarfs. Serum LH and FSH are elevated in gonadal dysgenesis after the age of puberty, whereas the concentration of these hormones is very low in pituitary dwarfism.

Patients with deprivation or psychosocial dwarfism are characterized by deficient growth, mental subnormality, polyphagia and polydipsia. These patients have been reported to have transient growth hormone deficiency which regresses rapidly on removal from unfavorable home conditions.

A group of patients of Oriental Jewish origin with growth failure and clinical signs of isolated growth hormone deficiency were described by Laron as having normal or elevated serum growth hormone concentration with deficient production of somatomedin.

Some metabolic and skeletal disorders associated with growth deficiency and having characteristic clinical and biochemical abnormalities are described in Chapter 10.

ISOLATED GROWTH HORMONE DEFICIENCY

This is a rare disease closely related to pituitary dwarfism, and may be regarded as a variant of this disease. The onset of the disease is in the first, second or third year of life. The primary manifestation is stunted growth that becomes more conspicuous as the patient grows older; other signs of pituitary dwarfism may also be present. In contrast to the latter, however, normal sexual development does occur at puberty. The diagnosis is based on laboratory findings indicating growth hormone (GH) deficiency. Serum GH concentration is very low, 0 to 2 ng/ml, and does not increase during insulin-induced hypoglycemia. Serum LH and FSH in the first years of life are low, as is usual in children, but rise to normal adult values after puberty. The pituitary stimulation test, using LH-releasing hormone, facilitates differentiation of isolated GH deficiency from pituitary dwarfism in early childhood. No response of serum LH to LH-RH administration is seen in pituitary dwarfism whereas in patients with isolated growth hormone deficiency LH-RH provokes a rise in serum FSH and LH concentrations. There are occasional cases which appear to be typical pituitary dwarfs in the first two decades but who mature sexually with considerable delay.

Fig. 1. A 14-year-old female with delayed puberty. There is no evidence of sexual maturation. Growth is stunted (130 cm, 51 in.). Chromatin pattern is positive; bone age 11 years. Normal response to insulin-induced hypoglycemia. Serum LH is 3 mIU/ml and FSH 2 mIU/ml. Sexual maturation was achieved 2 years later.

Fig. 2. A 16-year-old female with Turner's syndrome showing short stature, lack of secondary sex characteristics, broad shoulders. Chromosome constitution is 45,X. Elevated serum LH (47 mIU/ml) and FSH (36 mIU/ml), and typical roentgen manifestations were found.

Fig. 3. A 19-year-old female with juvenile hypothyroidism. Stunted growth (137 cm, 54 in.), puffed face with double chin and feminine sex characteristics are seen. Serum T_4 is 0.5 μg/dl and serum TSH is 56 μU/ml.

Figs. 4A and 4B. A 19-year-old patient with isolated growth hormone deficiency. Height greatly stunted at 119 cm (47 in.). Normal feminine body proportions and sexual development; menstrual cycles commenced at 12 and are regular. Face childlike with prominent cheeks. Serum growth hormone undetectable; no response in serum HGH to insulin and L-dopa administration. Serum LH is 12 mIU/ml and FSH is 10 mIU/ml.

PLATE 32

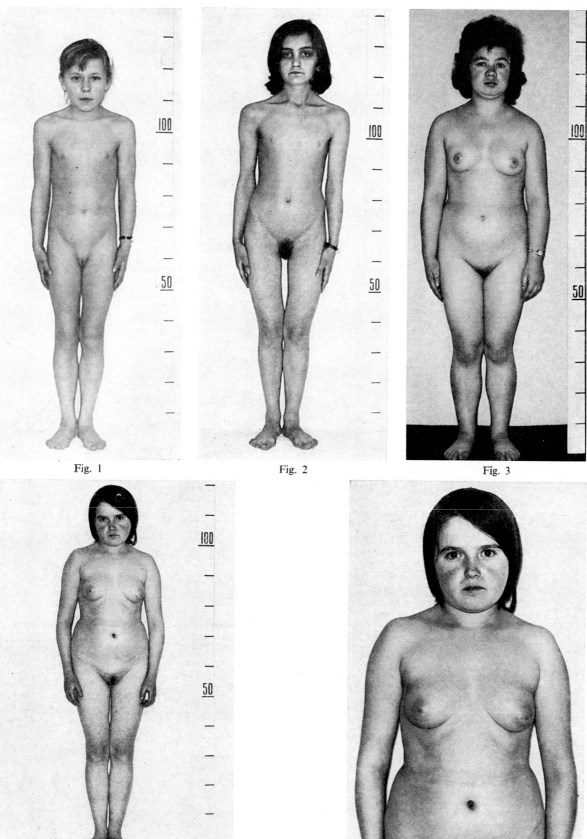

Fig. 1

Fig. 2

Fig. 3

Fig. 4A

Fig. 4B

DELAYED GROWTH AND PUBERTY

(CONSTITUTIONAL DELAY IN GROWTH AND PUBERTY)

Delayed growth associated with delay in the onset of sexual development is a frequent disturbance in males, but of rare occurrence in females. In some patients, case history indicates prematurity or some chronic diseases in early life. In others there is a familial tendency toward delayed growth and onset of puberty.

Growth does not cease entirely but continues at a slower rate, the difference in development usually being noticed at school age when compared to that in normal children. At puberty patients complain of lack of sexual development. At this period physical examination reveals short stature (15 to 25 cm below average) and underdeveloped genitalia of the same size as in younger, normal males. Without treatment the patients attain normal height and sexual maturity between the ages of 17 and 22 years. There are no abnormalities revealed in laboratory findings. Basal serum GH is normal, and there is a rapid rise to high concentrations (10 to 100 ng/ml) during the insulin-induced hypoglycemia.

Roentgen studies of the skeleton show a 2- to 5-year delay in bone age that is proportional to the delay in height; thus bone age equals height age. No other changes are found. In particular, the skull has the dimensions of that found in males 2 to 5 years younger but shows no underdevelopment of the facial bones that is typical of pituitary dwarfism.

Roentgenograms of the hand and wrist are also helpful in differentiating among delayed puberty, primordial dwarfism, familial short stature and Turner's syndrome. The bone age is retarded in delayed puberty, while it is normal in the other diseases.

Fig. 1. A 17-year-old male with delayed growth and sexual maturation. Normal response of serum HGH to insulin hypo-glycemia (rise to 24 ng/ml). Serum LH 5 mIU/ml, after LH-RH administration, 32 mIU/ml. Several years observation showed a gain in height of up to 170 cm; complete sexual development.

Fig. 2. A 14-year-old male with delayed puberty and stunted growth. Serum HGH after insulin administration 36 ng/ml. Normal response of serum LH (43 mIU/ml) and FSH (26 mIU/ml) in LH-RH stimulation test.

Fig. 3. Roentgenogram of the hand of the patient shown in Fig. 2 shows a delay in bone age of 10 years.

Fig. 4. Results of HGH during insulin tolerance test (0.1 U/kg of body weight) in delayed puberty and pituitary dwarfism. In delayed puberty there is a normal increase in serum HGH during insulin hypoglycemia, while no response occurs in pituitary dwarfism.

PLATE 33

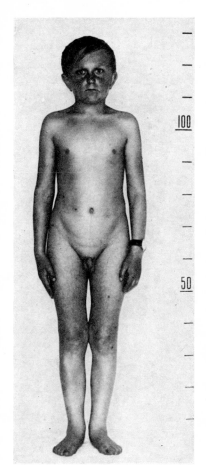

Fig. 1

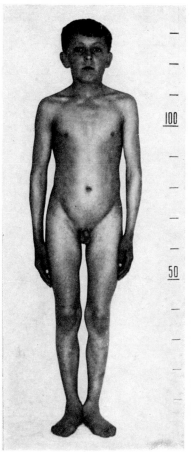

Fig. 2

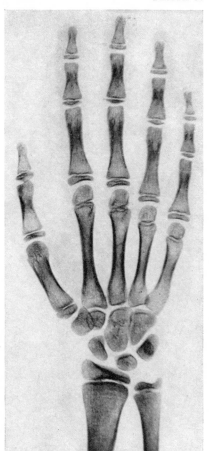

Fig. 3

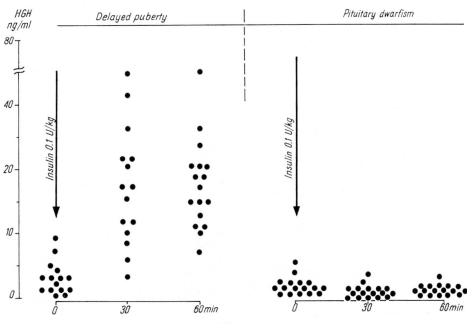

Fig. 4

ANOREXIA NERVOSA

Anorexia nervosa is a disease found in young single females the onset of which is at the age of 13 to 25 years. The main signs and symptoms are amenorrhea and psychogenic aversion to food leading to self-starvation and striking emaciation. The onset of the disease is usually preceded by a psychic trauma, or by a strong desire in obese patients to lose weight. The patients have a distorted, implacable attitude toward eating, food and their weight.

In the first months of the disease there is a rapid loss of weight leading to extreme emaciation. Later, despite minute intake of food, the weight remains at a nearly constant level of 31 to 35 kg owing to decreased metabolism and activity. Severe constipation is very common. A feeling of cold may be present.

The patients perform their usual tasks, claim they feel well and that they "eat quite sufficiently," although they are known to hoard their food. On physical examination they present a picture of striking emaciation, with complete atrophy of the subcutaneous fat and muscles that leaves the bones prominent. The skin is dry and scaly; in the late stages of the disease the whole body is generally covered by lusterless, gray, downy hair. The body temperature drops below normal; the hands and feet are cold and blue. The breasts remain fairly normal, and the sexual hair, especially in the pubic area, is preserved. The face looks some years older, though there are no wrinkles as in hypopituitarism. Ankle edema may develop.

The pulse is slow, 40 to 60 beats/min; the blood pressure is lowered. Serum triiodothyronine is decreased but serum TSH concentration remains normal and serum reverse T_3 is elevated. The basal metabolic rate is definitely lowered, in the hypothyroid range; serum cholesterol is low and ECGs as well as reflexograms do not show changes typical of hypothyroidism.

Figs. 1A and 1B. Gross emaciation in a 19-year-old patient with anorexia nervosa exhibiting aged appearance; protruding ribs and other bones; sunken abdomen; muscle atrophy. There is normal breast development; no loss of pubic hair. Height 167 cm; weight 33 kg.

Fig. 2. Forearm of a patient with anorexia nervosa shows fat and muscle atrophy, dry scaly skin and downy, curly hair typical of prolonged starvation.

Fig. 3. Grayish skin covered by downy hair on a patient with anorexia nervosa.

PLATE 34

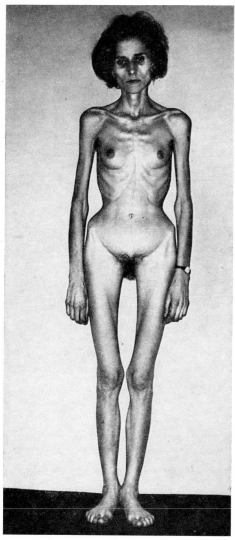

Fig. 1A

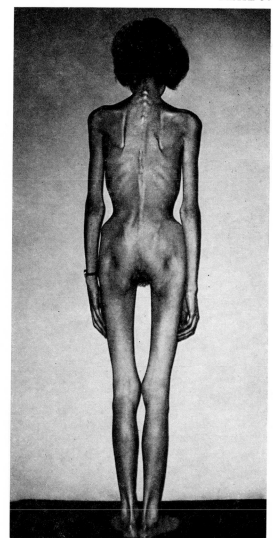

Fig. 1B

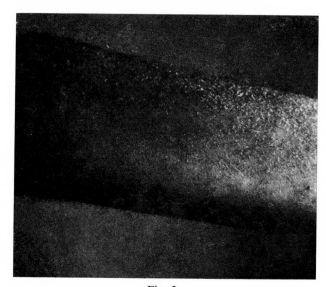

Fig. 2

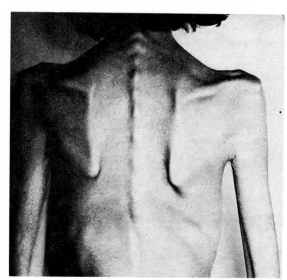

Fig. 3

The urinary 17-ketosteroids and 17-hydroxycorticoids are normal or slightly lowered but not as much as in hypopituitarism. There is no taste hypersensitivity. Hypokalemia is found in some patients, especially in those experiencing frequent regurgitation. The serum LH and FSH are lowered. In most patients there is a rapid rise in serum FSH after intravenous LH-releasing hormone administration. The vaginal smears show estrogen deficiency and lack of cyclic changes.

All signs and symptoms disappear when the patients start to eat normal amounts of food; in this period there may be episodes of bulimia and spontaneous or self-induced vomiting. When not treated patients are prone to infections and pulmonary tuberculosis, which may prove fatal.

HYPERPROLACTINEMIA

(GALACTORRHEA AND AMENORRHEA)

Hyperprolactinemia, the excessive secretion of pituitary prolactin, is present in many endocrine disorders. Common causes of hyperprolactinemia include pituitary tumors such as chromophobe adenomas, tumors associated with acromegaly or Cushing's disease, hypopituitarism of any etiology, hypothalamic lesions (especially those affecting the median eminence), encephalitis, basal meningitis or primary hypothyroidism with either amenorrhea or precocious puberty. Of rare occurrence are ectopic tumors secreting prolactin. Transient hyperprolactinemia may be induced by several drugs, i.e., oral contraceptives, rauwolfia derivatives, chlorpromazine and other drugs. Hyperprolactinemia is usually accompanied by galactorrhea and amenorrhea and has been previously described under the eponyms of Chiari-Frommel, del Castillo and Forbes-Albright syndromes. The Chiari-Frommel syndrome means persistent or transient lactation, amenorrhea and ovarian atrophy after pregnancy. On the other hand, Forbes-Albright syndrome occurs without antecedent pregnancy; the patients have galactorrhea, menstrual disturbances and frequently also signs of a pituitary tumor secreting prolactin.

Laboratory studies reveal markedly increased serum prolactin, low serum LH and FSH, atrophic or intermediate vaginal smears. In cases involving pituitary tumors, roentgenograms of the skull may show enlargement of the sella turcica. Administration of bromergocryptine (CB 154, Sandoz) is effective in suppressing galactorrhea. The course of the disease depends on the etiology. In some cases the signs and symptoms disappear spontaneously or after several months of therapy. In other cases, however, manifestations of acromegaly, Cushing's disease or hypopituitarism may develop.

Fig. 1A. A 16-year-old female with anorexia nervosa. Height 159 cm; weight 32 kg. Striking emaciation; atrophy of the subcutaneous fat and muscles; prominent bones can be seen. The breasts and pubic hair are well preserved.
Fig. 1B. Same patient shows complete regression of changes after treatment.

PLATE 35

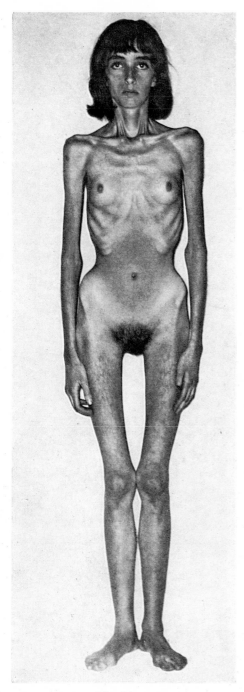

Fig. 1A

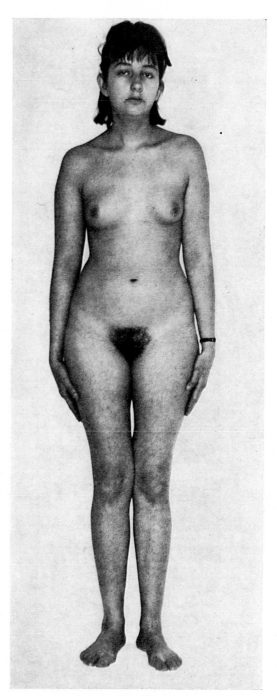

Fig. 1B

II. THE NEUROHYPOPHYSIS

DIABETES INSIPIDUS

Diabetes insipidus is a disease which results from disturbances in the neurohypophyseal system leading to a deficiency in antidiuretic hormone (vasopressin) and consequent polydypsia, polyuria and low specific gravity of the urine. The disease affects both sexes equally and generally starts between the ages of 10 and 40 years. It persits indefinitely unless hypopituitarism develops, in which case the symptoms regress. Vasopressin deficiency may result from damage to the hypothalamus or the neurohypophysis by suprasellar or intrasellar tumors, trauma, fractures of the base of the skull, inflammatory changes or scars. In the idiopathic form, degenerative changes in the hypothalamic nuclei are probably responsible.

Symptoms

1. Increased thirst that is only temporarily quenched by the intake of large amounts of cold water.
2. Polyuria in the range of 6 to 20 liters/24 hr.
3. Nocturia, disturbing sleep. The patients are forced to urinate and drink water several times through the night.
4. Feeling of dryness in the mouth.
5. Husky voice when water intake is insufficient.
6. Feeling of cold.

Signs

1. No physical signs are usually evident.
2. During restriction of water intake, there is dryness of mucous membranes, dryness of the skin, hoarseness of the voice.
3. Lowered body temperature, infrequently.

Laboratory Findings

1. Increased volume of urine from 6 to 20 liters/24 hr of a low specific gravity (1.001 to 1.005).
2. Deprivation of water does not diminish urine flow; polyuria continues, and body weight drops.

Fig. 1. Urinary volume before and after treatment in patients with diabetes insipidus. In untreated cases urinary volume is greatly increased, usually to between 7 and 12 liters/day. After intramuscular injections of pitressin tannate (5 to 10 U/24 hr), the urine volume is reduced to normal. Oral administration of chlorpropamide (250 to 500 mg/24 hr) or clofibrate (750 mg/24 hr) is followed by reduction in urine volume in over 50% of cases.

Fig. 2. Response to 5% sodium chloride (NaCl) infusion in hydrated patients with diabetes insipidus and control subjects (Carter-Robbins test), showing mean values of 3 tests. First, both groups were given water orally (20 ml/kg body weight) and water losses were replaced. After the patients attained a urine flow above 5 ml/min, infusion of hypertonic NaCl was started. In control subjects this was followed by a drop in urine volume. No response in urine flow was found in patients with diabetes insipidus.

Fig. 3. Results of plasma vasopressin radioimmunoassay in 4 patients with diabetes insipidus and 6 control subjects, before and after smoking 2 cigarettes. Plasma vasopressin rose decidedly in control subjects, whereas it remained undetectable in cases of diabetes insipidus.

Fig. 4. Results of urinary vasopressin radioimmunoassay in 3 patients with diabetes insipidus and 4 control subjects during hypertonic NaCl infusion. A considerable rise in urinary arginine vasopressin occurred in control subjects, whereas there was no response in urinary AVP in the patients.

PLATE 36

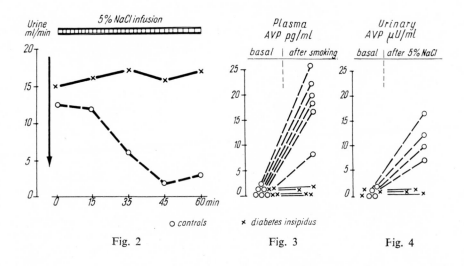

Fig. 1

○ before treatment   ● on treatment

Fig. 2

Fig. 3

Fig. 4

○ controls   × diabetes insipidus

3. Intravenous administration of hypertonic salt solution does not decrease the urine flow; the specific gravity of the urine remains low (under 1.008).

4. Administration of vasopressin promptly decreases the urinary output and raises its specific gravity.

5. Low plasma vasopressin concentration during water deprivation, salt loading or cigarette smoking, which raises plasma vasopressin in healthy subjects.

VASOPRESSIN EXCESS
(HYPERSECRETION OF ANTIDIURETIC HORMONE)

An excess of antidiuretic hormone associated with hyponatremia is rarely seen in patients with carcinoma of the lung or disorders of the central nervous system.

Symptoms, Signs and Laboratory Findings

1. Anorexia, nausea, vomiting.
2. Weakness, apathy, confusion, coma.
3. Hyponatremia; hypoosmolality of serum.
4. Increase in urinary sodium; the urine is hypertonic in relation to the plasma.
5. Increased plasma vasopressin concentration despite water loading.
6. Regression of hyponatremia and of clinical manifestations on water restriction.
7. No signs of renal, cardiac or adrenal disease.

Chapter 2

THE THYROID

THYROTOXICOSIS

(HYPERTHYROIDISM)

Thyrotoxicosis (hyperthyroidism), the excessive secretion of thyroid hormones, occurs in various clinical forms. The most common is Graves' disease (Basedow's disease) that occurs most frequently in women in the third and fourth decade of life, less frequently in men and children. The disease is characterized by thyrotoxicosis associated with diffuse thyroid enlargement, exophthalmos and other ocular changes, myopathy and presence in serum of the long acting thyroid stimulator (LATS) and LATS-protector.

A second form of thyrotoxicosis, toxic adenoma, is produced by an autonomously hyperfunctioning adenoma of the thyroid; it appears in a younger age group. In this form, a small round nodule, usually 2 to 4 cm in diameter, may be palpable. Thyroid nodule is smooth and firm and moves freely upwards when swallowing. Cardiovascular manifestations predominate the clinical picture, whereas ocular manifestations and muscle weakness do not occur; LATS activity is usually not detectable.

Toxic multinodular goiter is usually a complication of non-toxic multinodular goiter, and occurs predominantly in females over age 50. Tachycardia, atrial fibrillation, heart failure and muscle weakness are common manifestations; on the other hand, infiltrative ophthalmopathy is not present.

Thyrotoxicosis exhibits numerous clinical symptoms and affects many organs and tissues, especially skin, cardiovascular system, nervous system, alimentary tract, muscles, and eyes.

Fig. 1. Face of a 28-year-old patient with thyrotoxicosis of recent onset. Wide palpebral fissures and staring eyes give an expression of surprise. The thyroid is enlarged. Serum thyroxine 21 μg/dl, serum triiodothyronine 560 ng/dl, ^{131}I uptake is 88%.

Fig. 2. Face of a 49-year-old patient with Graves' disease showing characteristic eye changes: exophthalmos, wide palpebral fissures, and stare; furrows appear between the eyes. Serum thyroxine 15.8 μg/dl, ^{131}I uptake is 82%.

Fig. 3. Thyrotoxicosis. Note widened palpebral fissures, frightened expression of the eyes, thinned facies in a 48-year-old patient.

Fig. 4. A 50-year-old patient with Graves' disease. Marked swelling of the neck due to diffuse thyroid enlargement. Edema of the lower lids. Widened palpebral fissures. Fixed, staring expression of the eyes. Thinning of the scalp hair.

PLATE 1

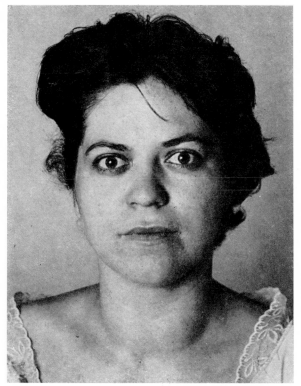

Fig. 1

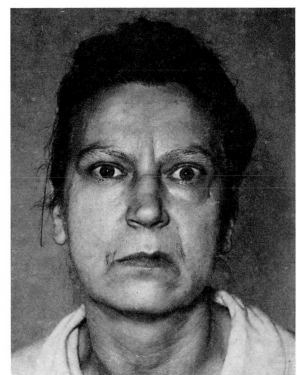

Fig. 2

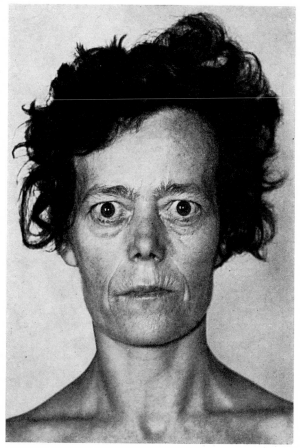

Fig. 3

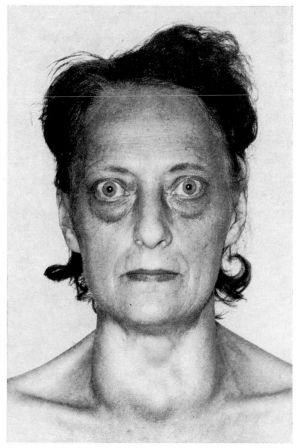

Fig. 4

Symptoms

1. Excessive irritability, anxiety, patients are easily upset; inability to relax.
2. Insomnia.
3. Heart palpitations; easy fatigability; dyspnea on exertion.
4. Constant feeling of heat, even in cold weather. Extreme discomfort in hot weather.
5. Progressive loss of weight despite a good or voracious appetite.
6. Frequent stools or diarrhea.
7. Excessive sweating.
8. Enlargement or protrusion of eyes.
9. Thyroid enlargement, with sensation of pressure on the neck.
10. Muscular weakness; weak knees when descending stairs.
11. Irregular and sparse menstruations in females.
12. Emotional instability; tendency to unprovoked weeping.
13. Excessive thirst.
14. Failing concentration; rapid flow of thoughts.
15. Falling hair.
16. Occasional abdominal pain resembling acute abdomen.

Signs

1. Restlessness: patients perform many unnecessary movements, cannot sit still.
2. Leanness; loss of subcutaneous fat.
3. Skin is pink, thin, smooth without any eruptions; excessively warm and moist. Occasional hyper-pigmentation or vitiligo.
4. The face is thin and has a scared or restless expression.
5. Eye changes: stare, widened palpebral fissures, exophthalmos, sometimes lid edema.
6. Diffuse or nodular thyroid enlargement, sometimes with vascular murmurs over the gland.
7. Tachycardia. The heart rate nearly always is accelerated (100 to 150 beats/min) even at rest or in sleep. Systolic murmurs are common. In older patients atrial fibrillation is frequent.
8. Tendency to hypertension. Widened pulse pressure; an increase in systolic and decrease in diastolic pressure.
9. Loss of the usual downy hair on the extremities. In females, axillary hair is frequently lost and hair on the scalp is thinned.
10. Fine, rapid trembling of the upper extremities, of the tongue, sometimes of the whole body.
11. Rapid, nervous speech.
12. Brisk, accelerated tendon reflexes.
13. Muscle atrophy and weakness.

Fig. 1. A 60-year-old patient with Graves' disease. Note advanced eye changes and fixed stare typical of the disease. Ferocious look accentuated both by widened fissures and furrows between the eyebrows.

Fig. 2. A 52-year-old patient with Graves' disease displays marked protrusion of the eyeballs, widened palpebral fissures, squint, lid lag.

Fig. 3A. Considerably emaciated face of a 32-year-old patient with thyrotoxicosis. Asymmetric protrusion of the eyeballs gives an incongruous appearance. Insignificant goiter present.

Fig. 3B. The same patient after 6 months treatment with antithyroid drugs. The thyroid is now enlarged. Weight gain 8 kg. Note normal appearance of the face and eyes.

PLATE 2

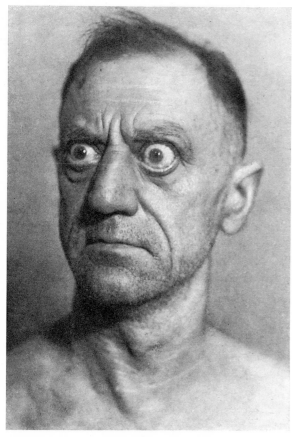

Fig. 1

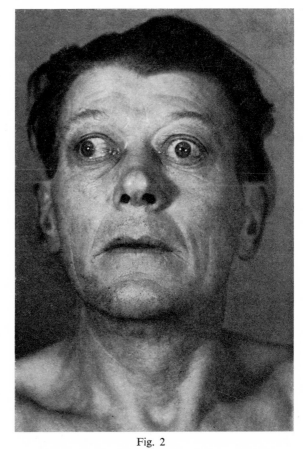

Fig. 2

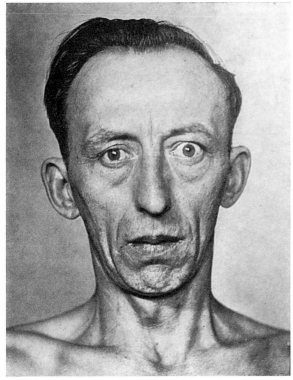

Fig. 3A

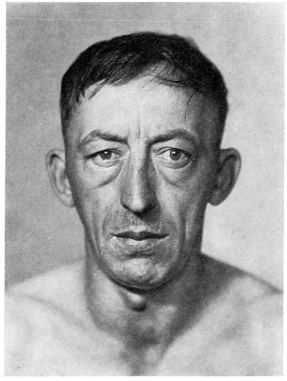

Fig. 3B

Ocular Manifestations of Graves' Disease

The ocular manifestations of Graves' disease may be divided into two distinct categories, mild and severe. The latter often referred to as infiltrative ophthalmopathy, or progressive exophthalmos. In its mild form, patients sometimes complain of photophobia and increased lacrimation. Ocular manifestations consist of retraction of the eyelids, widening of the palpebral fissures, stare, proptosis and lid lag. When the patient looks downward, the upper lid movement lags behind the globe, thus exposing more of the sclera (von Graefe's sign). These eye changes give the patient's face a frightened, astonished or staring expression. Slight edema of the lids may be present. The ocular manifestations are closely related to thyrotoxicosis and gradually regress after successful treatment, with the exception of exophthalmos, which may persist for several years.

The Skin

Changes in the skin are one of the classic manifestations of thyrotoxicosis. The skin is moist and warm, smooth and pleasant to the touch, and of a pinkish hue. Any eruptions on the shoulders of the patients disappear when hyperthyroidism develops. The skin alterations result from dilatation of the peripheral vessels and increased sweating. The skin temperature is raised, especially at the periphery.

The downy hair on the extremities and the axillary hair become sparse or, in some females, are completely lost. Similarly, the hair of the scalp thins, and the remaining hair is very soft and fine. Premature graying is common. Vitiligo and redness of the palms are more frequent than in general population.

Fig. 1. A 36-year-old patient with Graves' disease. Widened palpebral fissures, retracted eyelids and protruding eyeballs give a staring appearance. Slight swelling of the eyelids is also present.
Fig. 2. Eyes of a 40-year-old patient with Graves' disease. Frightened look due to exophthalmos and lid lag.
Fig. 3. Fine tremor of the hands — a very common sign in thyrotoxicosis.

PLATE 3

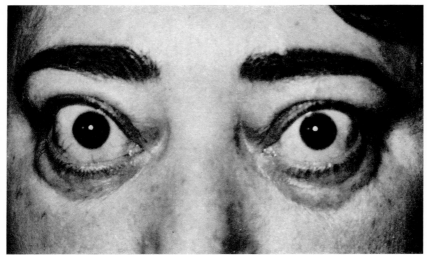

Fig. 1

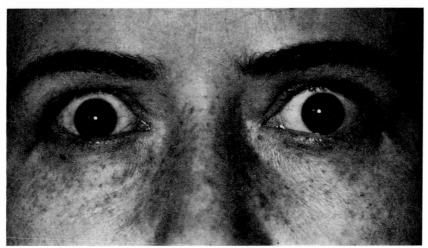

Fig. 2

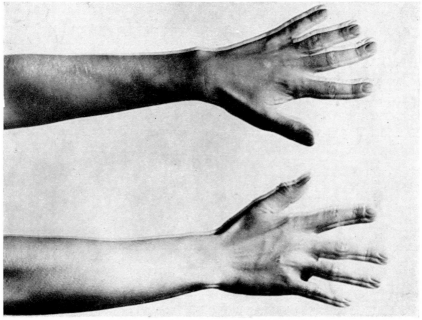

Fig. 3

The Circulation

Nearly all patients with thyrotoxicosis complain of dyspnea on exertion and palpitations that are exaggerated by excitement. The heart rate is accelerated, usually to between 100 and 130 beats/min. In older patients atrial fibrillation, or flutter, may develop, at first spasmodically, but later becoming continuous. The heartbeats and apical impulses are strong; the sounds are loud. Systolic murmurs over the pulmonic area are common; after treatment they disappear, together with other heart abnormalities. There is frequently an increase in the systolic blood pressure usually to between 160 and 180 mm, with simultaneous drop of the diastolic pressure amounting to between 50 and 80 mm. Thus, the difference between the systolic and diastolic pressure is increased.

In some older patients, especially those who have suffered previous heart damage or atrial fibrillation, congestive heart failure may develop; it is usually resistant to administration of digoxin but regresses once the thyrotoxicosis is controlled.

Electrocardiograms in thyrotoxicosis almost always show sinus tachycardia. In some cases there are signs of right atrial and left ventricular hypertrophy, in other cases atrioventricular fibrillation, or flutter. Fluoroscopy and kymography reveal the heart contractures to be exaggerated, and there is sometimes a widening of both truncus and main branches of the pulmonary artery.

The carotid arteriogram is altered, showing an almost perpendicular upstroke of the percussion wave with an acute peak. There is a rapid downward deflection toward a deepened incisura, almost reaching the isoelectric line and followed by a distinct dicrotic wave. Hemodynamic studies show an increase in cardiac output and in stroke volume. The pulse wave velocity is also increased. The circulation time is shortened.

Figs. 1A to 1C. Standard leads from ECGs of 3 patients with thyrotoxicosis show increased voltage of P waves in lead II, a frequent occurrence in this disease.

Fig. 2. ECG of a 62-year-old patient with thyrotoxicosis shows atrial fibrillation common in older patients.

Fig. 3. ECG of a 48-year-old patient with thyrotoxicosis illustrates atrial flutter.

88

PLATE 4

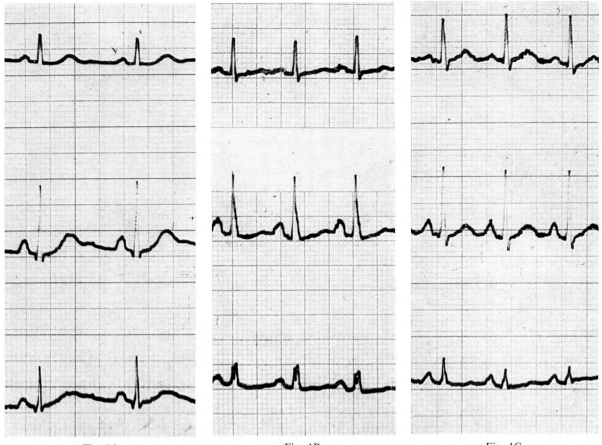

Fig. 1A   Fig. 1B   Fig. 1C

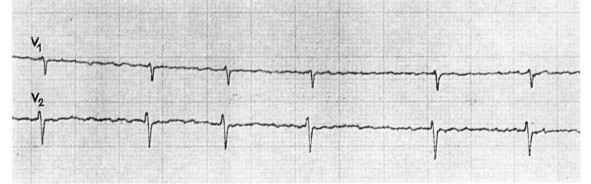

Fig. 2

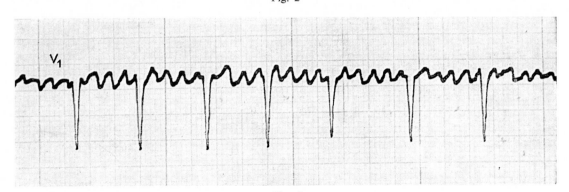

Fig. 3

Thyroid Scintiscanning

This technique allows precise localization of radioiodine accumulation in the thyroid. The scintiscanning is useful in a proper evaluation of solitary nodules since it detects areas of increased or decreased radioiodine accumulation; thus discrimination can be made between "hot" and "cold" nodules. The former secretes an excess of thyroid hormones and is a potential cause of thyrotoxicosis. In contrast, "cold" nodules are more likely to be malignant. Thyroid scintiscanning is helpful in revealing substernal goiter, ectopic thyroid tissue and functioning metastases of thyroid carcinoma.

Fig. 1. Scintiscan of a normal thyroid showing uniform distribution of radioactive iodine.

Fig. 2. Scintiscan of thyroid of a patient with toxic adenoma shows a "hot" nodule in the left lobe. Radioactive iodine accumulates solely in the hyperactive nodule.

Fig. 3. Scintiscan of a female with thyrotoxicosis and diffuse thyroid enlargement shows marked increase in size and concentration.

Fig. 4. Thyroid scintiscan of a female with thyroid enlargement and adenoma shows lack of radioiodine accumulation in the lower pole of this lobe due to a "cold" nodule.

PLATE 5

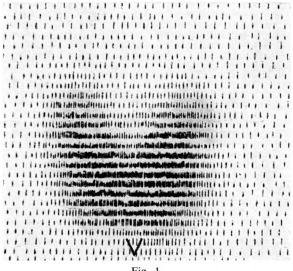

Fig. 1

Fig. 2

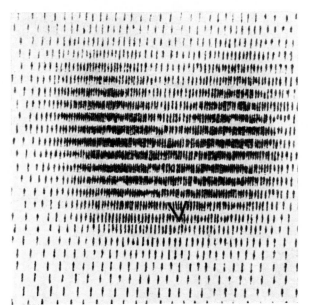

Fig. 3

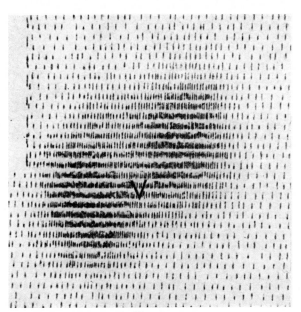

Fig. 4

Laboratory Findings

1. High serum triiodothyronine concentration above 300 ng/dl (N = 80 to 200 ng/dl).
2. High serum thyroxine concentration above 12 μg/dl in the majority of patients; normal values occur in cases with T_3 toxicosis. Free thyroxine markedly elevated. High normalized thyroxine level.
3. Low plasma TSH concentration. No response to thyrotropin-releasing hormone. After intravenous injection of 0.2 mg TRH, the serum TSH remains low (0 to 5 μU/ml), while in control subjects it rapidly rises (N = 8 to 28 μU/ml).
4. Increased ^{131}I uptake of from 70% to 95% (N = 25% to 60%).
5. Triiodothyronine uptake ratio increased.
6. No suppression of the ^{131}I uptake after triiodothyronine administration.
7. Presence of LATS in the serum.
8. ECG: sinus tachycardia, increased voltage of P wave in the standard lead II. Atrial fibrillation in older patients.
9. Increased basal metabolic rate.
10. Decreased cholesterol level.
11. Increased serum thyroglobulin concentration.
12. Reflexogram: shortened reflex time.

Fig. 1. Serum triiodothyronine concentration in thyrotoxicosis, in hypothyroidism and in control subjects. In all thyrotoxic patients the serum T_3 concentration is considerably elevated above 300 ng/dl.

Fig. 2. Serum thyrotropin concentration in stimulation tests using TRH in thyrotoxic and control subjects. The latter show a definite rise in serum TSH 20 and 30 min following administration of 0.2 mg TRH iv, whereas in the former there is no response to TRH, and the serum TSH level remains low (0 to 5 μU/ml).

Fig. 3. Results of ^{131}I uptake in thyrotoxic and control subjects. The uptake is accelerated and increased in cases of thyrotoxicosis.

Fig. 4. Effective thyroxine ratio (normalized serum thyroxine index) in thyrotoxicosis, in hypothyroidism and in control subjects. In thyrotoxic patients the ratio definitely increases; it is lower in hypothyroidism.

PLATE 6

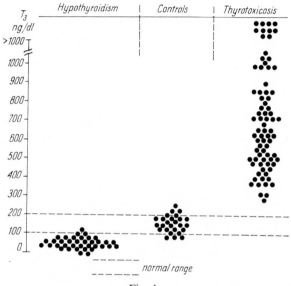

Fig. 1

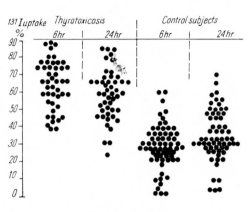

Fig. 3

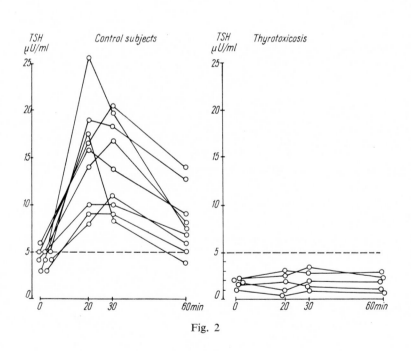

Fig. 2

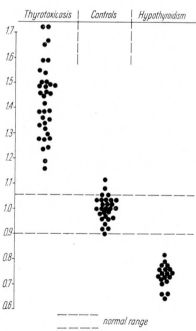

Fig. 4

INFILTRATIVE OPHTHALMOPATHY

(PROGRESSIVE EXOPHTHALMOS)

This is a serious eye condition associated with Graves' disease, though its course is independent of thyrotoxicosis and may even progress after thyroid function has been restored to normal. In ophthalmopathy, hyperthyroidism is usually mild; the thyroid is only slightly enlarged and ocular manifestations dominate the clinical picture.

Etiology is still unknown; exophthalmos-producing substance and LATS are reported to be present in the serum of the persons afflicted. The usual symptoms associated with infiltrative ophthalmopathy are watering eyes, photophobia, sandiness and headaches. Exophthalmos is usually masked by marked edema of the eyelids. Chemosis, conjunctivitis, paralysis of eye muscles, limited eye movement, failure of the upper and lower eyelids to apposition, double vision and some diminished visual acuity are characteristic of the disease. As the disease progresses entropion, corneal ulceration and panophtalmitis may occur. Extraocular muscle weakness inhibits eye movement, especially the upward gaze; patients are unable to look upward without tilting their heads. Many patients are considerably handicapped by the disease for several months. The manifestations usually regress gradually in subsequent years.

Extensive periorbital edema, marked exophthalmos and extraocular muscle weakness with limitation of upward gaze are typical of infiltrative ophthalmopathy and differ from the stare and lid retraction found in the mild form of eye changes of Graves' disease, though transitional forms may occur.

Fig. 1. Pronounced pouches due to periorbital edema, chemosis and conjunctivitis in a male with infiltrative ophthalmopathy associated with mild hyperthyroidism.

Fig. 2. Infiltrative ophthalmopathy which developed several months after the onset of Graves' disease. There is marked edema of the conjunctiva and eyelids, and paralysis of external eye muscles. The patient is unable to look upward.

Fig. 3. Periorbital edema, striking chemosis and conjunctivitis in a 54-year-old female with insignificant hyperthyroidism.

PLATE 7

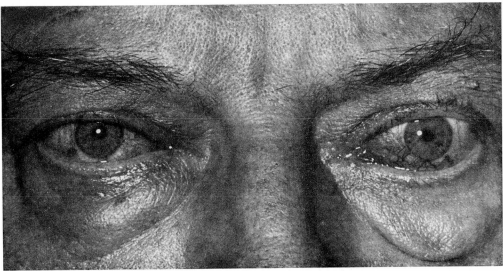

Fig. 1

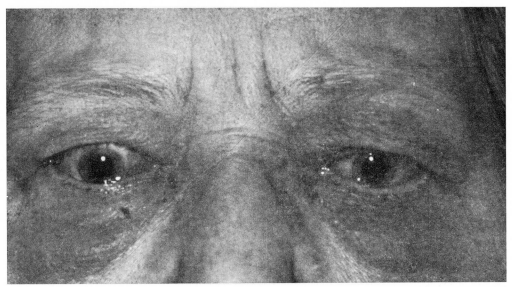

Fig. 2

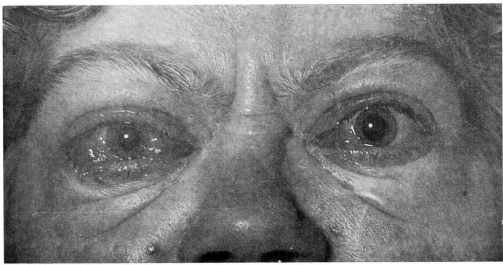

Fig. 3

LOCALIZED PRETIBIAL MYXEDEMA

Localized pretibial myxedema is the term used to indentify rare skin changes, localized in the antero-lateral region of the lower legs, that occur before, during or after thyrotoxicosis. In both calves there is a firm swelling elevated above the surface of the skin, usually oval in outline, and of a pink color. The pores of the affected skin are enlarged and thus the skin resembles an orange peel; the skin is sometimes hairless.

The changes are bilateral, and for the most part, symmetric; they may last for several years or regress spontaneously. The pathogenesis of this syndrome is obscure; however, a frequent association with ophthalmopathy of Graves' disease suggests a common etiologic factor. Histologically, mucinous infiltrations extending deeply into the dermis and similar to skin changes in myxedema are found, hence the term pretibial myxedema.

THYROID ACROPACHY

This is a rare disease of unknown etiology nearly always associated with Graves' disease and pretibial myxedema. The main characteristics are: clubbing of the fingers and toes, swelling of the soft tissues and periosteal new bone formation of the phalanges and, occasionally, other distal bones. The periosteum of the affected bones is thickened and has lacy, frothy, bubbled appearance.

Fig. 1. Face of a 50-year-old patient with infiltrative ophthalmopathy. Exophthalmos, chemosis, and conjunctivitis are present; thyroid function remains normal. Pretibial myxedema also present.

Fig. 2. A 50-year-old patient with Graves' disease shows manifestations of infiltrative ophthalmopathy, asymmetric exophthalmos, periorbital edema and conjunctivitis, especially on the left side.

Fig. 3. Hand of a patient with infiltrative ophthalmopathy of Graves' disease presenting signs of thyroid acropachy, clubbing of the fingers and swelling of the soft tissues.

Figs. 4A and 4B. Lower legs of 2 male patients showing changes typical of pretibial myxedema: localized edema of pink color, and in Fig. 4B — loss of hair: the pores are accentuated and slightly elevated, all these changes resembling an orange peel.

PLATE 8

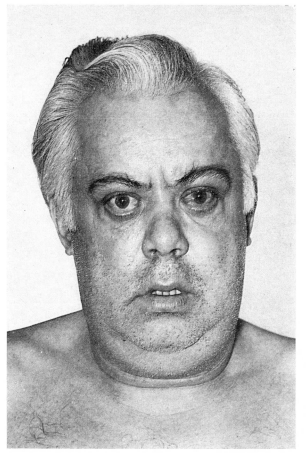

Fig. 1

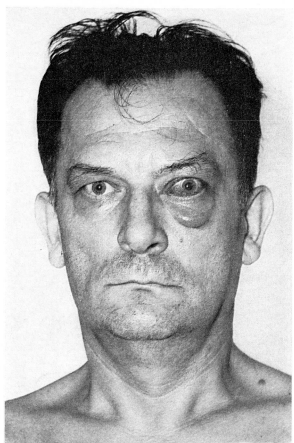

Fig. 2

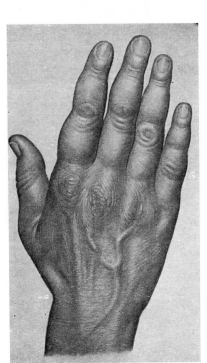

Fig. 3

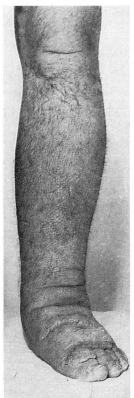

Fig. 4A

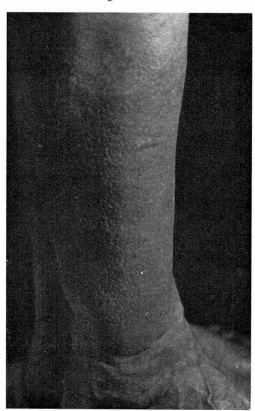

Fig. 4B

HYPOTHYROIDISM

(MYXEDEMA)

Hypothyroidism is a chronic disease which results from a deficiency in thyroid hormones. It is 10 times as common in females as in males and occurs in all age groups. It occurs most often, however, between the ages of 40 and 60. Because of the insidious onset, slow progression of the clinical manifestations and unspecific initial symptoms, some patients remain undiagnosed for many years. Hypothyroidism is caused by loss or atrophy of thyroid tissue (thyroprivic hypothyroidism) of unknown etiology, or by the end stage of autoimmune thyroiditis. Hypothyroidism may follow total, or occasionally subtotal, thyroidectomy (postablative hypothyroidism) or destruction of thyroid tissue by radioiodine (postradioiodine hypothyroidism). Hypothyroidism may also result from biochemical abnormalities in the synthesis of thyroid hormones that are associated with goiter (goitrous hypothyroidism).

Fig. 1. A 30-year-old patient with hypothyroidism. Note edema of upper lids and cheeks. Lips are thick and cyanotic. There is double chin.

Fig. 2. Face of 36-year-old patient with hypothyroidism of recent origin. The face is bloated, blepharoptosis is present, as is cyanosis on lips and cheeks (the so-called "malar flush").

Fig. 3. A 51-year-old patient with hypothyroidism. The face is pale and puffed; the upper lids are markedly swollen.

Fig. 4. Face of a 57-year-old patient with myxedema is markedly swollen, especially the cheeks and nose, and there is a double chin. The upper eyelids droop; the palpebral fissures are narrow, the eyebrows drawn up and angular and the forehead wrinkled.

PLATE 9

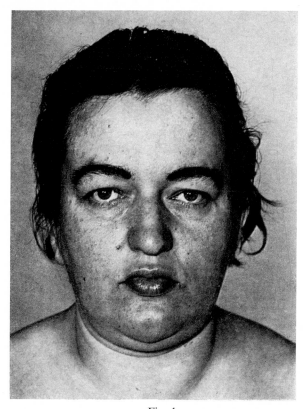

Fig. 1

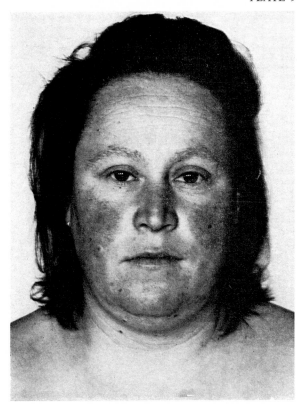

Fig. 2

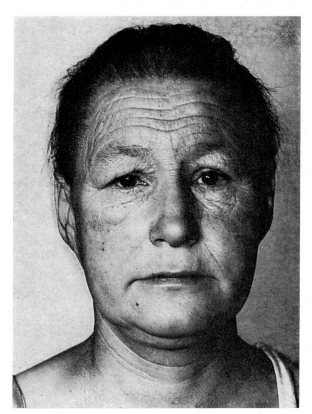

Fig. 3

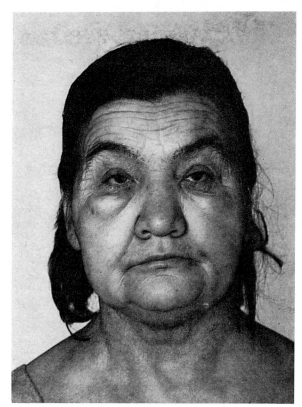

Fig. 4

Symptoms

1. Weakness.
2. Fatigability; dyspnea on exertion.
3. Lethargy; drowsiness; failing concentration.
4. Sensation of cold, even in warm weather; extreme sensitivity to cold.
5. Edema of lids, face and hands, usually more pronounced in the morning.
6. Numbness and paresthesia of the fingers.
7. Pains in the limbs; difficulty in walking.
8. Dryness of the skin, despite ointment application; elbows, knees, occasionally hands appear dirty, even after careful washing.
9. Constipation.
10. Increase in weight despite poor appetite and reduced intake of food.
11. Huskiness in voice; inability to sing.
12. Impairment of hearing.
13. Menorrhagia; dysmenorrhea in females; occasional sterility.
14. Nervousness.
15. Failing memory.
16. Falling hair.

Fig. 1. Face of a 48-year-old patient with hypothyroidism is pale and swollen; cyanosis present on the cheeks, tip of the nose and chin.

Fig. 2. A 61-year-old patient with hypothyroidism exhibiting marked edema of the upper and lower lids, nose and cheeks. The upper lids are swollen and drooping; the eyes are dark and have a weepy look; the palpebral fissures are considerably narrowed.

Fig. 3. Coarse hair which does not retain a wave, swollen cheeks and eyelids and double chin in a 45-year-old patient with hypothyroidism.

Fig. 4. Face of a 66-year-old patient shows advanced myxedema. Puffy forehead, nose, cheeks and chin; angularly lifted eyebrows, swollen upper lids, dark weepy eyes; narrowed fissures; cyanotic lips and cheeks; coarse hair are presenting manifestations.

PLATE 10

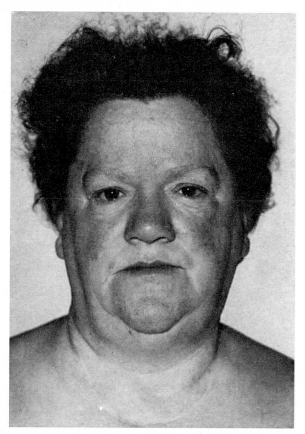

Fig. 1

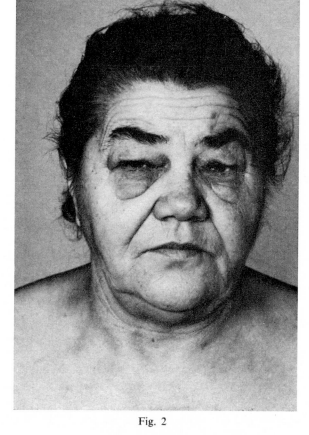

Fig. 2

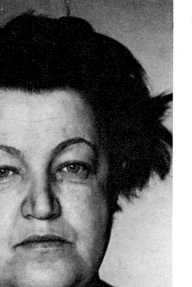

Fig. 3

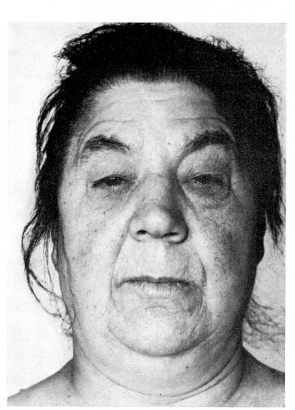

Fig. 4

Signs

1. Myxedema, puffy features.
2. Sluggish movements; unsteady walk.
3. Skin dry, coarse and scaly.
4. Skin pale, with yellowish tint.
5. Bloated face with somnolent expression; cyanosis of lips and cheeks.
6. Eyes: palpebral ptosis and edema, narrowed palpebral fissures, weepy appearance. Eyebrows lifted upwards, thinned at periphery.
7. Slow speech; huskiness in voice; articulation slurred.
8. Lusterless brittle hair that will not curl; partial baldness.
9. Loss of axillary hair and body hair in females.
10. Broad neck, double chin, supraclavicular fat pads. Scar on the neck in postthyroidectomy patients.
11. Heart sounds feeble; bradycardia.
12. Obesity in the majority of patients.
13. Protuberant abdomen.
14. Lowered body temperature.
15. Deafness.
16. Delayed reflexes in tendons.

Fig. 1. A 42-year-old male with hypothyroidism. Acromegaly was suspected because of enlarged hands and feet and changes in the face. The upper eyelids and cheeks are puffed; the lips thick. Serum HGH 2 ng/ml, thyroxine 1.2 μg/dl, triiodothyronine 50 ng/dl, ^{131}I uptake is 4%.

Fig. 2. A 60-year-old male with hypothyroidism. The face and especially the eyelids are puffed; the palpebral fissures are narrowed.

Figs. 3A and 3B. Induced hypothyroidism in a 65-year-old patient with intractable angina after three myocardial infarctions. A. Before radioiodine treatment. B. After radioiodine administration which resulted in myxedema. The face is bloated, lips cyanotic; the upper and lower lids are markedly swollen. Narrow palpebral fissures give the face a sleepy appearance.

PLATE 11

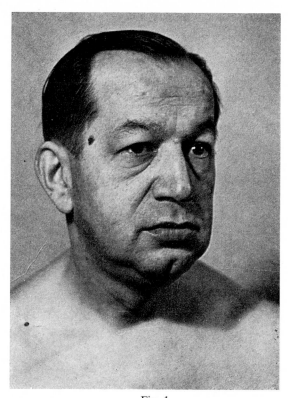

Fig. 1

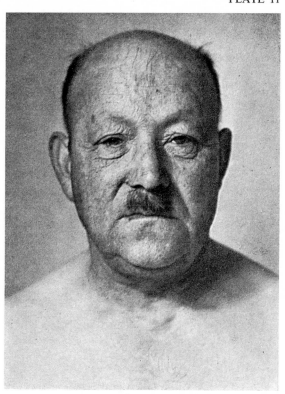

Fig. 2

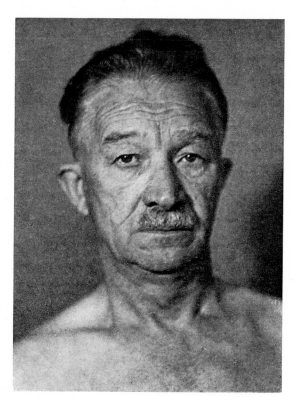

Fig. 3A

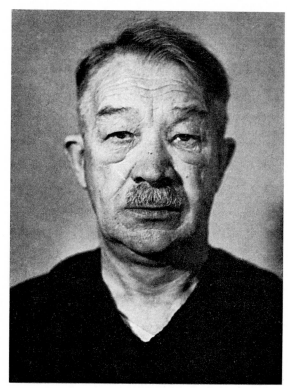

Fig. 3B

The Face

Edema of the face and eyelids is a common symptom. On physical examination the face is often puffed and bloated, becoming broader and more rounded. Individual characteristics disappear as the protruding parts of the face are distorted by myxedema; the similarity of one patient to another increases. The folds of the skin, especially the nasolabial folds, become less distinct. The narrowed palpebral fissures, bloated face and complete lack of animation give the face a somnolent expression. The nose is broad, and its bridge disappears in the edema of the surrounding tissues, giving an impression of widely set eyes. The lips thicken and have a cyanotic appearance. The facial skin is dry, pale and sometimes sallow. In many cases there is cyanosis on the tip of the nose, on the cheeks and chin, sometimes of a very dark hue like a malar flush.

Fig. 1A. A 29-year-old patient with pronounced muscle weakness and hypothyroidism undiagnosed for several years. The face is slightly puffed, the upper lids droop giving a sleepy appearance.

Fig. 1B. Face of the same patient after 2 months treatment with thyroxine. Complete change in appearance; the palpebral fissures become normal, puffiness disappears.

Fig. 2A. A 62-year-old patient with myxedema. Marked edema of the face; cyanotic lips, cheeks and nose; narrow fissures, somnolent look. The hair is stiff, without luster and does not retain a wave.

Fig. 2B. The same patient after 3 months replacement therapy. Disappearance of edema and cyanosis. Healthy appearance. The hair is easy to manage.

PLATE 12

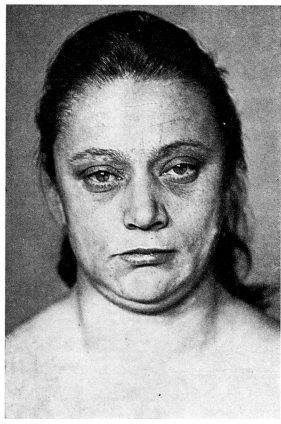

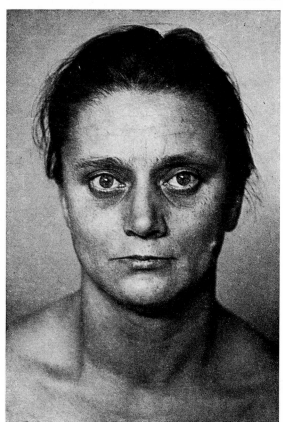

Fig. 1A

Fig. 1B

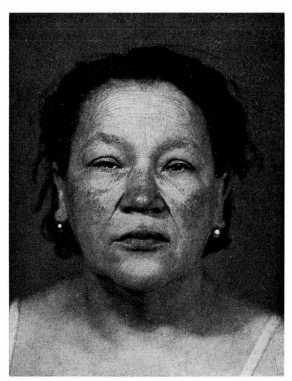

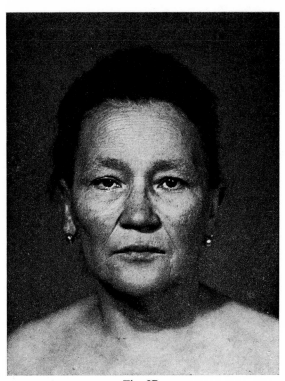

Fig. 2A

Fig. 2B

The Eyes

Narrowing of the palpebral fissures, a common sign, is caused by blepharoptosis, i.e., drooping of the upper eyelids, and their edema. The upper and lower lids become puffed, as does the base of the nose on occasion. In some cases the upper lids are uniformly swollen; in others they hang loosely like a curtain with numerous folds, overhanging the lid margin. In many patients the eyes are dark and have a tearful look. The dark eyes are caused by a narrowing of the palpebral fissures that prevents light from reaching the eyes in a quantity such as is normal when the fissures are wide open, as well by the puffy upper lids that shadow the eyes.

The tearful look of the eyes is probably the result of the flow of tears being disturbed due to a swelled nasolacrimal canal, and to some extent from edema of the bulbar conjunctiva. The bags under the eyes tend to increase the impression of weepiness.

The eyebrows are lifted as if drawn up, and sometimes change their normal arch shape, become angular and gable-like. The patient may wrinkle the forehead and raise the eyebrows in an effort to lift the drooping upper lids. The eyebrows are coarse, dull and sparse, especially at their outer parts.

After proper treatment all ocular signs disappear; the eyebrows lower and regain shape, the palpebral fissures widen; the eyes appear lighter and livelier; edema of the lids and nose vanishes.

Fig. 1. Dark, weepy eyes of a 58-year-old female with hypothyroidism; enormous swelling of upper and lower lids, angular eyebrows, drooping eyelids and narrow fissures.

Fig. 2. Pouched eyes of a 66-year-old male with myxedema. Marked swelling of lids; upper lids hang loosely and overshadow the lid margins; narrowed fissures.

Fig. 3. Eyes of a 36-year-old female with hypothyroidism. Marked blepharoptosis; thickened lids; weepy look.

PLATE 13

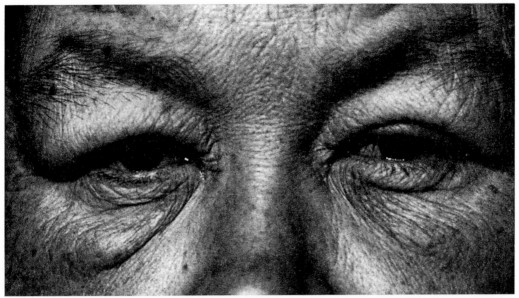

Fig. 1

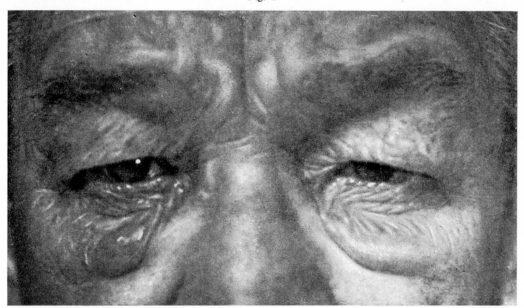

Fig. 2

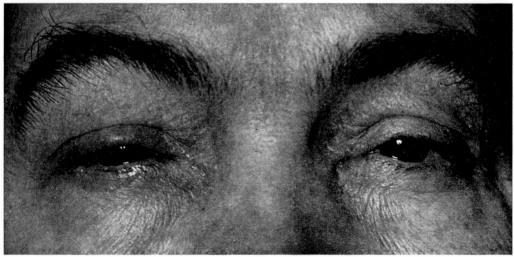

Fig. 3

The Skin

The skin is nearly always pale, cold and dry due to a decrease in sweating, sebaceous activity and defective peripheral circulation. Sometimes it is coarse and scaly, and may peel. In some cases there is hyperkeratosis; the skin is grayish and looks dirty, particularly on the knees and elbows. The skin temperature is lowered. In myxedema coma it is so low that it cannot be measured by the use of a normal thermometer.

Fig. 1. Loss of hair on forearms of a 50-year-old patient with hypothyroidism.
Fig. 2A. Dorsum of hand of a 58-year-old patient with hypothyroidism; the skin is thickened, dry and scaly.
Fig. 2B. The same area of the hand. Larger magnification shows a brany peeling.
Fig. 3A. A 58-year-old patient with hypothyroidism and vitiligo. Advanced baldness seen. The hair is brittle, coarse and does not retain a wave.
Fig. 3B. The same patient after one year on replacement therapy with thyroxine. Note regrowth of lost hair.

PLATE 14

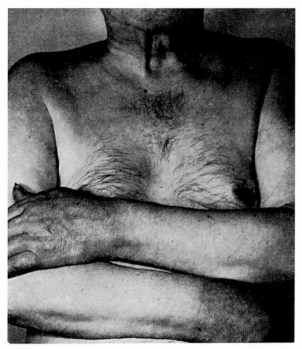

Fig. 1

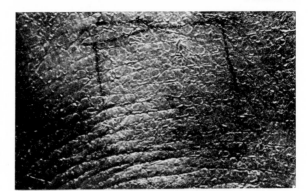

Fig. 2A

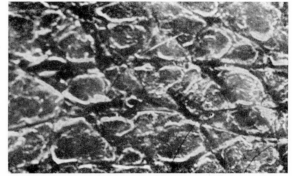

Fig. 2B

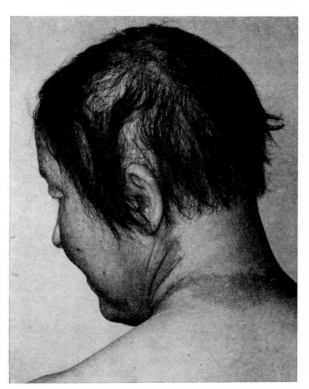

Fig. 3A

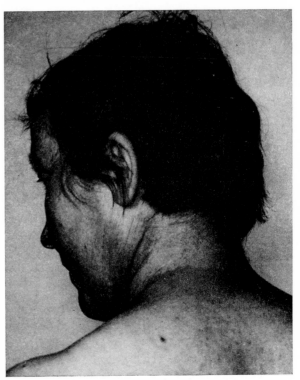

Fig. 3B

The Hands

Numbness and stiffness of the fingers, tingling sensations, and swelling of the hands are usual complaints of patients with hypothyroidism.

On physical examination the fingers are thick and of diminished flexibility. Often there is puffiness of the fingers and on the dorsa of the hands. This myxedema is firm and does not pit on pressure. The skin is always dry, sometimes scaly, usually thickened, and not transparent when compared to the dry and atrophic skin of aged persons in whom the veins on the dorsa of the hands are visible. The thickened, dry skin occasionally has a fish scale appearance or looks leathery. Some patients lose their body hair.

Following treatment the puffiness disappears; the skin becomes loose, forming numerous wrinkles on the dorsa of the hands. At this time the patients may complain of itching. Later, the skin becomes smooth, the veins visible again. Men regain their lost hair.

Fig. 1. Hand of a 55-year-old female with hypothyroidism. Thick, puffed dorsa of the hands, swollen fingers; dry and shiny skin.

Fig. 2. Hand of a 60-year-old patient with hypothyroidism exhibiting slight puffiness, dry scaly skin, atrophic epidermis.

Fig. 3A. Hand of a 48-year-old patient with hypothyroidism. The skin is dry with a leathery appearance; fingers are slightly swollen.

Fig. 3B. The same hand after 4 months treatment with thyroxine. The skin is smooth; the veins visible, no swelling in fingers.

PLATE 15

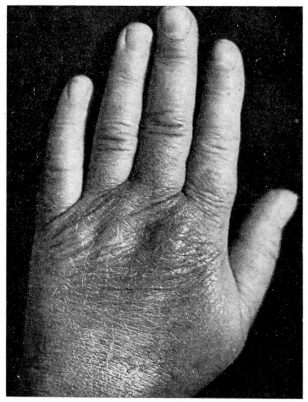

Fig. 1

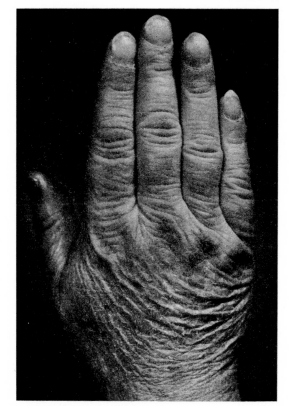
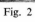

Fig. 2

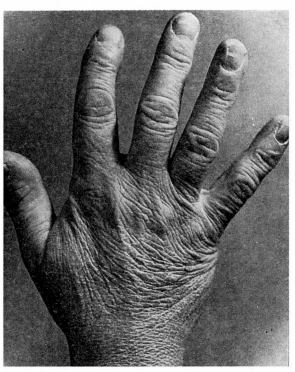
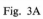

Fig. 3A

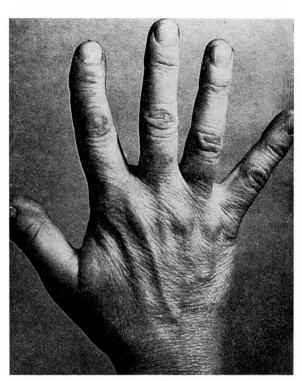

Fig. 3B

The Heart

The chief complaints of many patients are easy fatigability, dyspnea on exertion, inability to perform physical work and edema. Such symptoms suggest a diagnosis of heart disease; cyanosis and feeble heart sounds seem to confirm this. For this reason some patients are unsuccessfully treated for a mistaken diagnosis of heart disease, while hypothyroidism remains undiagnosed.

In patients with long standing hypothyroidism, physical examination reveals that the area of cardiadullness on percussion is increased and that heart sounds are feeble on auscultation.

Roentgen examination of the chest reveals a generalized enlargement of the cardiac shadow with feeble pulsations. These weak cardiac pulsations, which may be a sign of pericardial effusion, are best demonstrated by roentgenokymography or electrokymography. After appropriate treatment, the cardiac size and pulsations return to normal in the majority of patients.

Electrocardiograms in hypothyroidism almost always reveal flattening or inversion of T waves in standard and left precordial leads; a decreased voltage of QRS complexes, lowering of ST segments, QT prolongation and sinus bradycardia are also frequently seen.

Fig. 1A. Chest roentgenogram of a 50-year-old patient with long term hypothyroidism. Note marked enlargement of the cardiac shadow.

Fig. 1B. Chest roentgenogram of the same patient after 5 months of replacement therapy. Cardiac size and shape have returned to normal.

Fig. 2A. Arteriogram of the cervical artery shows dome-shaped systolic plateau with small, hardly visible dicrotic notch.

Fig. 2B. Cervical arteriogram in a patient with thyrotoxicosis reveals changes typical of this disease: sharp systolic plateau and deep dicrotic notch.

Fig. 3. ECG of a 48-year-old patient with long standing hypothyroidism showing typical abnormalities: low voltage of QRS, flat T waves and sinus bradycardia.

Fig. 4A. ECG of a patient who recently experienced onset of hypothyroidism. Typical negative, or markedly flattened, T waves are seen in the standard and left precordial leads.

Fig. 4B. ECG of the same patient after 3 months thyroxine therapy shows complete disappearance of abnormalities.

PLATE 16

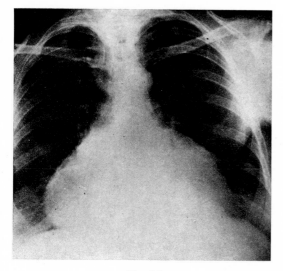

Fig. 1A

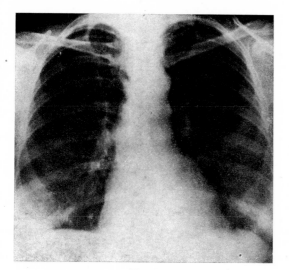

Fig. 1B

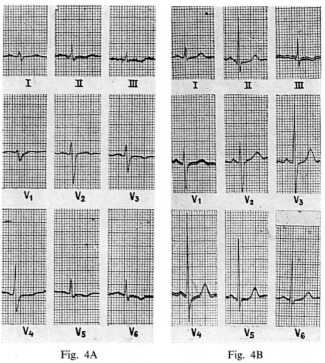

Fig. 4A   Fig. 4B

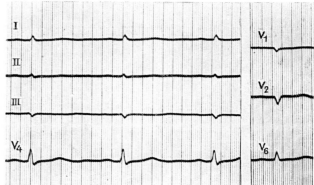

Fig. 3

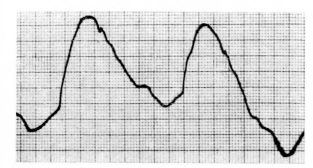

Fig. 2A

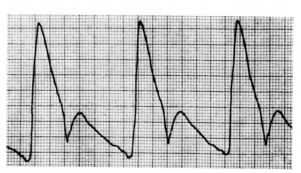

Fig. 2B

Laboratory Findings

1. Low serum thyroxine concentration.
2. High plasma TSH concentration (20 to 500 μU/ml), an early and constant finding in primary hypothyroidism.
3. Low serum triiodothyronine concentration.
4. ^{131}I uptake very low.
5. In 80% of cases hypothyroid reflexogram.
6. Basal metabolic rate lowered.
7. Protein-bound iodine decreased.
8. T_3 uptake ratio decreased.
9. Serum cholesterol elevated.
10. ECG abnormalities: inverted or flat T waves, low QRS voltage, depressed ST segment, bradycardia.
11. Roentgen findings: enlarged heart with feeble pulsations.
12. Blood sedimentation rate increased.
13. Deficient response in serum HGH to insulin-induced hypoglycemia.
14. Anemia.
15. Increased carotene concentration in the serum.
16. EEG: slowing of the basic rhythm and low voltage.
17. Frequent achlorhydria.

Fig. 1. Serum thyroxine concentration in 42 cases of hypothyroidism as determined by radioimmunoassay. The T_4 concentration is very low, 0 to 3 μg/dl.

Fig. 2. Results of serum triiodothyronine radioimmunoassay in 56 patients with hypothyroidism. The serum T_3 concentration is lowered, ranging usually from 20 to 70 ng/dl (N = 80 to 200 ng/dl). In a few cases the T_3 values overlap the normal range.

Fig. 3. Results of TSH radioimmunoassay in 46 patients with primary hypothyroidism, in control subjects and in 10 patients with secondary hypothyroidism in the course of hypopituitarism. In all patients with primary hypothyroidism TSH levels are definitely elevated (22 to 500 μU/ml) while in secondary hypothyroidism they are low (0 to 5 μU/ml).

Fig. 4. Results of ^{131}I uptake in patients with hypothyroidism and in control subjects. In all untreated patients with hypothyroidism, ^{131}I uptake is below 10%. In control subjects, ^{131}I uptake amounts to from 25% to 60%; in a few subjects the up take is in the hypothyroid range. In some cases where hypothyroidism occurred following radioiodine therapy for Graves' disease, the ^{131}I uptake is within the normal range.

PLATE 17

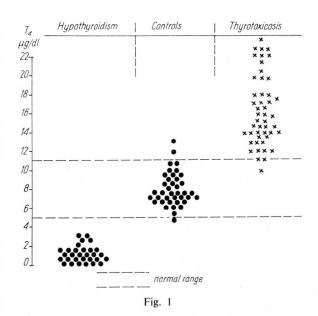

Fig. 1

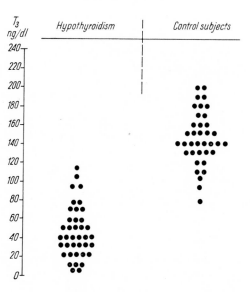

Fig. 2

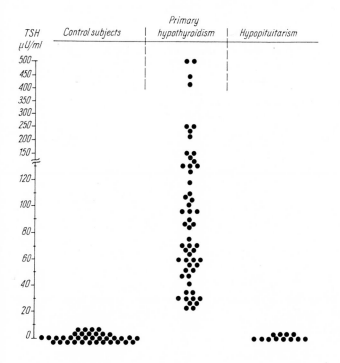

Fig. 3

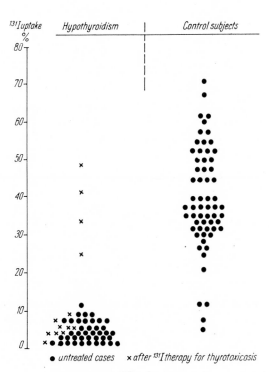

Fig. 4

115

INCIPIENT HYPOTHYROIDISM

In patients under regular medical observation after thyroidectomy, radioiodine therapy and post-thyroiditis it is possible to detect early stages of hypothyroidism. The manifestations of incipient hypothyroidism are negligible, for instance, feeling of cold paresthesia of fingers, swelling of the hands and face may be the only symptoms. On examination there are only faint physical signs, drooping and occasional puffiness of the eyelids, insignificant dryness of the skin and/or hoarseness of the voice.

At this stage laboratory findings are helpful in diagnosing hypothyroidism. Elevated serum TSH, low serum thyroxine that gradually decreases, electrocardiographic abnormalities consisting of flattened or inverted T waves confirm the diagnosis.

The Reflexes

The tendon reflexes are diminished; the most characteristic feature is a striking prolongation of the reflex time. It can best be demonstrated by recording the Achilles tendon reflexes and measuring the time of the reflex and its relaxation phase. In normal subjects the mean reflex time is 0.25 sec (SD = 0.04) and the mean relaxation time is 0.17 sec (SD = 0.03). In 82% of cases with hypothyroidism the reflex time and the relaxation time are definitely prolonged above normal values. The voltage of the deflection in recordings of the Achilles tendon reflex is reduced; the contraction time is normal, while the relaxation phase is greatly prolonged.

Fig. 1A. ECG of patient shown in Fig. 1C (taken before radioiodine therapy) shows no abnormalities. The T waves are high and positive.

Fig. 1B. ECG of the same patient 5 months after radioiodine therapy reveals definite abnormalities: flat T waves in all standard and precordial leads.

Fig. 1C. A 38-year-old patient with incipient hypothyroidism, 9 months after radioiodine administration (10 mc) for thyrotoxicosis exhibits blepharoptosis and slight edema of the cheeks. Elevated serum TSH (32 μU/ml); other laboratory findings within normal range.

Fig. 2. A 31-year-old patient who developed hypothyroidism 6 months after treatment with ^{131}I for thyrotoxicosis. Edema of the eyelids and palpebral ptosis are the only clinical findings. ECG abnormal. Reflexogram shows prolonged relaxation phase. Serum thyroxine 3 μg/dl, ^{131}I uptake 42%.

Figs. 3A to 3C. Reflexograms of a normal subject (*B*) and in a case of hypothyroidism (*C*).

PLATE 18

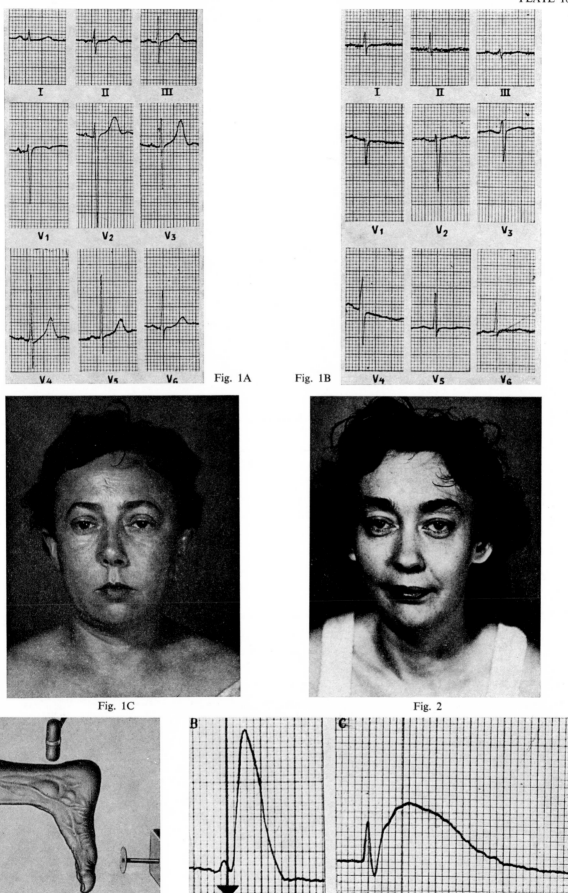

Fig. 1A

Fig. 1B

Fig. 1C

Fig. 2

Fig. 3A

Figs. 3B and 3C

CONGENITAL HYPOTHYROIDISM

(CONGENITAL MYXEDEMA; CRETINISM)

Congenital hypothyroidism is an infrequent disease that may be caused by an absence of thyroid gland tissue, by faulty growth and development of the thyroid at the base of the tongue or upper part of the neck, or by an inborn enzymatic defect in the synthesis of thyroid hormones. Cases of athyreotic hypothyroidism occur only sporadically throughout the world, while a high familial incidence of endemic goitrous hypothyroidism (goitrous cretinism) is found in regions deficient in iodine such as the Alps, Andes and Himalayas. The disease, more common in young females than in young males, is characterized by stunted growth, delayed physical and mental development, sluggishness, puffy features and other manifestations.

Fig. 1. General appearance of a 4-year-old female with congenital hypothyroidism. Stunted growth (81 cm, 32 in.). Note enlarged head; swollen face; broad, flat nose; open mouth and protruding tongue, swellings in the supraclavicular area; short, broad neck; dry, grayish skin; edema of the hands and feet. The patient cannot stand unsupported; cannot walk or speak. Serum thyroxine 1.5 μg/dl, TSH 86 μU/ml. Bone age is 3 months. First lumbar vertebral body is deformed; no ossification centers are found in the femoral heads.

PLATE 19

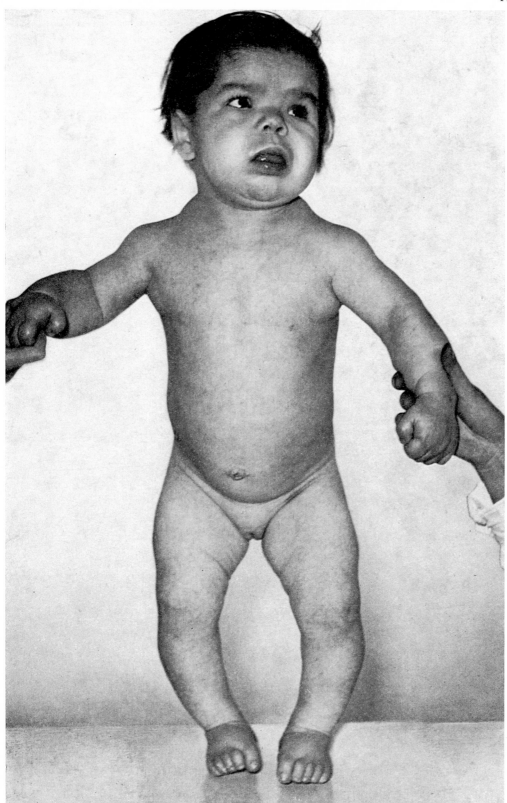

Fig. 1

Symptoms

1. Stunted growth, a constant finding even in mild cases.
2. Disinterest in food; despite low food intake, the patients look overweight or are of normal weight.
3. Lack of activity; sluggishness, drowsiness, no interest in surroundings.
4. Impairment of mental development; marked delay in speech ability.
5. Slow, unsteady walk.
6. Hoarse, low-pitched cry.
7. Persistent constipation.
8. Delayed dentition.

Fig. 1. Advanced generalized myxedema in a 14-year-old untreated patient. The face is greatly swollen and of cretinous appearance; an enlarged tongue protrudes from the open mouth. The large head embedded in supraclavicular edema rests directly on the trunk. Protruding abdomen; enormous myxedematous changes. The patient has difficulties in standing and walking. Height 102 cm (40 in.). Bone age 6 months. Stippled ossification centers of the femoral heads.

Fig. 2. A 13-year-old untreated patient with congenital goitrous hypothyroidism. Height 106 cm (42 in.). Note cretinoid facial features, short neck and protruding abdomen with umbilical hernia. Bone age 1 year. Epiphyseal dysgenesis; the femoral heads reveal multiple irregular ossification centers.

Fig. 3. A 6-year-old female with congenital hypothyroidism and insignificant manifestations. Delayed growth the only complaint. Height 98 cm (39 in.). The face is round, cheeks slightly puffed, and abdomen is large. Serum thyroxine 2 μg/dl, serum TSH 48 μU/ml. Bone age 6 months, no epiphyseal centers of the femoral heads present.

Fig. 4. A 12-year-old patient with untreated hypothyroidism. Note large head, swollen face, short neck, protruding abdomen with umbilical hernia; lower extremities flexed at the hip and knee joints.

PLATE 20

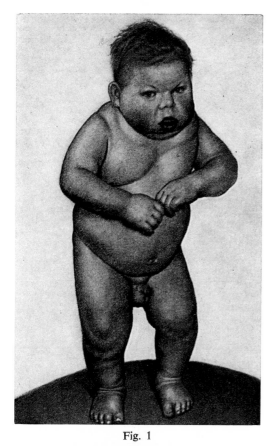

Fig. 1

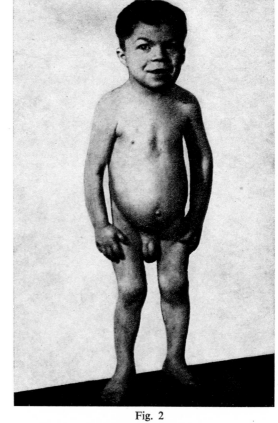

Fig. 2

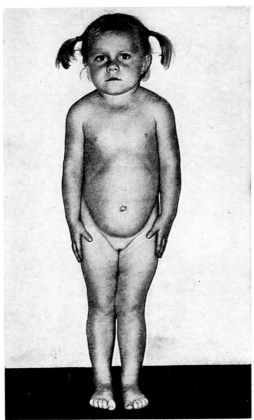

Fig. 3

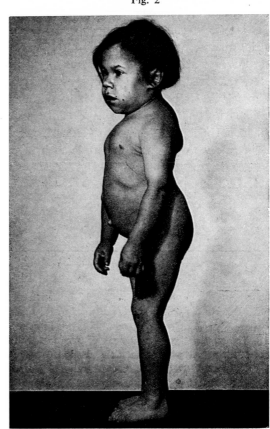

Fig. 4

Signs

1. Short stature; dwarfism.
2. Persistence of childlike body proportions; short extremities; stocky trunk; large head.
3. Pale, cyanose, puffy face.
4. Protuberant abdomen (potbelly); umbilical hernia.
5. Dry, thickened, grayish skin.
6. Supraclavicular pads. Loose folds of thickened skin and subcutaneous tissue.
7. Downy hair, usually on the nape of the neck and on the back.
8. Characteristic posture: lumbar lordosis; prominent buttocks; slightly flexed knees.
9. Skin pale with yellowish tinge due to hypercarotinemia.
10. Husky, hoarse, deep voice; delayed development of speech.

Fig. 1A. A 6-year-old female with congenital hypothyroidism. Large head, swollen face, narrowed palpebral fissures, broad and puffed neck, large protruding abdomen with umbilical hernia, short extremities are shown. Height 96 cm (38 in.). Bone age 3 months. No ossification centers of the femoral heads are present; L_1 vertebral body is deformed; marked retardation in mental development.

Fig. 1B. The same patient after 3 years of treatment with thyroxine which resulted in rapid growth spurt and complete regression of all pathologic manifestations. Mental development is delayed. Serum TSH after one month break in thyroxine therapy 46 μU/ml. Bone age now 8 years.

Fig. 2A. A 5-year-old patient with congenital hypothyroidism and insignificant manifestations. Growth and mental development delayed. Patient learned to walk in the third year and to talk in the fourth. Height 90 cm (35 in.); short neck; large abdomen; dry skin. Bone age 3 months; no ossification centers in the femoral heads.

Fig. 2B. The same patient after 3 months of thyroxine therapy resulting in increased alertness, stimulation of growth (3 cm) and weight loss.

PLATE 21

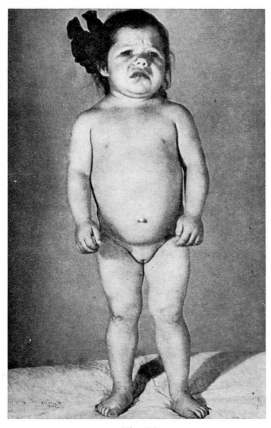

Fig. 1A

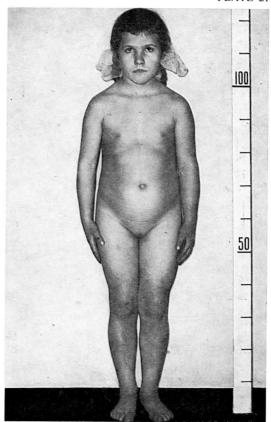

Fig. 1B

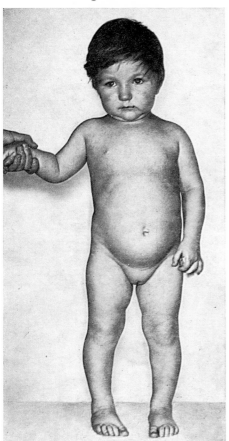

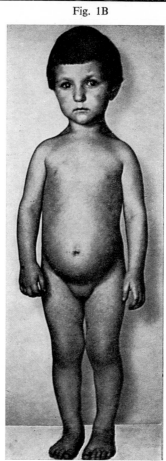

Fig. 2A   Fig. 2B

The Head and Neck

The head is large in comparison to the body. In typical cases the face is broad, rounded and bloated, with puffed cheeks. The nose is short and flattened with nostrils tilted upward giving the face a "piglike" expression. The base of the nose is underdeveloped; the eyes appear to be wide apart. The palpebral fissures are narrowed; the upper lids dropped; the eyebrows lifted upwards. The blepharoptosis hinders the ability to see forward so that the patients must tilt the head backwards. The lips are swollen and blue. The face is pale and sometimes slightly yellow, but the cheeks — like the lips — are cyanosed.

In some cases the face has a cretinous expression owing to the enlarged tongue which protrudes from the half-opened mouth. Other patients have a dull appearance. In some patients the facial appearance is inconspicuous, but the features are immature and the patients look younger than their years. The hair on the scalp is coarse, brittle, straight, dull and grows down on the forehead.

The neck is usually short and bull-like. In endemic goitrous cretinism there is a goiter, usually multi-nodular. The double chin, swollen supraclavicular pads and sloping shoulders efface the neck. There is a marked delay in the eruption of teeth and an increased susceptibility to decay.

Fig. 1. A 4-year-old female with congenital hypothyroidism. Manifestations include edema of the cheeks, coarse hair extending low on the forehead, flat nose with underdeveloped bridge and nostrils tilted upward, narrowed palpebral fissures, enlarged tongue protruding from the half-open mouth, broad neck, supraclavicular swellings.

Fig. 2. Face of a 12-year-old patient with untreated congenital hypothyroidism. Cheeks are puffy; the nose is flat, broad, with underdeveloped bridge; the skin is pale and grayish; the hair is coarse and does not retain a wave.

Fig. 3. Face of a 5-year-old female with congenital hypothyroidism does not differ from healthy children. The cheeks are slightly puffed; the nose is broad and flat. Marked stunting of growth; height 94 cm (37 in.). Bone age 6 months. Serum TSH 32 μU/ml.

Fig. 4. Face of a 6-year-old patient with congenital hypothyroidism has a normal appearance. Growth and development delayed. Typical roentgenographic findings: bone age 6 months, stippled femoral heads. Serum thyroxine 2.8 μg/dl. Dramatic improvement and stimulation of growth on thyroxine therapy.

PLATE 22

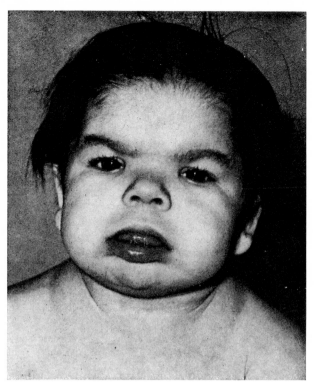

Fig. 1

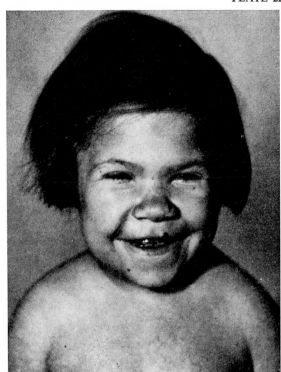

Fig. 2

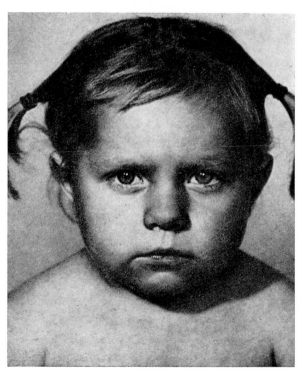

Fig. 3

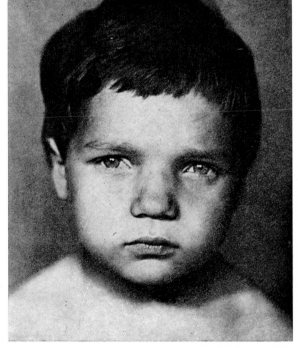

Fig. 4

The Hands

The hands are broad and pudgy with short fingers. If the patient remains untreated, the fingers become broader but remain short. In some cases the dorsa of the hands and fingers are puffed. In other cases the skin on the hands is dry and thick. Sometimes it is abundant, forming folds, or has a leathery appearance.

The Skin

The skin is cool and dry and has a dusky grayish look due to impaired peripheral circulation and diminished sweating; sometimes it is scaly. The temperature of the skin is low; frostbite is common.

There is a persistence of infantile hair in the first months of life. In older children downy hair on the back is occasionally found.

The Chest and Abdomen

The chest is triangular in shape, retaining its proportions from early childhood. The upper ribs are markedly shorter than the lower. In chest roentgenograms the heart is frequently enlarged and shows feeble pulsations.

Reduced intestinal activity and constipation are encountered in nearly all the patients. There is potbelly; the protuberance and enlargement of the abdomen are due chiefly to poor muscle tone. There is often an umbilical hernia.

Fig. 1A. A 6-year-old patient with congenital hypothyroidism showing marked puffiness of the cheeks and neck; edema of the upper lids; narrowing of the palpebral fissures; short and flat nose with undeveloped bridge; the nostrils tilt upward; the swollen, cyanotic lips. The skin is pale and grayish; the hair is coarse and dull and grows low on the forehead. The position of the head is tilted backwards to enable the patient to look straight ahead.

Fig. 1B. The same patient after 6 months treatment with thyroxine shows complete change in facial appearance. Edema has disappeared; the nose is longer, narrower; the palpebral fissures are of normal width; double chin has disappeared; the neck is longer. The hair is elastic and shiny.

Fig. 2A. Face of a 12-year-old patient with hypothyroidism. There is slight puffiness in the cheeks, and drooping of the upper lids. Cyanotic tint on the cheeks and lips. Broad, short neck. Dull hair. Serum thyroxine 1.8 μg/dl, serum TSH 22 μU/ml. Bone age 5 years; height 122 cm. Mental development normal.

Fig. 2B. The same patient after one year treatment with thyroxine resulting in growth stimulation and increased animation. Puffiness of the cheeks, blepharoptosis and cyanosis has disappeared; the palpebral fissures are wider; the hair is smooth and shiny; the neck longer.

Fig. 3A. Hand of a 12-year-old patient with untreated congenital hypothyroidism is broad and short; the skin is dry, rough and scaly.

Fig. 3B. Hand of the same patient after 10 months replacement therapy; the fingers are longer; the skin fine and smooth.

PLATE 23

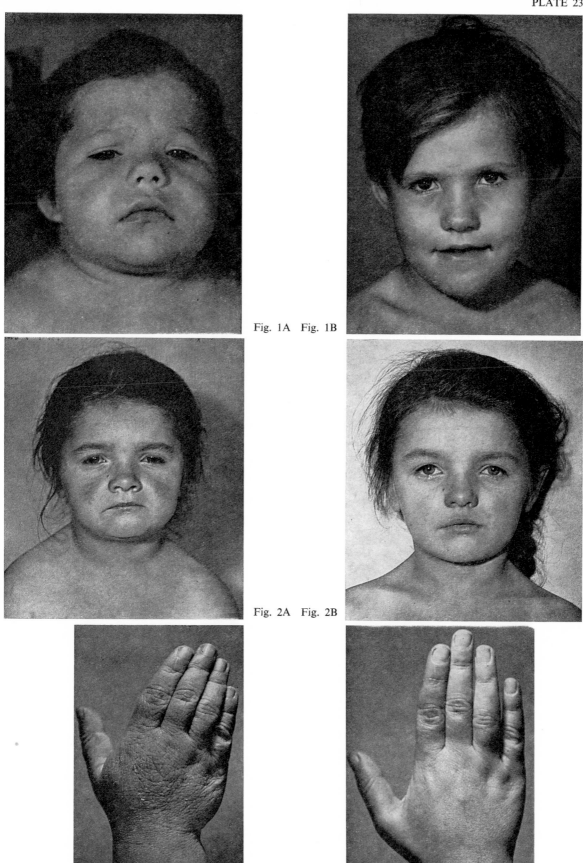

Fig. 1A   Fig. 1B

Fig. 2A   Fig. 2B

Fig. 3A   Fig. 3B

The Muscles

Slow progress in motor achievement, delayed walking, and easy fatigability are constant symptoms. On physical examination the muscles appear hypertrophied, but their strength is much reduced, as demonstrated by dynamometry. The movements are sluggish. In nearly all the patients Trendelenburg's sign is positive, indicating a weakness of the gluteal muscles. The patients start walking at the age of 3 to 6 years, are unable to hop on one leg, and have particular difficulties in climbing downstairs, so that they are obliged to use the rails. The legs are slightly flexed at hips and knees. The gait is unsteady and is accompanied by a limp or shuffle.

The Spine

Changes in the spine are frequently seen in roentgenograms. Some patients show kyphosis with the apex at the first or second lumbar vertebra; in other patients the back is flat owing to lack of normal curvature of the spine.

Fig. 1. A 7-year-old patient with congenital hypothyroidism. Extremities short compared to the trunk; head rather large; neck short. Conspicuous enlargement and protrusion of the abdomen due to poor muscle tone; puffiness of the cheeks, hands and legs.

Fig. 2. A 4-year-old patient with congenital hypothyroidism exhibiting a large head, short lower extremities, and kyphosis (apex at the first lumbar vertebra).

Figs. 3A and 3B. A positive (A) and negative (B) Trendelenburg's sign. Trendelenburg's sign is positive in almost all patients with congenital hypothyroidism.

Fig. 4A. Spine roentgenogram of the patient from Fig. 2 shows deformed vertebral body of L_1 and a bent spine. The deformed body is wedge-shaped with undeveloped upper and lower anterior parts.

Fig. 4B. Roentgenogram of the same patient after one year therapy with thyroxine shows anteroposterior growth of the deformed body. The anterior surface remains wedge-shaped.

PLATE 24

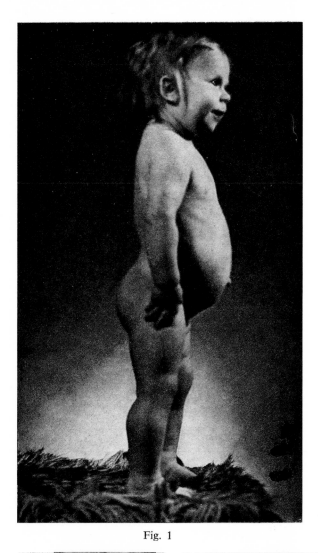

Fig. 1

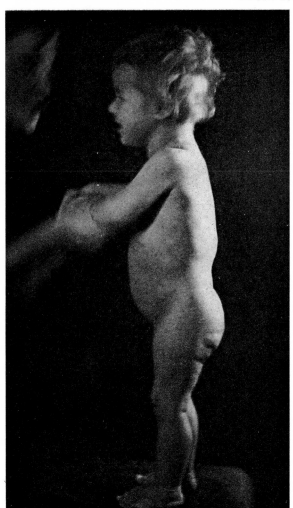

Fig. 2

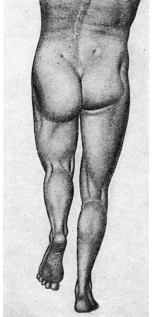

Fig. 3A

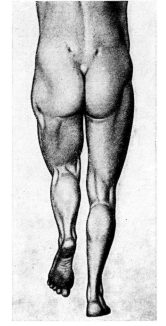

Fig. 3B

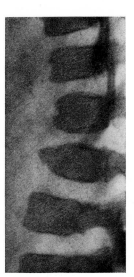

Fig. 4A

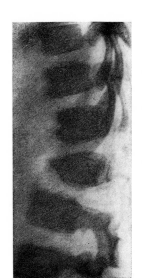

Fig. 4B

Roentgen Manifestations

In all cases characteristic changes are found. Roentgenograms of the hand and wrist taken during the first few years of life reveal the following abnormalities: delayed bone age, sign of roentgen vacuity, i.e., an increased space between the long bones caused by the presence of uncalcified ossification centers of the carpal bones and epiphyses, and a greater delay in bone age than in the height age. Subsequently, differences in maturation of carpal bones and of the epiphyses of long bones are often evident: the carpal bone maturation is less delayed than the epiphyseal maturation. Pseudoepiphyses at the metacarpal bases and increased density of terminal plates of long bones are sometimes observed.

A further feature is epiphyseal dysgenesis, best seen in the hip joints; the femoral heads are formed from multiple ossification centers of irregular size and shape. On the lateral roentgenograms of the lumbar spine the deformity of the first or second vertebral body is noted in half the patients. The anterior part of the deformed body is undeveloped and has a wedge- or steplike shape. The remaining vertebral bodies are flattened and the intervertebral spaces widened.

In the skull, development and pneumatization of the paranasal sinuses and mastoid cells are absent or much delayed; the fontanels remain open, and the sella turcica is sometimes enlarged. In a few patients an increased density of the base is noted.

In all cases of congenital hypothyroidism at least some of the above described findings are seen, thus the roentgen examination is of assistance in diagnosis. Control roentgenograms of the hand and wrist are helpful in evaluation of treatment. A proper dosage of thyroid preparations corresponds with a proportional increase in the height and in bone age. A more rapid advance of the bone age than the height age indicates an overdose, whereas slow progress in height and bone age points to insufficient doses of the drugs.

Fig. 1. Roentgenogram of the hand and wrist of a 5-year-old patient with congenital hypothyroidism shows marked delay in bone maturation; bone age 3 months. The long bones are widely spaced due to the presence of cartilagenous bone centers, a sign of roentgen vacuity.

Fig. 2. Roentgenogram of the hip joint in a 7-year-old male with congenital hypothyroidism. The femoral head is formed from several irregular, flattened ossification centers instead of one circular center. The femoral neck is greatly shortened and broadened resulting in coxa vara.

Figs. 3A to 3C. Ossification of the femoral head in a patient with congenital hypothyroidism. *A.* At age 5, before treatment, no ossification center is seen. *B.* At age 6, after one year on replacement therapy, several small, completely irregular ossification centers are now evident. *C.* At age 8, after 3 years of replacement therapy, the femoral head is well formed, semicircular, only slightly flattened.

PLATE 25

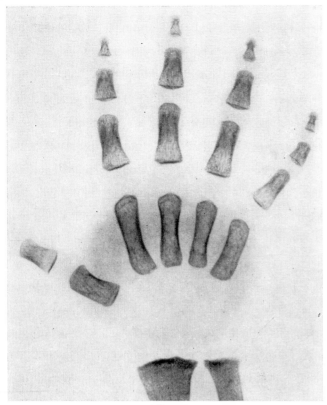

Fig. 1

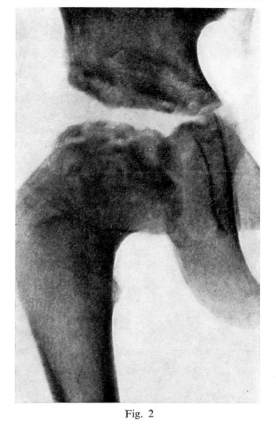

Fig. 2

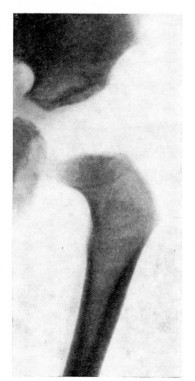

Fig. 3A

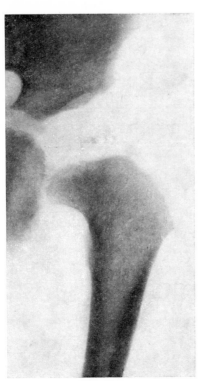

Fig. 3B

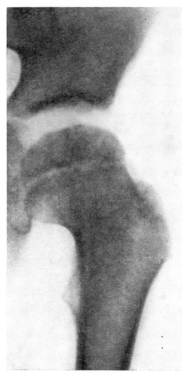

Fig. 3C

ENDEMIC CRETINISM

Endemic cretinism appears in areas of severe iodine deficiency such as the Alps, Andes and Himalayas where endemic goiter is common. The term cretin is used to describe patients retarded in stature and mental development who frequently have impairment in hearing and speech, and motor abnormalities. The clinical picture of endemic cretinism is not uniform; some of the cretins have goiter while others do not. In some cases there are symptoms and signs of hypothyroidism (myxedematous cretinism). Others do not appear to be hypothyroid, however, mental deficiency and skeletal changes indicate that thyroid deficiency must have been present in fetal or early postnatal life.

In typical cases several defects are evident: imbecility, short stature, abnormal gait, clumsiness of movements, flexion at the knees and hip joints, typical facial changes, low forehead and low hairline, flattened saddle nose, strabismus, enlarged tongue and protruding teeth. Hormonal studies usually reveal low serum thyroxine, normal serum triiodothyronine and elevated TSH concentration. Radiographic abnormalities comprise coxa valga, flattening of the femoral heads, delayed skeletal maturation and, in some cases, epiphyseal dysgenesis. Other patients have mental deficiency and deafmutism or motor abnormalities but do not differ in appearance from healthy relatives. This form of the disease is described as "nervous endemic cretinism."

Fig. 1. Face of a 25-year-old cretin from Esperanza in the high Andes area showing low forehead, flat and broad nose with depressed bridge, and protruding teeth. The patient was imbecile, experienced walking difficulties due to pronounced contractures at hip and knee joints forcing him to move on all fours.

Fig. 2. A 15-year-old patient with juvenile hypothyroidism with her healthy 9-year-old sister. Differences in habitus are evident. The height of the patient is 123 cm (48 in.). The face is round and slightly puffed, the neck is short, the shoulders sloping. Fat has accumulated on the trunk. The healthy sister is 131 cm (52 in.) tall, has an oval face, longer neck, is thin and has longer extremities.

Fig. 3. A 16-year-old female with juvenile hypothyroidism and normal mental development. Height 128 cm (50 in.). Swollen face, double chin, swollen neck and supraclavicular areas, sloping shoulders, protruding abdomen and short extremities are seen.

Fig. 4A. Face of a 32-year-old patient with untreated juvenile hypothyroidism. History reveals that growth ceased at about age 12. Mental development normal; muscle weakness. The face is enormously swollen and the palpebral fissures narrowed due to ptosis and edema of the eyelids.

Fig. 4B. Same patient after one year treatment with thyroxine and testosterone. Note complete change of facial features and disappearance of edema. The palpebral fissures are wider, the lips narrower, the face thinner, the neck longer.

132

PLATE 26

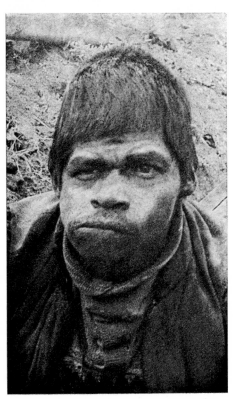

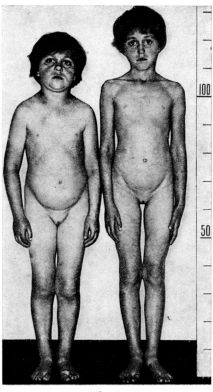

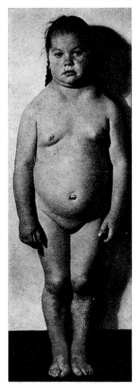

Fig. 1   Fig. 2   Fig. 3

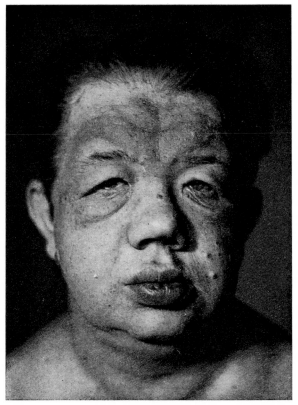

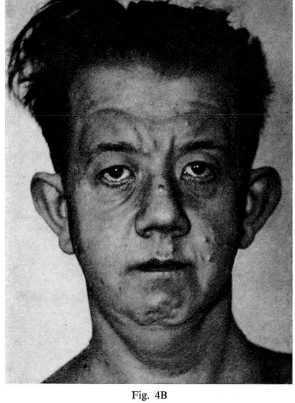

Fig. 4A   Fig. 4B

JUVENILE HYPOTHYROIDISM

Hypothyroidism appears very infrequently in childhood and adolescence. The manifestations are mild, hence the disease can remain undiagnosed for several years. A constant sign is impairment in growth, usually accompanied by a delay in sexual maturation. Mental development is normal. The patients may be somnolent and apathetic. Occasionally, dryness of the skin and generalized myxedema involving the face, neck, abdomen, hands and feet are present. Laboratory studies show the same changes as those found in hypothyroidism in adults. Serum TSH is greatly elevated in all cases; serum thyroxine and triiodothyronine are lowered. The ECG shows negative or flattened T waves in standard and left precordial leads, unusual in healthy children and adolescents. Recordings of the ankle reflex show a prolongation of the relaxation phase in the majority of patients.

Roentgen manifestations include a delay in bone age; however, when patients reach sexual maturation the bone age advances and epiphyseal fusion occurs. Radiography of the hand reveals the metacarpals and phalanges to be short and broad. The ossification centers of the iliac crest do not fuse with the wings, even in patients over the age of 30.

With adequate replacement therapy all clinical manifestations of hypothyroidism disappear, and linear growth is stimulated in younger patients. Serum TSH concentration, electrocardiographic abnormalities and prolonged tendon reflexes revert to normal.

Fig. 1A. A 36-year-old patient with untreated juvenile hypothyroidism. Height 138 cm (54 in.); stocky build. Short extremities. Pelvic roentgenogram showed no fusion of the ossification centers of the crest with the iliac wing. Serum TSH elevated to 46 μU/ml.

Fig. 1B. Same patient. Note puffed cheeks, upper lids and chin; broad neck; numerous skin folds on the forehead; coarse brittle hair.

Fig. 1C. Hand of the same patient is short and broad with stubby fingers. The skin is thick, dry and leathery.

Fig. 1D. Trendelenburg's sign in the same patient is positive. Despite muscle hypertrophy there is pronounced muscle weakness, that affects the gluteal muscles also.

PLATE 27

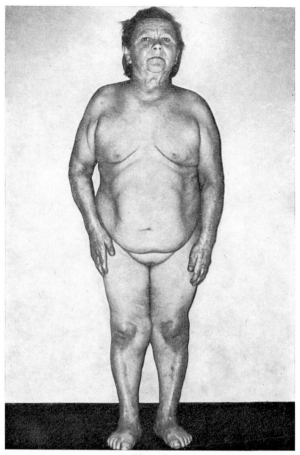

Fig. 1A

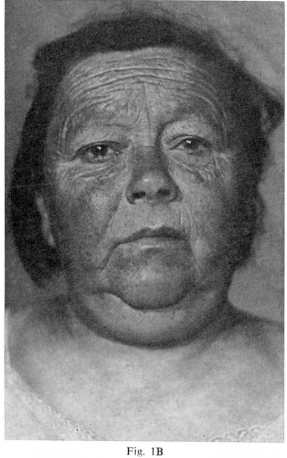

Fig. 1B

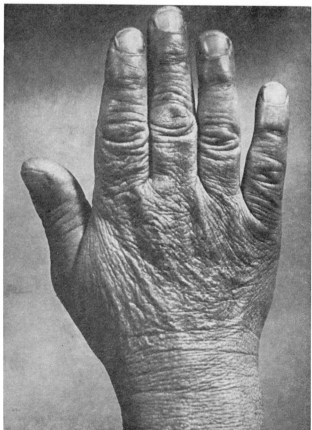

Fig. 1C

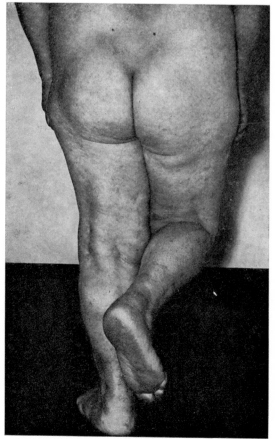

Fig. 1D

SIMPLE GOITER

(NONTOXIC GOITER)

Simple goiter is thyroid enlargement not associated with abnormal thyroid function, i.e., thyrotoxicosis or hypothyroidism, nor does it result from inflammation or neoplasia. The disease is common in females, less frequent in children and males. Rather, iodine deficiency in food and water, dietary goitrogens and subtle biosynthetic defects within the thyroid gland are regarded as etiologic factors.

In the majority of cases the only manifestation is swelling of the neck. On examination there may be diffuse enlargement of the thyroid gland (diffuse goiter), which itself is soft, painless, and mobile; on swallowing it moves upward. In other cases one or several nodules may be palpable in the thyroid gland (nodular goiter).

In rare cases involving large goiters, displacement or compression of the trachea and esophagus occurs. There may be a feeling of tightness, a choking sensation, stridor and swallowing difficulties. Simple goiter, which occurs during adolescence or pregnancy, later regresses in some patients; in others, it persists. In adolescent females, appearance of simple goiter may precede thyrotoxicosis.

Laboratory tests of thyroid function give results within normal limits; serum triiodothyronine, thyroxine, TSH, ^{131}I uptake and PBI are all normal. An increased serum TSH concentration usually indicates a preliminary stage of hypothyroidism.

Fig. 1. A female exhibiting nontoxic nodular goiter. A small nodule, 3 cm in diameter, is present in the isthmus. Thyroid function tests are within normal range.

Fig. 2. A 17-year-old female showing diffuse enlargement of the thyroid. Tests of thyroid function (T_4, T_3, TSH) reveal no abnormalities.

Fig. 3. Multinodular and cystic nontoxic goiter in a 72-year-old patient.

Fig. 4. Diffuse multinodular colloid goiter in a 61-year-old female. No signs of thyrotoxicosis are present.

136

PLATE 28

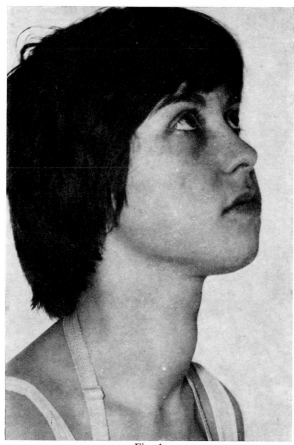

Fig. 1

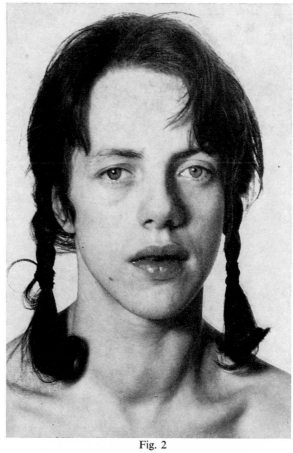

Fig. 2

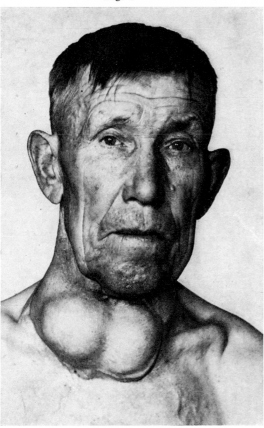

Fig. 3

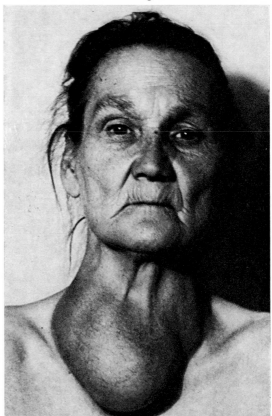

Fig. 4

Retrosternal goiter. Retrosternal goiter is an infrequent variant of simple goiter. There are generally no symptoms if the goiter is small but it may be incidentally found on roentgen examination of the chest that reveals retrosternal extension of a goiter, round or oval shadow behind the sternum. The goiter moves upwards during swallowing and, in addition, may cause displacement or narrowing of the trachea.

As the goiter enlarges it may cause pressure symptoms such as cough, hoarseness, stridor, feeling of suffocation and occasional dysphagia. When patients raise both arms to the side of the head, congestion of the face and respiratory distress are evident.

Fig. 1. Retrosternal and multinodular nontoxic goiters in a 50-year-old patient. Varicose veins (resulting from collateral circulation) and thyroid enlargement are seen.

Fig. 2. Retrosternal goiter, duration 13 years, in a male patient. There is tremendous collateral circulation on chest and neck; swollen face.

Fig. 3. Chest roentgenogram showing huge retrosternal goiter with compression and tracheal displacement.

Fig. 4. Chest roentgenogram reveals a substernal adenomatous goiter and tracheal displacement.

PLATE 29

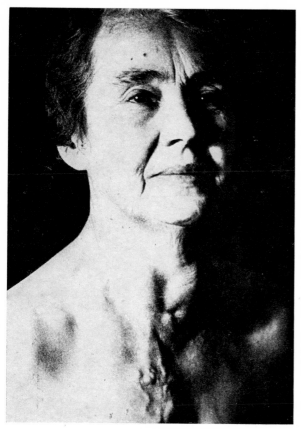

Fig. 1

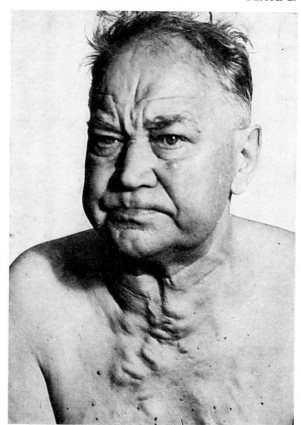

Fig. 2

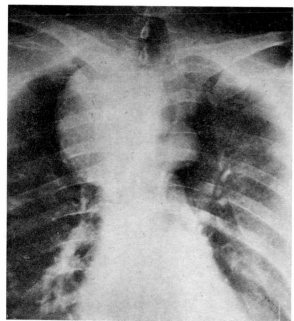

Fig. 3

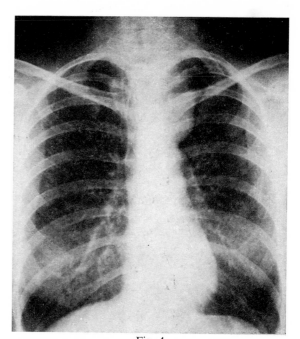

Fig. 4

CANCER OF THE THYROID

The symptoms of the cancer are not characteristic. Enlargement of the thyroid gland, sometimes preceded by goiter, may be the first symptom. Subsequent pressure symptoms such as cough, difficulty in swallowing, choking and hoarseness appear. When an irregular, hard nodule is found in the thyroid, cancer is suspected — especially when it is fixed to surrounding tissue. Enlarged cervical lymph nodes may indicate metastasis. Vocal cord paralysis associated with hard and fixed goiter is also an important indication of thyroid carcinoma. Laboratory findings are not characteristic; anemia and increased sedimentation rate occur in advanced stages of the disease. Roentgenoscopy frequently reveals displacement of the trachea or esophagus, and may also disclose metastases in the lungs or bones. Thyroid scintiscan reveals a "cold" nodule, i.e., the ^{131}I uptake of a malignant nodule is lower compared to normal thyroid tissue. Diagnosis of thyroid cancer is confirmed by histologic study.

MEDULLARY CARCINOMA OF THE THYROID

Medullary carcinoma of the thyroid is composed of C cells that secrete excessive amounts of the calcitonin. In addition, the tumor may be the source of other substances including histaminase, 5-hydroxytryptamine, ACTH and prostaglandins.

The diagnosis of medullary carcinoma may be confirmed by hormonal assay, very high plasma calcitonin concentration, and an exaggerated calcitonin response to calcium infusion. In half the patients increased histaminase activity is found. After successful removal of the tumor the plasma calcitonin level reverts to normal.

Fig. 1. Bloated face of a 52-year-old patient with cancer of the thyroid. Scar on the neck from total thyroidectomy. Hyperpigmentation of the skin after X-ray irradiation is seen.

Fig. 2. Diffuse thyroid enlargement and bulge in the supraclavicular fossa in a patient with thyroid carcinoma.

Fig. 3A. The tumor removed from the patient shown in Fig. 1 is of hard consistency and appears shiny and lard-like on cross section.

Fig. 3B. Photomicrograph of tumor shown in Fig. 3A. Malignant cells had infiltrated the muscle fibers.

PLATE 30

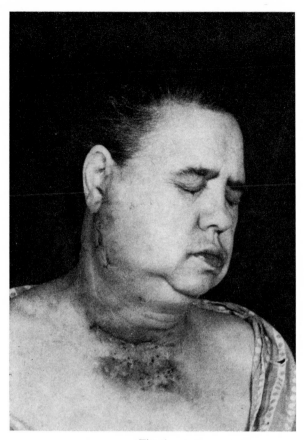

Fig. 1

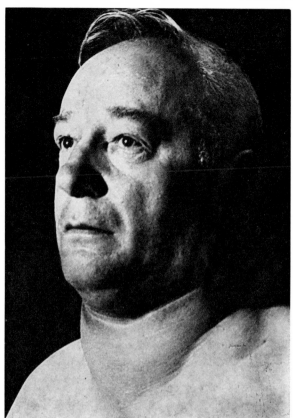

Fig. 2

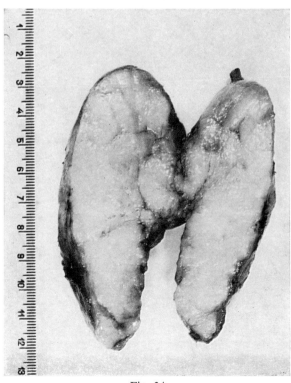

Fig. 3A

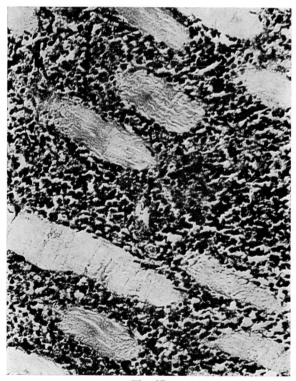

Fig. 3B

141

ACUTE THYROIDITIS

The disease appears rarely in the course of septicemia, in infectious diseases such as typhoid, or as a result of local infection. The primary manifestations are fever, painful enlargement of the thyroid, pain on swallowing and hoarseness. The sedimentation rate increases, and leukocytosis occurs.

SUBACUTE THYROIDITIS
(DE QUERVAIN'S DISEASE)

This is a rare disease of unknown etiology. Symptoms include pains in the neck radiating to the ear, difficulty in swallowing, fever, swelling and hardening of the thyroid. In the early stages of the disease the levels of serum thyroxine, triiodothyronine and thyroglobulin rise; ^{131}I uptake, however, decreases. The sedimentation rate is elevated. Diagnosis based on clinical manifestations can be confirmed by histologic studies of the thyroid that show granulomatous pseudotubercles, giant cells and areas of degeneration with subsequent fibrosis.

HASHIMOTO'S DISEASE
(STRUMA LYMPHOMATOSA)

Hashimoto's disease is a chronic inflammatory condition in the thyroid gland associated with enlargement of the thyroid and development of thyroid antibodies. It is predominant in females. The primary symptom is painful, symmetrical enlargement of the thyroid which, on palpation, is hard. Occasional difficulties in swallowing and coughing may occur due to pressure on the trachea and esophagus. In some patients the clinical manifestations are so slight that the disease remains undiagnosed and a high titer of thyroid antibodies may be the only indication of past involvement. Persons with Hashimoto's disease almost invariably have a high titer of thyroid antibodies directed against thyroglobulins, microsomal fractions, colloid antigens or the nuclear components of thyroid cells. The antibodies are detectable by several immunologic techniques such as complement-fixation (for microsomal fraction), tanned red cells or coated latex particles (for thyroglobulin) or fluorescent techniques (with the use of fixed or unfixed thyroid tissue). Other laboratory findings include increased sedimentation rate, abnormal hepatic function tests, temporarily raised levels of thyroxine and triiodothyronine and increased radioiodine uptake. Diagnosis may be confirmed by thyroid biopsy. Histopathology reveals interfollicular infiltrations by lymphocytes and plasma cells, oxyphilic granules in the cytoplasm of the follicular epithelium, fibrosis and hyalinization. Many patients with Hashimoto's disease eventually develop hypothyroidism.

Fig. 1. Histologic appearance of the thyroid in Hashimoto's disease. Extensive lymphocyte infiltrations and lymphoid follicles are seen (H+E, ×44).

Fig. 2. Interfollicular infiltrations by lymphocytes that compress the thyroid follicles in another patient with Hashimoto's disease (H+E, ×130).

Fig. 3. Multinuclear cells found in the thyroid tissue in Hashimoto's disease. In the middle of the figure a giant multinuclear cell is seen with nuclei in semicircular arrangement (H+E, ×44).

Fig. 4. Infiltration of lymphocytes and plasma cells. Note presence of giant multinuclear cells in the thyroid tissue of a patient with Hashimoto's disease.

PLATE 31

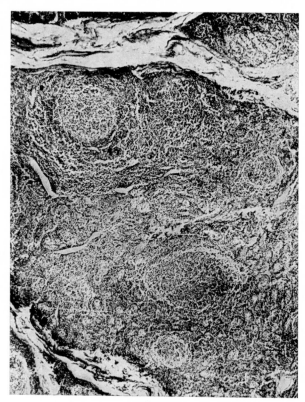

Fig. 1

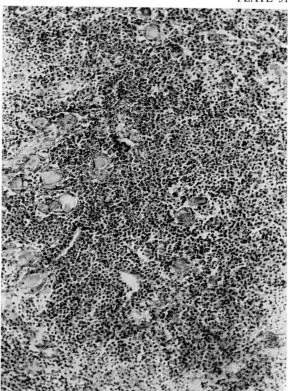

Fig. 2

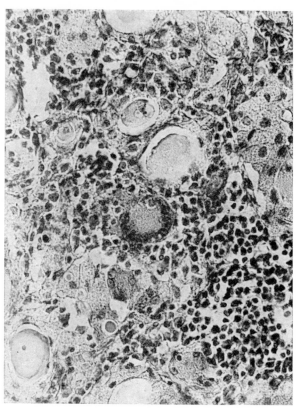

Fig. 3

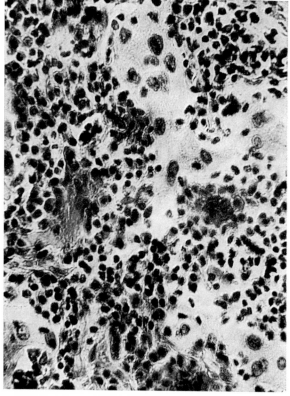

Fig. 4

RIEDEL'S THYROIDITIS

(LIGNEOUS THYROIDITIS)

This is an extremely rare disease that appears predominantly in adult females. Its progression is very slow. The primary manifestation is an iron-hard, irregular goiter with compression or displacement of adjacent structures — the trachea and esophagus. Subtotal thyroidectomy relieves pressure and permits histologic differentiation from thyroid malignancy. In Riedel's thyroiditis histology reveals extensive scar formation, the glandular tissue being replaced by dense, fibrous tissue. Hypothyroidism often develops in subsequent years.

Chapter 3

THE ADRENALS

CUSHING'S DISEASE

(CUSHING'S SYNDROME; HYPERCORTISOLISM)

Cushing's disease, or Cushing's syndrome, results from excessive secretion of cortisol by the hypertrophic or neoplastic adrenal cortex. The term Cushing's disease usually refers to overproduction of ACTH by the pituitary with subsequent bilateral hyperplasia of the adrenal cortex, while the term Cushing's syndrome refers to adrenocortical adenoma or carcinoma that secrete excessive amounts of cortisol.

The actual cause of Cushing's disease is not yet fully understood, whether the primary disorder is inappropriate release of corticotropin releasing hormone by the hypothalamus, or adenoma of the anterior pituitary with excess of ACTH. It should be emphasized that surgical removal of the adrenal glands results in disappearance of all signs and symptoms, and that all manifestations of Cushing's syndrome may be produced by a prolonged administration of large amounts of cortisol.

The disease progresses with time, and if not treated may prove fatal as a result of cardiac failure, cerebral hemorrhage, renal failure or infection. The disease is more frequent in females than in males; it is rarely seen in children. The primary clinical manifestations are truncal obesity, rounding and redness of the face, muscle wasting, hirsutism, hypertension, osteoporosis and sexual dysfunction.

Fig. 1A. A 13-year-old male with Cushing's syndrome. Note rounding of the face; excessive fat on the trunk; protruding abdomen; extensive purplish striae on the abdomen; slender upper extremities.

Fig. 1B. Same patient shows rounding of the face and plethora. Note presence of acne; low hairline; shortening of neck; puffy cheeks overshadowing the ears and shrunken mouth resembling fish mouth. Palpebral fissures are narrowed due to fat accumulation.

Fig. 2A. A 12-year-old male with Cushing's syndrome. The face is round and reddish with a double chin, the cheeks prominent. Blood pressure 165/90. Bilateral hyperplasia of adrenals found during surgery. Urinary 17-hydroxycorticoids 25 mg/24 hr.

Fig. 2B. Same patient 5 months after bilateral subtotal adrenalectomy. All signs and symptoms of Cushing's syndrome have disappeared. Note changes in facial appearance: the shape is now triangular; the ears are visible; fat deposits on the cheeks are gone. Urinary 17-hydroxycorticoids have dropped to 7 mg/24 hr. Blood pressure 120/80.

PLATE 1

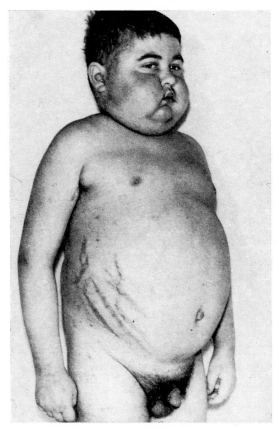

Fig. 1A

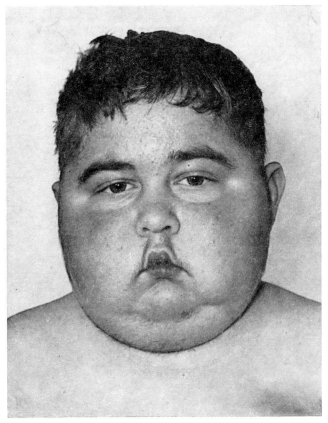

Fig. 1B

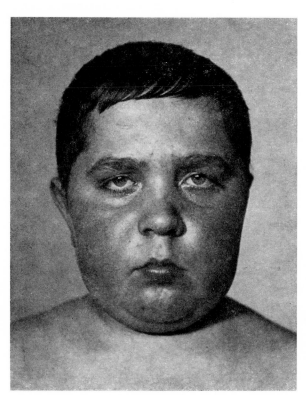

Fig. 2A

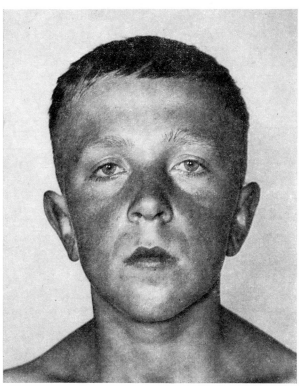

Fig. 2B

Symptoms

1. Weakness; fatigability; inability to perform heavy work in early stages of the disease; in severe cases the patients are confined to bed.
2. Muscle weakness most evident when climbing.
3. Pains in the limbs and lumbosacral region that may lead to difficulties in walking.
4. Headaches; vertigo.
5. Amenorrhea and sterility in females. Loss of libido and potency in males.
6. Weight gain.
7. Depression or other psychic changes.

Fig. 1. A 38-year-old patient with Cushing's syndrome. Round and red face, truncal obesity; large, protruding abdomen with cutaneous striae are seen.

Fig. 2. A 49-year-old patient with Cushing's disease. Rounded dark red face, enormous abdomen, pronounced muscle atrophy present. Plasma cortisol 320 ng/ml; urinary 17-hydroxycorticoids 31 mg/24 hr.

Fig. 3. A 30-year-old patient with Cushing's disease. Rounded face, marked hirsutism; protruding abdomen; truncal obesity; extensive ecchymoses on the breasts, abdomen and extremities. Blood pressure 230/120. Urinary 17-hydroxycorticoids 29 mg/24 hr.

Figs. 4A and 4B. A 32-year-old patient with Cushing's disease. Round, red face, short neck, fat pads in the supraclavicular areas and on the back of the neck (buffalo hump). Marked obesity of the trunk, protruding abdomen. Numerous ecchymoses and bruises on the trunk and lower extremities. Edema of the legs. Elevated plasma cortisol 290 ng/ml, and urinary 17-hydroxycorticoids.

Fig. 5. A 57-year-old patient with Cushing's disease. Note protruding abdomen, accumulation of fat on back of neck. Extremities are thin, the muscles atrophic. Numerous ecchymoses. Advanced osteoporosis of the spine and skull on roentgen examinations. Elevated urinary 17-hydroxycorticoids 33 mg/24 hr. Bilateral adrenal hyperplasia was found on surgical exploration.

PLATE 2

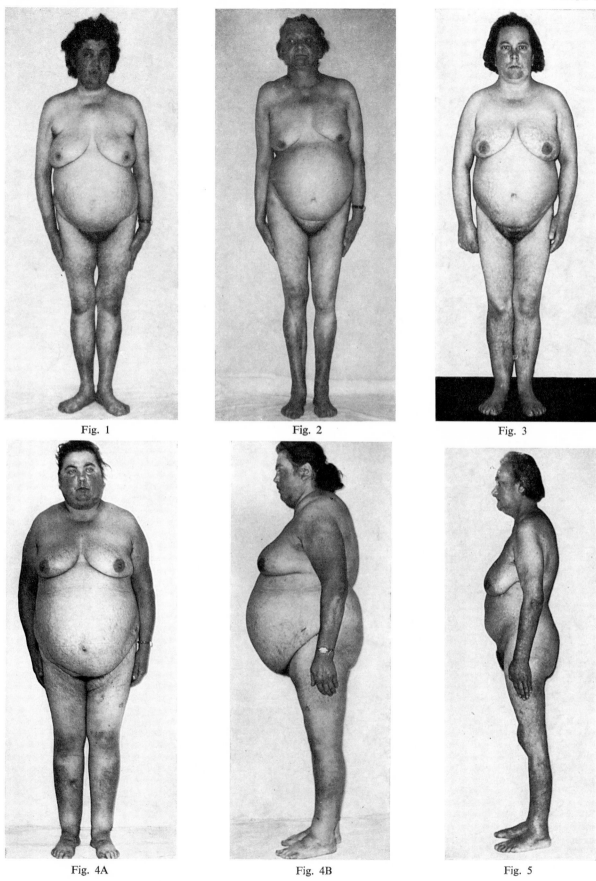

Fig. 1   Fig. 2   Fig. 3

Fig. 4A   Fig. 4B   Fig. 5

Signs

1. Rounding of the face, plethora.
2. A peculiar type obesity affecting only the trunk, face and neck.
3. Muscle-wasting, primarily in the extremities and gluteal area.
4. Dryness of the skin; hypertrichosis; purplish striae of the skin in some cases.
5. Hypertension.
6. Hirsutism in females, occasional clitoral hypertrophy.
7. Shortening of the spine; cervicodorsal kyphosis.
8. Cessation of growth, delay in sexual maturity in children and adolescents.

Fig. 1. A 19-year-old patient with Cushing's syndrome. Note facial rounding, double chin, narrowed palpebral fissures; hair extending low on the forehead.

Fig. 2. Face of a 28-year-old patient shows rounding, plethora; excessive fat accumulation on the cheeks obscures the ears. Darkening of the scalp hair and eyebrows. Hirsutism on the chin and above the upper lip. Dilated capillary vessels.

Figs. 3A to 3C. Face of a 13-year-old patient with Cushing's syndrome shows changes characteristic of the disease: round face, prominent cheeks, drooping corners of the mouth (*A*). *B*. Partial regression of facial changes 3 months after removal of adrenal adenoma. Fat accumulation of the cheeks regresses. *C*. Face of the same patient, 12 months after removal of the adenoma. Complete disappearance of manifestations.

PLATE 3

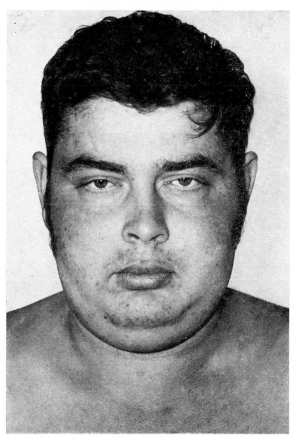

Fig. 1

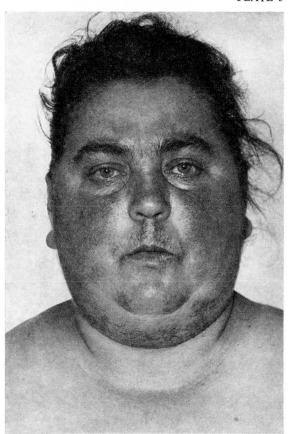

Fig. 2

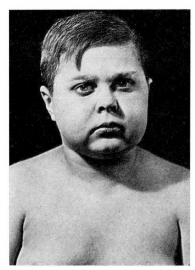

Fig. 3A

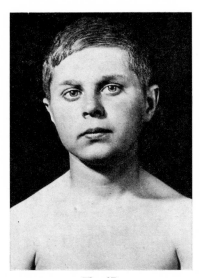

Fig. 3B

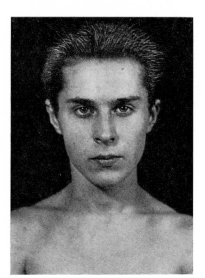

Fig. 3C

The Face

Changes of the face constitute the primary signs of the disease. The face becomes round and red, hence is compared to a full moon. Individual characteristics of the face disappear, and the patient becomes un-recognizable — even to his family — after an interval of several months. The cheeks are excessively puffed and filled with fat, so that the ears are almost invisible. The nose appears smaller since it, too, is embedded in fat. Fat accumulation in the lids narrows the palpebral fissures. The mouth shrinks; its outer corners droop, giving it a horseshoe shape.

The skin of the face has an unpleasant appearance; it is dry, plethoric, and nearly always exhibits eruptions or acne. The capillary vessels of the cheeks and nose are markedly dilated. In females excessive hair appears on the chin, upper lips and sides of the cheeks. There is frequently double chin and broadening of the neck.

The hair grows low on the forehead, reaching almost to the eyebrows, is generally without luster and is lifeless; its color is darker than before the onset of the disease. The eyebrows also darken, as if colored with soot, and meet over the bridge of the nose. Sometimes the entire face is covered with graish lanugolike hair.

Fig. 1A. Face of a 20-year-old patient with Cushing's syndrome shows characteristic changes: rounding, plethora, double chin, oily skin, drooping corners of the mouth. Hair lacks luster and is difficult to comb. Urinary 17-hydroxycorticoids 28 mg/24 hr; blood pressure 190/105. Osteoporosis of the spine is present.

Fig. 1B. Face of the same patient 4 months after removal of the adrenocortical adenoma demonstrates complete regression of symptomatic features. The hair is glossy and easy to comb; blood pressure 125/80; urinary 17-hydroxycorticoids 7 mg/24 hr. Back pains have disappeared, though osteoporosis persists.

Fig. 2A. A 12-year-old patient with Cushing's disease exhibits typical bloated, plethoric moon face with acne and hirsutism, The scalp hair and the eyebrows have darkened. Double chin, fat pads in supraclavicular areas are present. Blood pressure 170/90.

Fig. 2B. Same patient 19 months later, after bilateral subtotal adrenalectomy. Plethora, moon face and double chin have disappeared; hirsutism has regressed; the hair is lighter and glossy; the eyebrows are thinner; supraclavicular fossa are seen. Blood pressure 120/80.

152

PLATE 4

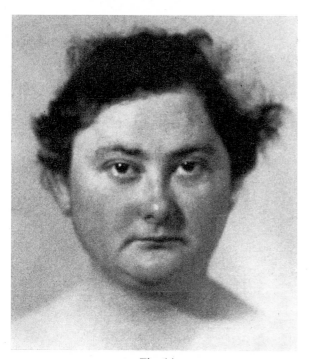

Fig. 1A

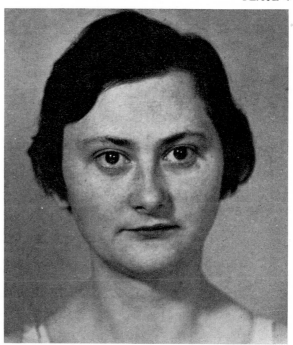

Fig. 1B

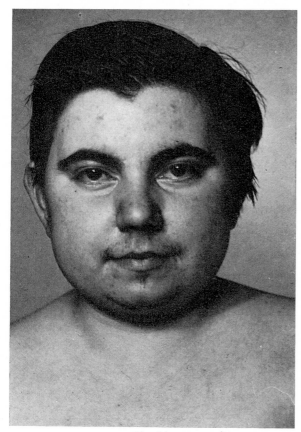

Fig. 2A

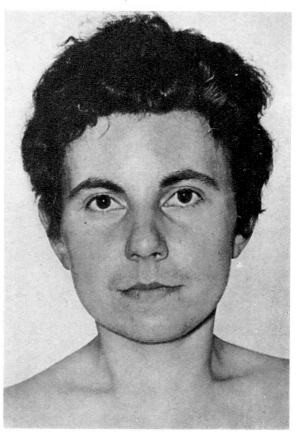

Fig. 2B

The Skin and Subcutaneous Fat

The skin is dry, thin and sometimes coarse to the touch due to keratosis pilaris. In some patients purplish striae develop on the abdomen, breasts, thighs and upper arms. The striae are wide, and the skin is loose in the affected areas. After successful treatment the striae whiten and shrink. Ecchymoses and bruises are frequently seen. There may be a mosaic mottling of the legs (cutis marmorata). The healing of wounds is impaired.

Subcutaneous fat is excessive on the face, neck and trunk, while the extremities are spared of obesity. Fat pads occur under the chin, in the supraclavicular regions and at the cervicodorsal angle of the spine (buffalo hump).

Hypertension and Cardiovascular Changes

Hypertension is present in nearly all cases. The vessels are brittle and tend toward cutaneous ecchymoses; slight injuries cause subcutaneous hemorrhages. The hypertension and negative protein balance lead to early heart muscle damage. This is demonstrated in electrocardiographic examination where signs of left ventricular strain can be seen, i.e., negative T waves in lead I, and left precordial leads and depressed ST segments in these leads.

In about half the patients the ECG reveals prolongation of the QT interval, flat or negative T waves, depressed ST segments and the presence of U waves — findings typical of hypokalemia. Laboratory tests reveal evidence of lowered potassium concentration in the serum. On administration of potassium the changes regress.

Fig. 1. Hand of a 35-year-old patient with Cushing's syndrome. The skin is dry and thin.
Fig. 2. Back of 38-year-old patient with Cushing's syndrome. Note fat accumulation on the trunk, gluteal muscle atrophy, buffalo-type obesity.
Fig. 3. Forearm of a 35-year-old patient with Cushing's syndrome showing extensive muscle wasting. The skin is dry with numerous ecchymoses and subcutaneous hemorrhages. Vein puncture constantly causes subcutaneous hemorrhage.
Fig. 4. Closeup view of the back of the hand shows atrophic and dry epidermis.

PLATE 5

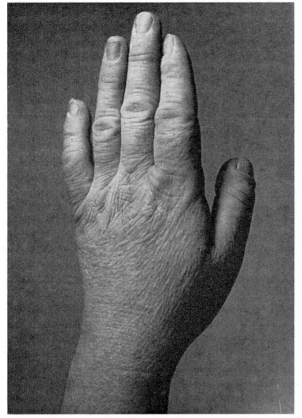

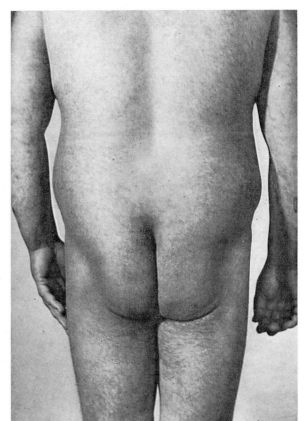

Fig. 1

Fig. 2

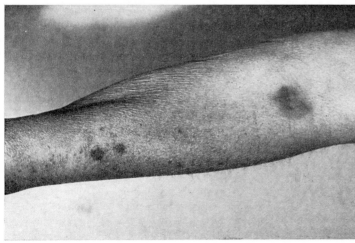

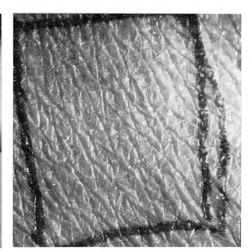

Fig. 3

Fig. 4

Roentgen Manifestations

The radiographic changes in Cushing's syndrome reveal decreased bone density (osteoporosis) chiefly affecting the spine, pelvis and ribs. The bones of the extremities are involved to a lesser degree and rather infrequently. Painless and spontaneous fractures of the ribs and compression fractures of vertebral bodies frequently occur; the compressed vertebral bodies show marginal condensations. The vertebral bodies are flattened or concavoconcave, while the intervertebral spaces are markedly widened and convex. The skull may also be affected and shows decreased bone density of patchy distribution, mainly in frontal and parietal bones.

Extraperitoneal gas insufflation with subsequent roentgenograms and tomograms of the adrenal area and adrenal venography are of assistance in the differential diagnosis of adrenal hyperplasia and tumor, as well as in locating the tumor.

Fig. 1. Spine roentgenogram of a 20-year-old patient with Cushing's syndrome shows extensive osteoporosis; the vertebral bodies are translucent, markedly flattened with marginal condensation; the intervertebral spaces are enlarged.

Fig. 2. Spine roentgenogram of a 42-year-old male shows decreased density of the vertebral bodies and marked flattening of L_2 caused by fracture.

Fig. 3. Rib fractures in a 38-year-old female with Cushing's syndrome.

Fig. 4. Roentgenogram of the foot of a 13-year-old male with Cushing's syndrome reveals advanced osteoporosis. The bones are translucent, with complete loss of trabecular structure. The outline of the bones is dense, as if pencil-contoured.

156

PLATE 6

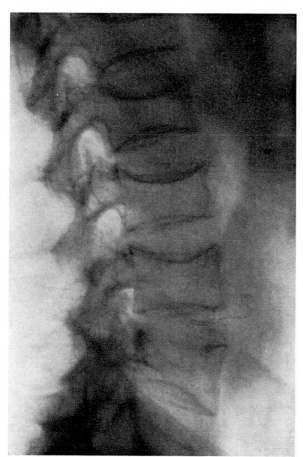

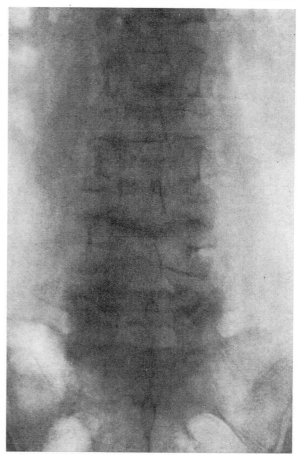

Fig. 1

Fig. 2

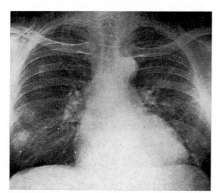

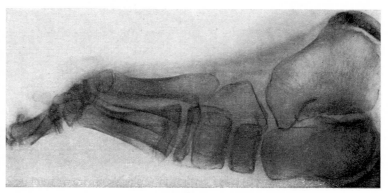

Fig. 3

Fig. 4

Laboratory Findings

1. Most important: high plasma cortisol concentration without diurnal variations. The plasma cortisol remains elevated in the afternoon, with no drop as is seen in normal subjects.
2. Increased urinary cortisol and 17-hydroxycorticoids.
3. Dexamethasone suppression test: administration of dexamethasone (0.5 mg every 6 hours, for two days) will suppress plasma cortisol to less than 4 μg/dl in normal subjects whereas plasma cortisol remains above this level in Cushing's syndrome.
4. Relatively high plasma ACTH concentration in patients with adrenocortical hyperplasia.
5. Diabetic glucose tolerance test.
6. Deficient HGH response to insulin-induced hypoglycemia.
7. Occasional leukocytosis (from 10,000 to 20,000 in 1 mm^3); lymphopenia (15% or less); eosinopenia (less than 50 in 1 mm^3); polycythemia; increase in sedimentation rate.
8. Hypokalemia and hypochloremia; occasional alkalosis and alkaline urine, more frequent in ectopic ACTH syndrome.

Fig. 1. Basal levels of plasma cortisol in Cushing's syndrome before and after bilateral subtotal adrenalectomy.

Fig. 2. Urinary 17-hydroxycorticoids in patients with Cushing's syndrome and in control subjects.

Fig. 3. Results of urinary cortisol radioimmunoassay in patients with Cushing's syndrome and in control subjects.

Figs. 4A and 4B. *A*. Results of serum HGH radioimmunoassay during insulin tolerance test in untreated patients with Cushing's syndrome. There is no rise in HGH concentration during insulin-induced hypoglycemia as is seen in normal subjects. *B*. Results of HGH assays in the same patients after successful surgery. Normal increase in serum HGH concentration following insulin-induced hypoglycemia in the majority of patients.

PLATE 7

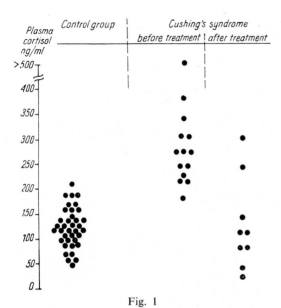

Fig. 1

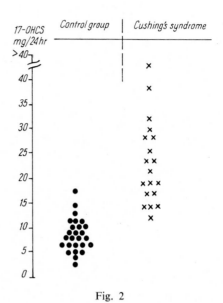

Fig. 2

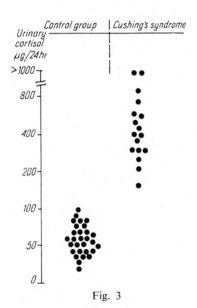

Fig. 3

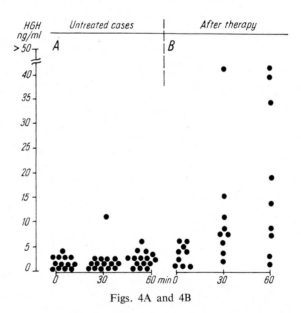

Figs. 4A and 4B

Differentiation of Bilateral Adrenal Hyperplasia and Tumor

The following tests assist in differential diagnosis:

1. Dexamethasone suppression test with high doses of dexamethasone (2 mg every 6 hours, for 2 days) reveals a decrease in plasma cortisol in adrenal hyperplasia. The absence of cortisol suppression indicates the presence of a tumor.
2. Adrenal vein sampling reveals higher plasma cortisol on the side of the tumor and suppressed cortisol level (corresponding to that of peripheral blood) on the opposite side.
3. Adrenal venography and retroperitoneal gas insufflation are helpful in roentgen visualization and localization of the tumor.
4. Adrenal scanning with ^{131}I iodocholesterol is useful in evaluating adrenal tumor (unilateral cholesterol uptake) or hyperplasia (bilateral increased uptake).

Fig. 1. Large adenoma of the left adrenal.

Fig. 2. Roentgenogram (after retroperitoneal gas insufflation) showing large circular shadow above the left kidney in a 32-year-old patient with Cushing's syndrome. The presence of tumor was verified at surgery.

Fig. 3. Grossly enlarged adrenal gland removed from a 20-year-old patient with Cushing's syndrome.

Fig. 4. Well-encapsulated adenoma of adrenals causing Cushing's syndrome. The patient recovered after removal of the tumor.

PLATE 8

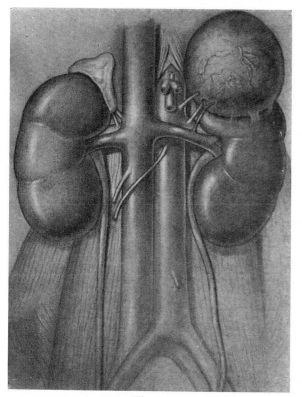

Fig. 1

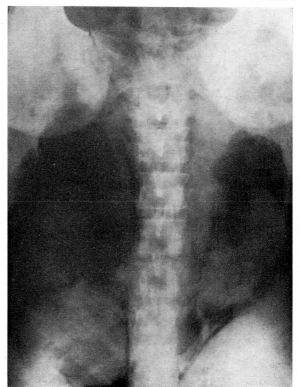

Fig. 2

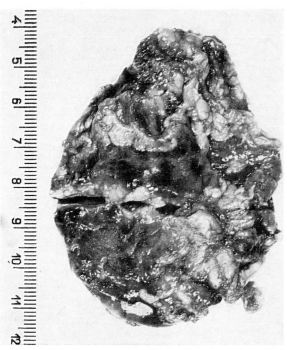

Fig. 3

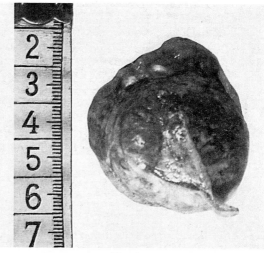

Fig. 4

ECTOPIC ACTH SYNDROME

Excessive secretion of ACTH and subsequent hypercortisolism may result from ACTH production in ectopic sites by various kinds of malignant tumors of which the most common are oat-cell carcinoma of the lung, carcinoma of the pancreas and thymus. The clinical picture somewhat resembles Cushing's syndrome in that muscular weakness and wasting, hypertension, atrophic changes of the skin, hypokalemia and excessive secretion of cortisol are present. However, obesity, rounding of the face and cutaneous striae are usually absent because of advancing malignancy. Hormonal studies show high plasma cortisol and urinary 17-OHCS, elevated plasma ACTH concentration and failure to suppress plasma cortisol by large doses of dexamethasone. The ectopic ACTH syndrome may be a part of multiple endocrine adenomatosis.

Figs. 1A to 1C. A 20-year-old male with ectopic ACTH syndrome, oat-cell carcinoma of the lung (verified 2 years later at autopsy), associated with bilateral adrenocortical hyperplasia. Characteristic manifestations evident: round face, shortened neck, fat accumulation on the trunk, protruding abdomen, kyphosis, purplish striae on the hips and extremities, advanced muscle atrophy, slender limbs, lanugo-like hair on the back. Urinary 17-hydroxycorticoids 27 mg/24 hr. Blood pressure 210/110. Roentgenograms revealed extensive osteoporosis of the spine.

Fig. 2A. Full, moon face of the patient shown in Fig. 1. Prominent cheeks with dilated capillary vessels and double chin are present. Fat accumulation on upper lids narrows the palpebral fissures. Hair darkens and grows low on forehead, extending down to the eyebrows, which are also darkened and joined.

Fig. 2B. Same patient after successful bilateral subtotal adrenalectomy. Note regression of manifestations: face is thin, ears easily seen, hair is lighter and has regained its luster, the hairline has receded. Urinary 17-hydroxycorticoids 5 mg/24 hr.

PLATE 9

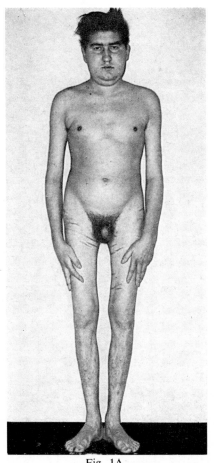
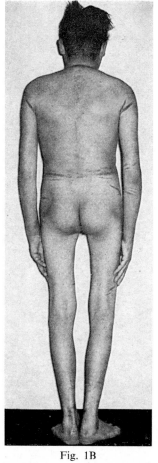
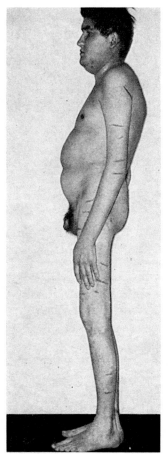

| Fig. 1A | Fig. 1B | Fig. 1C |

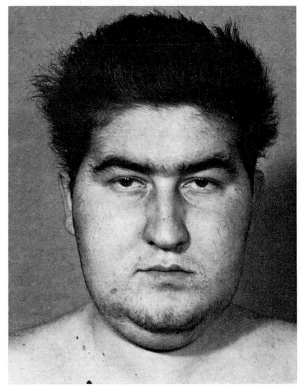
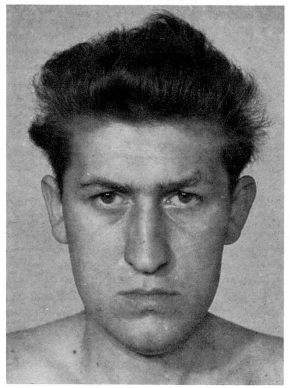
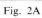

| Fig. 2A | Fig. 2B |

CONGENITAL ADRENAL HYPERPLASIA

(ADRENOGENITAL SYNDROME)

Congenital adrenal hyperplasia is a congenital disorder of the adrenal cortex due to enzymatic blocks and resulting in cortisol deficiency with subsequent rise in ACTH secretion, adrenocortical hyperplasia and excessive secretion of adrenal androgens. In children, the clinical findings consist of precocious puberty in males and accelerated growth and pseudohermaphroditism in females.

Several enzymatic blocks in congenital adrenal hyperplasia have been described and all are transmitted as an autosomal recessive trait. Deficiency of 21-hydroxylase is the most common variant that accounts for over 90% of the patients. The disease is characterized by deficient synthesis of cortisol leading to increased ACTH secretion, excess of plasma 17-hydroxyprogesterone and its urinary metabolite pregnanetriol as well as increased dehydroisoandrosterone and 17-ketosteroids. Two forms, a mild, caused by a partial block and severe, with complete enzymatic block, are distinguished. Most common is the former and its manifestations are listed below.

Partial Deficiency of 21-Hydroxylase

Signs and Symptoms in Young Males

1. Accelerated growth in the first years of life.
2. Strong muscle development with unusual muscular strength; young boys are capable of lifting from 50- to 70-kg weights.
3. Hyperpigmentation of the nipples.
4. Precocious sexual development; pubic hair appears between the ages of 2 and 7 years; the penis is enlarged, but the testes remain small. The voice changes between the ages of 5 and 8 years.
5. Early appearance of the male habitus; broad shoulders and narrow hips.
6. Acne is common in the first years of life.
7. Early cessation of growth between the ages of 10 and 13 years, resulting in short stature.
8. Sterility in adult patients due to immaturity of the testes resulting from suppression of pituitary gonadotropins.

Fig. 1. A 15-year-old female with congenital adrenogenital syndrome due to partial 21-hydroxylase deficiency showing heavy, muscular build; broad shoulders and narrow hips; poor breast development; excessive hair on face, abdomen and legs.

Fig. 2. A 22-year-old female with congenital adrenal hyperplasia (partial 21-hydroxylase deficiency) exhibits masculine body habitus, broad shoulders, narrow hips; marked hirsutism on the face, abdomen and lower extremities. Ambisexual genitals; lack of breast development despite 15-month treatment with estrogens. Short stature, 147 cm.

Fig. 3. A 16-year-old female with adrenogenital syndrome and hypertension, caused by 11β-hydroxylase deficiency. The patient was reared as a boy because of large clitoris resembling penis. Premature growth and development exhibited up to age 10, followed by cessation of further growth. Hypertension developed at age 14, and patient died two years later of malignant hypertension.

Fig. 4. Face of patient shown in Fig. 1. Note hair growth on upper lip and chin; severe acne on the cheeks.

Fig. 5. Face of a 30-year-old female with adrenogenital syndrome characterized by marked beard growth, broad mandible and heavy muscles.

PLATE 10

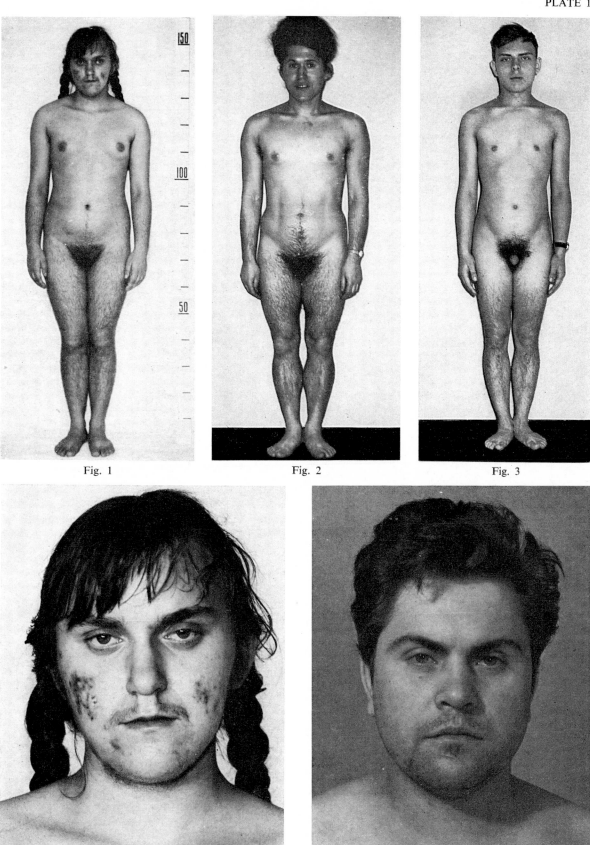

Fig. 1   Fig. 2   Fig. 3

Fig. 4   Fig. 5

Signs and Symptoms in Young Females

1. Ambiguous genitals, particularly clitoral enlargement, may be noted at birth; some infants therefore are mistakenly reared as boys.
2. Accelerated growth.
3. Strong muscle development and increased strength.
4. Appearance of male sex characteristics: development of sexual hair between ages 2 and 8 years, with a male escutcheon; generalized hirsutism in later years; beard growth between the ages of 10 and 15 years, later becoming thick and strong, thus requiring daily shaving. The voice becomes lower.
5. Oily, dense skin as in males; acne common.
6. Amenorrhea present in most cases; only scanty, irregular menstruations in others.
7. Occasional, slight breast development, or none.
8. Sterility in untreated patients.
9. Cessation of growth between ages of 10 and 12 years, with resulting short stature.
10. Male body habitus, broad shoulders and narrow hips; tendency to genu varum.
11. Scarcity of subcutaneous fat tissue.
12. Masculine features of the head: square face with strong muscular development, acne, hirsutism, receding hairline, and androgenic flush below the chin.

Fig. 1. Roentgenogram of hand of an 8-year-old female with congenital adrenogenital syndrome shows markedly advanced bone age of 15 years.

Fig. 2. Roentgenogram of the skull of a 15-year-old female with adrenogenital syndrome. Masculine characteristics of the skull are evident — large mastoid processes and broad mandible, which is thickened at angles.

Fig. 3. Roentgenogram of the ribs of an 18-year-old female with adrenogenital syndrome. Markedly accelerated calcification of the rib cartilages.

166

PLATE 11

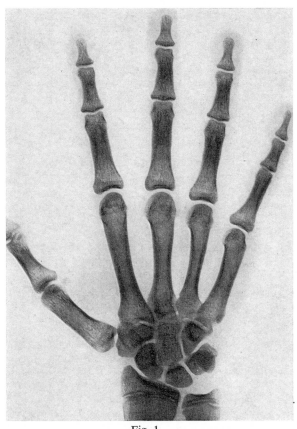

Fig. 1

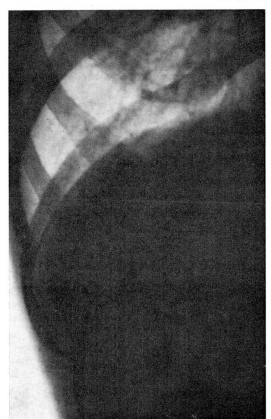

Fig. 3

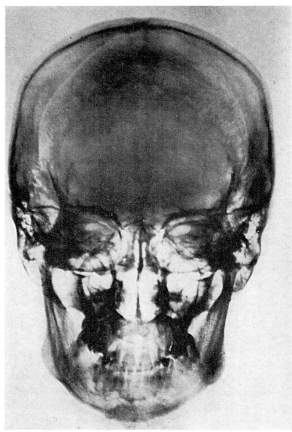

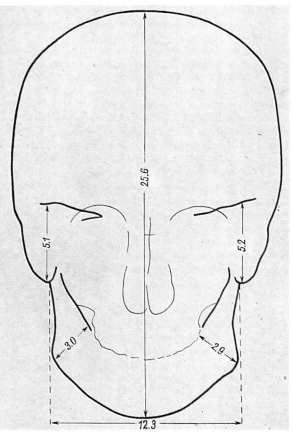

Fig. 2

Hormonal Findings

1. Elevated urinary 17-ketosteroids in patients over age 2 years. In infants the 17-ketosteroids may or may not be elevated.
2. Greatly elevated plasma 17-hydroxyprogesterone and urinary pregnanetriol.
3. Increased plasma 21-deoxycortisol.
4. Increase in urinary 17-ketogenic steroids.
5. Low plasma cortisol and urinary 17-hydroxycorticoids. Poor response of 17-hydroxycorticoid excretion to ACTH stimulation.
6. Dexamethasone suppression test is positive. After several days of dexamethasone administration there is a drop in 17-ketosteroid and 17-ketogenic steroid excretions.

Roentgen Manifestations

Accelerated skeletal growth and maturation are found in all patients between the ages of 2 and 10 years. At this time the bone age is accelerated in comparison to the height and chronologic ages. At about the age 10 years the epiphyses fuse prematurely with the shafts, usually resulting in decreased ultimate stature of the patients. The pneumatization of the paranasal sinuses is precocious; there is both precocious and excessive calcification of the rib and laryngeal cartilages in patients of both sexes.

An increase in bone density and thickness of the cortex of long bones in adrenogenital syndrome may be found when comparing radiograms of the hand of the patient along with the hand of a normal subject.

In female patients with adrenogenital syndrome the long bones appear slender and small in size. In contrast, radiograms of the female skull reveal male characteristics: the sagittal diameter, mastoid length, width of mandible and its angle are greater than normal and resemble those of a male skull.

In female patients the bony pelvis develops prematurely and presents typically female characteristics: a wide subpubic arch and a great rectangular sacrosciatic notch, the development being in accordance with the chromatin sex of the patients.

The radiograms of the hand and wrist are helpful in evaluating the effectiveness of hormonal therapy. Satisfactory results of cortisone treatment are characterized by a normal progress in skeletal growth and maturation.

Fig. 1. Genitalia of a 6-year-old male with adrenogenital syndrome show precocious sexual development, enlargement of the penis, appearance of the sexual hair and hyperpigmentation. The testes remain small.

Fig. 2. Urinary 17-ketosteroids in patients with congenital adrenogenital syndrome before and after cortisol administration. Definitely elevated levels of 17-ketosteroids dropped to normal after cortisol administration.

Fig. 3. Congenital adrenal hyperplasia. Enzymatic defects causing virilization: 21-hydroxylase deficiency (dotted outlined area indicates impaired formation of steroids) and 11β-hydroxylase deficiency (deficient synthesis of steroids within the shaded area). Double lined arrows show increased steroid secretion.

Fig. 4. Congenital adrenal hyperplasia. Enzymatic blocks causing hypertension: 11β-hydroxylase deficiency (Fig. 3) and 17α-hydroxylase deficiency. Dotted outlined areas indicate impaired synthesis of steroids; double lined arrows show increased steroid secretion.

PLATE 12

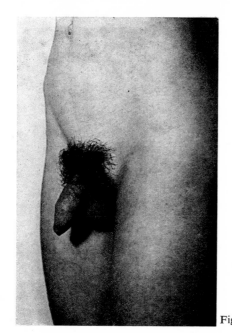

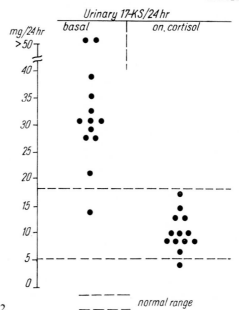

Fig. 1   Fig. 2

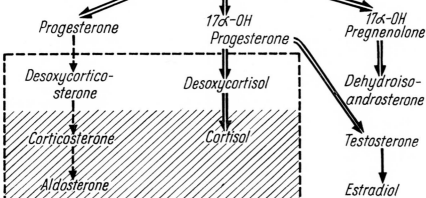

Fig. 3

Fig. 4

Complete Deficiency of 21-Hydroxylase

(Virilization with Salt-Losing Tendency)

The severe form of 21-hydroxylase deficiency is associated with deficiency of both cortisol and aldosterone, and subsequent hyperkalemia, sodium depletion, dehydration, hypotension, circulatory collapse and elevated plasma renin activity. The disease is easily diagnosed in female infants because of early masculinization of the external female genitals with formation of the urogenital sinus, partial fusion of the labioscrotal folds and clitoral hypertrophy; the sex chromatin in buccal smears is positive and there is a female karyotype. In boys the disease may not be properly diagnosed or even suspected and is frequently fatal. Only salt-wasting and familial occurrence may indicate the presence of this disease which can be confirmed by hormonal assay.

Deficiency of 11β-Hydroxylase

(Virilization with Hypertension)

In this form of congenital adrenal hyperplasia the deficiency of 11β-hydroxylase leads to low plasma cortisol and its urinary metabolite tetrahydrocortisol, elevation of plasma 11-deoxycortisol and 11-deoxycorticosterone and increased urinary 17-ketosteroids. In addition to accelerated growth, and virilization of female patients, there is also hypertension resulting from overproduction of deoxycorticosterone.

Deficiency of 3β-Hydroxysteroid Dehydrogenase

(Male or Female Pseudohermaphroditism and Adrenal Insufficiency)

This enzyme block causes deficient synthesis of cortisol, aldosterone and gonadal steroids. In both sexes the external genitalia are ambiguous but female patients exhibit less masculinization than in 21-hydroxylase deficiency. The mortality in early infancy is very high.

Deficiency of 17α-Hydroxylase

(Male Pseudohermaphroditism, Sexual Infantilism and Hypertension)

This variant is characterized by deficient synthesis of 17α-hydroxyprogesterone derivatives, cortisol, androgens and estrogens, but increased secretion of deoxycorticosterone and corticosterone. The manifestations consist of hypertension, hypokalemic alkalosis, lack of sexual maturation of female patients and pseudohermaphroditism in male patients. Hormonal assays reveal low plasma cortisol and urinary 17-hydroxycorticoids, elevated plasma ACTH, deoxycorticosterone and corticosterone. After the age of puberty plasma estrogens and testosterone remain very low and serum gonadotropins elevated.

Deficiency of 20α-Hydroxylase

(Congenital Lipoid Adrenal Hyperplasia)

This is a rare disease in which both the adrenals and gonads are incapable of synthesizing steroids. In male infants the external genitalia are female due to absence of testicular androgens. As a result of severe adrenal insufficiency most of the patients die in early infancy. Autopsy reveals greatly enlarged adrenals and enormous accumulation of lipids in the adrenal cortex and testes.

Fig. 1. Grossly enlarged adrenals in congenital adrenogenital syndrome (artist's rendering based on autopsy findings).

Fig. 2A. Scheme of internal and external genitals in adrenogenital syndrome. Enlarged clitoris and urogenital sinus are seen; the urethra and vagina have a common orifice.

Fig. 2B. Internal and external genitals in adrenogenital syndrome show marked clitoral hypertrophy, common duct of urethra and vagina. Female internal genitalia, i.e., uterus, ovary and fallopian tubes, are normal.

Fig. 3. External genitals of a 15-year-old female with adrenogenital syndrome showing marked hypertrophy of the clitoris and labia minora, excessive hair growth.

Fig. 4. Ambisexual genitals in an 18-year-old female with adrenogenital syndrome. Penis-like appearance of the clitoris, excessive hair growth are seen.

PLATE 13

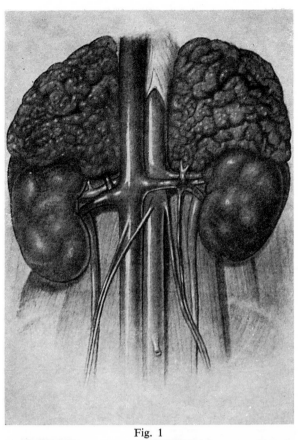

Fig. 1

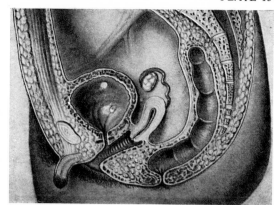

Fig. 2A

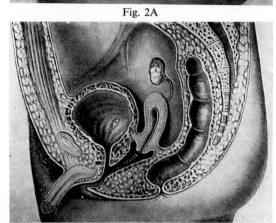

Fig. 2B

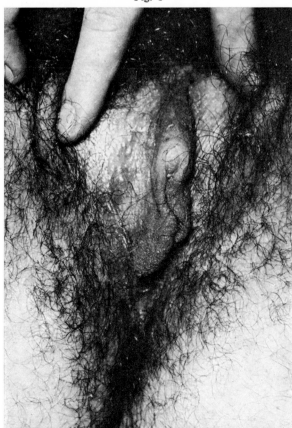

Fig. 3

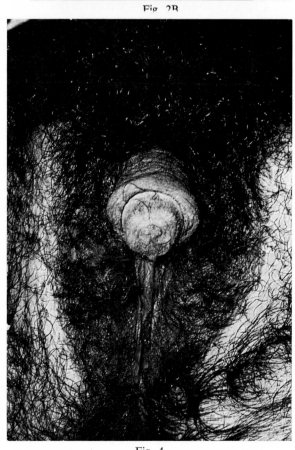

Fig. 4

MASCULINIZING ADRENOCORTICAL TUMORS IN ADULT FEMALES

Adenoma or adenocarcinoma of the adrenal cortex in adult females may secrete large quantities of androgens and lead to masculinization, secondary amenorrhea, sterility and regression of female sex characteristics.

Signs and Symptoms

1. Amenorrhea; sterility.
2. Hirsutism: appearance of hair on the face, chest, around the areolae, on the thighs; male escutcheon of pubic hair.
3. Acne; oily skin.
4. Greasy scalp hair with angular recession and partial baldness.
5. Low-pitched voice.
6. Hypertrophy of clitoris.
7. Increase in muscle strength.
8. Decrease in subcutaneous fat.

Laboratory Findings

1. Increased plasma and urinary testosterone.
2. Increased urinary 17-ketosteroids.
3. No response of 17-ketosteroids to dexamethasone suppression.
4. Low or low-normal serum LH; no midcycle peak of serum LH.
5. Vaginal smears: predominance of intermediate cells.
6. Roentgenograms and laminograms usually demonstrate the presence of an adrenal tumor.

Differential Diagnosis. In congenital adrenocortical hyperplasia, administration of dexamethasone is accompanied by a drop in urinary 17-ketosteroids to normal values within 2 days, while in masculinizing adrenal tumor 17-ketosteroids and plasma testosterone remain elevated. In masculinizing tumor of the ovary and in Stein-Leventhal syndrome pelvic pneumography shows enlargement of one or both ovaries, whereas in adrenocortical tumors the ovaries are of normal or reduced size. Transient forms of the disease exhibiting manifestations of virilizing adrenal tumor and Cushing's syndrome are seen in some cases. Surgical removal of the adrenocortical tumor leads to regression of masculinization, appearance of regular menstrual cycles and fertility. Partial baldness may persist indefinitely.

FEMINIZING ADRENOCORTICAL TUMORS IN ADULT MALES

Adrenocortical adenoma or adenocarcinoma may secrete estrogens and cause gynecomastia, atrophy of the testes, decrease in libido or impotence in adult male subjects. In young males the tumors evoke gynecomastia and accelerate growth and bone maturation with accompanying premature fusion of the epiphyses. The feminizing adrenal tumors are usually large and may be palpable or visible tomographically after retroperitoneal gas insufflation. Hormonal studies show elevated plasma and urinary estrogens; urinary 17-ketosteroids are usually also increased.

Some cases show signs of both feminizing adrenal tumor and Cushing's syndrome, i.e., hypertension, round face, muscle atrophy, osteoporosis. In these cases estrogens, plasma and urinary cortisol, and 17-hydroxycorticoids are elevated.

Fig. 1A. A 36-year-old female with marked virilization due to adrenal tumor. Manifestations include low-pitched voice; secondary amenorrhea; unusual muscular strength; loss of scalp hair, receding hairline; extensive facial hair growth.

Fig. 1B. Large adrenal tumor removed from the patient in Fig. 1A. All signs and symptoms regressed after removal of the tumor. The patient was in complete health for 12 years, then experienced a recurrence of the tumor.

Fig. 1C. Histopathology of the virilizing tumor in Fig. 1B showing marked pleomorphism and large distinct nuclei characteristic of adenocarcinoma.

Figs. 2A and 2B. Face of a 20-year-old female with virilizing tumor of the adrenals, before (*A*) and after (*B*) therapy. *A.* Secondary amenorrhea, hypertrichosis, clitoral hypertrophy. Thinning of scalp hair and extensive seborrhea occur. The hair becomes oily immediately after washing. Marked hypertrichosis of the face exhibited. *B.* The same patient 3 months after removal of the adrenocortical adenoma. Complete regression of all manifestations results in regular menstrual cycles, typical feminine appearance. Plasma testosterone before surgery 6.4 ng/ml, after removal of the adrenal adenoma 0.3 ng/ml.

PLATE 14

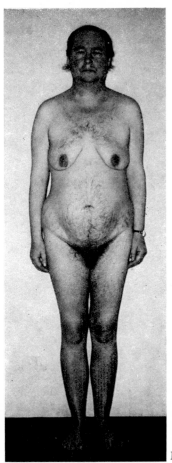

Fig. 1A

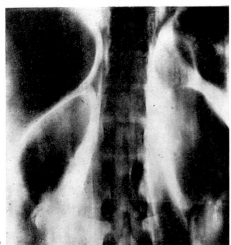

Fig. 1B

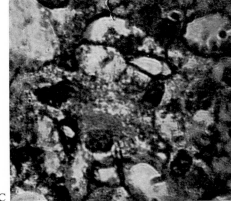

Fig. 1C

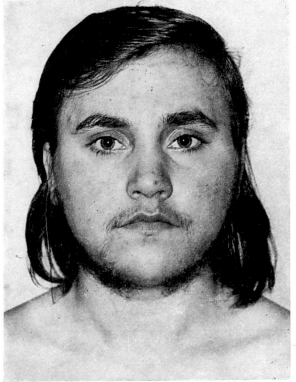

Fig. 2A

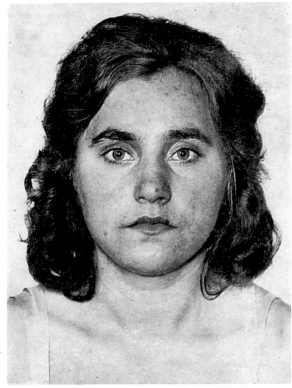

Fig. 2B

ACUTE ADRENOCORTICAL INSUFFICIENCY

(ADRENAL CRISIS; WATERHOUSE-FRIEDERICHSEN SYNDROME)

Acute adrenocortical insufficiency in the neonate results from acute adrenal hemorrhages which usually follow a prolonged and complicated labor. Manifestations include hyperpyrexia, tachypnea, cyanosis, petechiae, hemorrhagic lesions in the skin and convulsions leading to early death.

In children and adolescents massive adrenal hemorrhages, known as Waterhouse-Friederichsen syndrome, occur in the course of meningococcal septicemia.

Symptoms and Signs

1. Fever.
2. Abdominal pain, nausea, vomiting and diarrhea.
3. Purpura; numerous petechiae or subcutaneous hemorrhages.
4. Headache; increased irritability.
5. Stiffness of the neck and other meningeal signs.
6. Drop in blood pressure; collapse.
7. Prostration, convulsions and fatal coma.

Fig. 1A. A 17-year-old patient with acute adrenal insufficiency in the course of meningococcal infection. Confluent subcutaneous hemorrhages are seen on forehead and cheeks. Patient is unconscious.

Fig. 1B. Lower limbs of same patient showing intensive hemorrhagic lesions of the skin, and cyanotic coloration of the toes.

PLATE 15

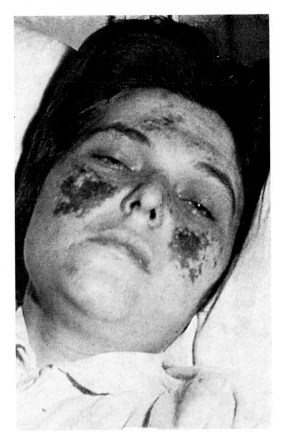

Fig. 1A

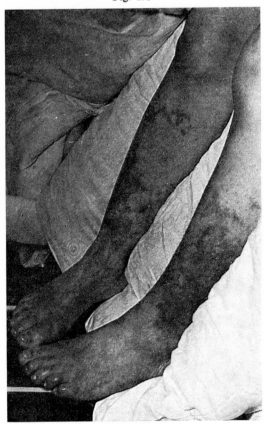

Fig. 1B

ADDISON'S DISEASE

(CHRONIC ADRENOCORTICAL INSUFFICIENCY)

Addison's disease, or chronic adrenal insufficiency, results primarily from destruction of both adrenal glands through tuberculosis, "primary" atrophy or neoplasia. The manifestations include progressive asthenia, weight loss and gastrointestinal disturbances, hypotonia and skin hyperpigmentation. These depend on the degree of deficiency of glucocorticoids and disappear during cortisol administration.

The disease usually occurs between the ages of 20 and 50 years, and gradually progresses. Even slight additional infections may cause a rapid deterioration known as adrenal crisis (acute adrenal insufficiency), which if not treated results in death.

Symptoms and Signs

1. Weakness may develop to such a degree that patients are confined to bed; easy fatigability on exertion; rapid muscular exhaustion.
2. Loss of appetite; decrease in weight — constant findings.
3. Nausea and vomiting; occasional abdominal pains and diarrhea.
4. Hyperpigmentation of the skin; darkened palmar creases.
5. Hypotonia, the systolic pressure usually under 100.
6. Increased irritability; nervousness; headaches; apathy.
7. Circulatory collapse; tremor and other signs of hypoglycemia.
8. Muscular cramps, usually in the calves.
9. Salt craving; patients prefer salty and sour food, and add salt to the meals.
10. Rapid aggravation of all manifestations during infection, surgery, water loading, after trauma and after insulin injection.
11. Loss of axillary hair in female patients.

Fig. 1. Hand and palm of a 40-year-old patient with chronic adrenal insufficiency. Definite darkening of the skin on the back of the hand and forearm, increased pigmentation of the palm creases. Palms and nails remain light.

Fig. 2. Hyperpigmentation of postsurgical scar in a patient with chronic adrenal insufficiency which developed following bilateral adrenalectomy for Cushing's syndrome.

Fig. 3. General appearance of a 20-year-old female with chronic adrenal insufficiency showing severe emaciation, definite darkening of the skin (sparing the palms), very dark nipples.

Fig. 4. Face of a 21-year-old patient with chronic adrenal insufficiency and vitiligo reveals very dark skin with spots devoid of pigment, giving a harlequin-like appearance.

Fig. 5. Close-up of skin on the back of the hand of a patient with chronic adrenal insufficiency. The skin is dry and very dark.

PLATE 16

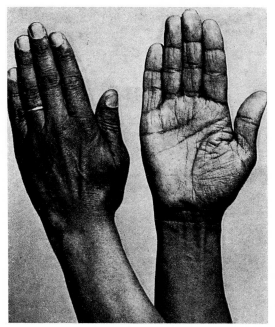

Fig. 1

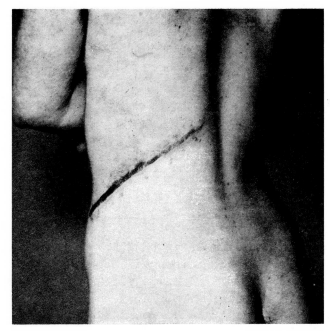

Fig. 2

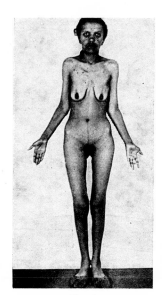

Fig. 3

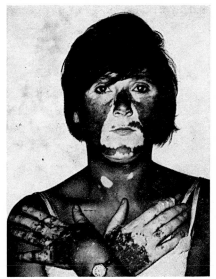

Fig. 4

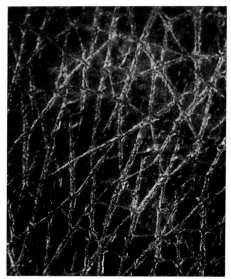

Fig. 5

Skin Changes

In Addison's disease the skin darkens considerably; in patients with dark eyes and hair the skin appears grayish brown; in blondes, hyperpigmentation is not as severe, and the skin is light brown. Furthermore, the skin is always dry, sometimes thin, atrophic, scaly at the elbows and knees, wrinkled on the face and hands. The unpleasant grayish brown hyperpigmentation of the skin is mainly seen in areas exposed to light such as face and hands, or which are subjected to friction such as knees, elbows and waist. The nipples and genital area are brown black. The palms, soles and nails are light pink and contrast markedly to the dark brown color of the flexion creases on the palms and surrounding skin. The scars may turn brown.

In one sixth of the cases vitiligo develops, then the skin has a harlequin appearance: white stains appear on a dark brown background. In some patients there are brown stains on the lips or bluish stains on the buccal mucosa or gums.

Body hair is lost in females and sparse in males; in the majority of females the axillary hair falls out. Simultaneously, due to lack of adrenal androgens, the function of the apocrine sweat glands ceases and the pH of axillary skin is acid instead of alkaline. The pubic hair remains; the menstruations are generally regular, but there is often infertility.

In males the sex hair is normal and the apocrine sweat gland function persists since the other source of androgens — the testes — are not affected.

Laboratory Findings

1. Low plasma and urinary cortisol.
2. Low or low-normal urinary 17-hydroxycorticoids.
3. ACTH stimulation test: lack of response in plasma cortisol and urinary 17-hydroxycorticoids after ACTH or Synacthen administration.
4. Very high plasma ACTH concentration.
5. Water loading test: impaired diuresis, inability to excrete diluted urine. After ingestion of water 1200 to 1500 ml, patients excrete less than half the amount of urine in the first 4 hours; the specific gravity of the urine is 1.008 to 1.030. When 100 mg cortisol is administered 4 hours prior to the test, the diuretic response to water load is markedly ameliorated.
6. Heightened taste sensitivity.
7. Hyponatremia, hypochloremia, occasional hyperkalemia. The ratio of serum sodium to potassium is decreased.
8. Increased sensitivity to smell.
9. Accelerated blood sedimentation rate.
10. Decrease in glomerular filtration rate. Increased blood urea is rare, and found in severe cases only.
11. Roentgen findings: heart smaller than average in all untreated cases; occasional calcifications in the adrenal area at the level of transverse processes of the first lumbar vertebra.
12. ECG: flattening of the T waves; occasional low QRS voltage in standard and left precordial leads; prolongation of the QT and PR intervals.
13. EEG: generalized slowing of the α-rhythm.
14. Increased plasma angiotensin II concentration.
15. Adrenal antibodies usually present in patients with primary atrophy of the adrenals.
16. Cortisol test: disappearance of taste and smell hypersensitivity; normal diuretic response in water loading test; normalization of ECG upon administration of cortisol 30 mg/day for several days.

Fig. 1. Plasma cortisol in chronic adrenal insufficiency before and after ACTH stimulation. Low basal plasma cortisol does not rise after intravenous administration of ACTH in patients with chronic adrenocortical insufficiency. There is a definite rise in plasma cortisol in normal subjects.

Fig. 2. Taste threshold for galvanic current in control subjects and in patients with chronic adrenal insufficiency. Latter exhibit a marked taste hypersensitivity enabling them to detect galvanic current ranging from 1 to 8 μA.

Fig. 3. Water loading test in 22 patients with chronic adrenal insufficiency reveals striking impairment of diuresis and high specific gravity of urine in untreated patients. Following cortisol administration there is a marked amelioration of diuresis.

Fig. 4. Results of plasma ACTH in Addison's disease and in control subjects. Grossly elevated plasma ACTH concentrations are found in all patients with chronic adrenal insufficiency.

PLATE 17

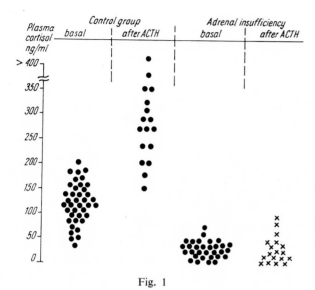

Fig. 1

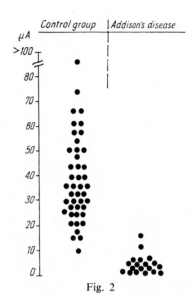

Fig. 2

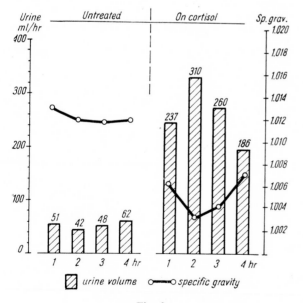

Fig. 3

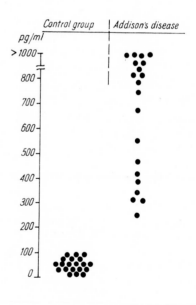

Fig. 4

PRIMARY HYPERALDOSTERONISM
(CONN'S SYNDROME; ALDOSTERONOMA)

Primary aldosteronism is caused by single or multiple adenomas and, rarely, hyperplasia of the adrenal cortex, which secrete excessive amounts of aldosterone. The principal manifestations are hypertension, polyuria, muscular weakness and hypokalemia. The disease is prevalent in females and usually occurs between the ages of 30 and 50 years.

Symptoms and Signs

1. Hypertension, both diastolic and systolic, is always present.
2. Headaches.
3. Polyuria; increased thirst.
4. Muscular weakness.
5. Periodic paralysis; lack of tendon reflexes.
6. Paresthesias of face and limbs.
7. Occasional tetany.

Laboratory Findings

1. Increased plasma and urinary aldosterone; failure to suppress aldosterone excretion in patients on a high sodium diet (200 mEq/day).
2. Low plasma renin activity. Even on a low sodium diet (10 mEq/day) the plasma renin activity remains low, while it increases markedly in normal subjects.
3. Hypokalemia is a very frequent finding associated with normochloremia or hyperchloremia.
4. Increased urinary potassium during salt loading. Patients maintained for 5 days on a high sodium diet (200 mEq Na/day and 100 mEq K/day) excrete large amounts of urinary potassium and develop hypokalemia.
5. ECG abnormalities typical of hypokalemia and hypertension: QT prolongation, flat or negative T waves, lowered ST segments, prolongation of the PR interval, appearance of the U wave and signs of left ventricular strain.
6. Polyuria; impairment of urine concentrating power during water deprivation or after Pitressin injection.
7. Alkaline pH of the urine.
8. Occasional hypernatremia.
9. Adrenal tumor not readily determined by roentgenography after retroperitoneal gas insufflation, as the tumor is usually small.
10. Adrenal vein catheterization for aldosterone assay and adrenal venography are helpful in locating the tumor.
11. Disappearance of all clinical manifestations and laboratory abnormalities after surgical removal of the adrenal tumor.

SECONDARY HYPERALDOSTERONISM

Secondary hyperaldosteronism appears in some edematous states such as nephrosis, hepatic cirrhosis, congestive heart failure, and in some cases of cyclic idiopathic edema. Additionally, it is always found in malignant hypertension, and occasionally in renovascular hypertension. Differentiation of secondary from primary hyperaldosteronism is important, as the treatment varies. Nephrosis, hepatic cirrhosis and heart failure are easily diagnosed because of typical clinical manifestations and edema; the serum potassium in these diseases is usually normal. Apart from certain clinical differences, malignant hypertension and renovascular hypertension are associated with a high plasma renin activity, while in primary hyperaldosteronism the renin activity is constantly low.

Fig. 1. Adrenal phlebography in a 26-year-old female with Cushing's syndrome and increased aldosterone secretion reveals the presence of a tumor in the right adrenal gland.

Figs. 2A and 2B. *A*. Aldosteronoma 22 mm in diameter removed from the left adrenal in a patient with Conn's syndrome; it was encapsulated and of pinkish hue. *B*. On cross section, the tumor proved to be canary yellow in color.

Fig. 3. ECG of same patient with primary aldosteronism shows prolongation of QT time, depression of ST segments resulting from hypopotassemia.

Fig. 4. Results of serum potassium concentration, 24-hr urine volume and arterial blood pressure in a case of primary aldosteronism before therapy and after surgery.

PLATE 18

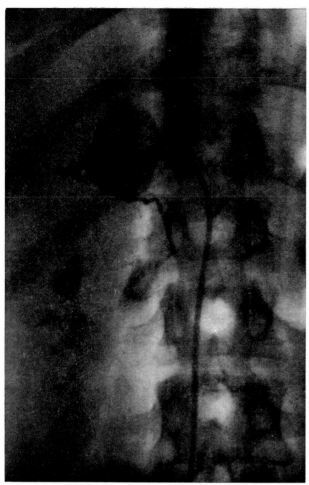

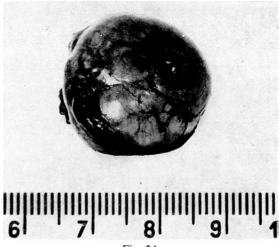

Fig. 2A

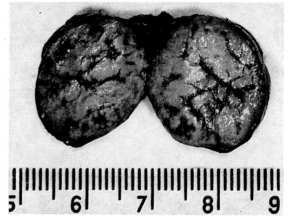

Fig. 2B

Fig. 1

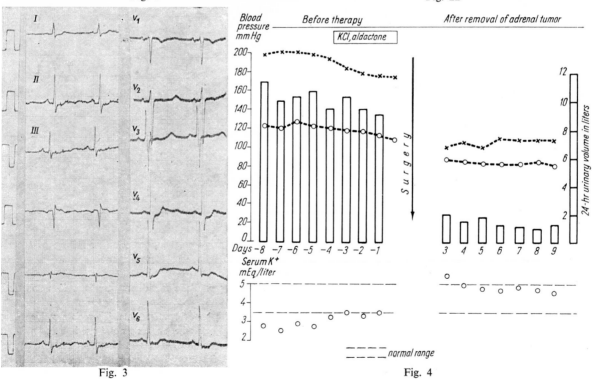

Fig. 3

Fig. 4

PHEOCHROMOCYTOMA

Pheochromocytoma is a tumor composed of chromaffin tissue. It is found in the adrenal medulla, and rarely in other sites such as the sympathetic chain in the abdomen or thorax, the bladder wall, testes or ovaries. Pheochromocytoma secretes large amounts of norepinephrine and epinephrine, causing paroxysmal or sustained hypertension.

Symptoms and Signs in Paroxysmal Hypertension

1. Headache.
2. Anxiety.
3. Palpitations.
4. Substernal pain; suffocating feeling in the chest.
5. Epigastric pain.
6. Profuse sweating.
7. Face pale or cyanotic.
8. Trembling; paresthesias.
9. Abrupt rise in blood pressure during attack.
10. Prostration and fatigue following the attack.

These manifestations appear suddenly and last from minutes to hours.

Symptoms and Signs in Sustained Hypertension

1. Headaches and vertigo.
2. Tremor.
3. Impairment of eye focusing; dilatation of the pupils
4. Occasional signs of malignant hypertension.

Laboratory Findings

1. Increased plasma and urinary catecholamines.
2. Increased urinary vanilmandelic acid.
3. Phentolamine test: systolic blood pressure drops 40 mm or more, and diastolic pressure drops 30 mm or more, in the first minutes following intravenous administration of 5 mg phentolamine (Regitine) — a characteristic of pheochromocytoma with sustained hypertension.

Fig. 1. Roentgenogram (after gas insufflation) in a 32-year-old patient with paroxysmal hypertension reveals an oval retroperitoneal tumor at the level of L_2 to L_4. On surgery the tumor proved to be a neuroblastoma arising from sympathetic ganglia.

Fig. 2. Possible sites (x) of catecholamine-producing tumors: in the adrenal medulla, sympathetic ganglia, spleen and testis (or ovary).

Fig. 3. Results of phentolamine (Regitine) and histamine tests in patients with pheochromocytoma. There is a sudden drop in blood pressure in response to phentolamine administration. Administration of histamine evokes a rapid rise in blood pressure accompanied by headache, flush and nausea. These pharmacologic agents produce no changes in blood pressure in control subjects. (From Melmon KL in Williams RH (ed) Textbook of Endocrinology, 5th Ed. WB Saunders Company, Philadelphia 1974, p. 311.)

PLATE 19

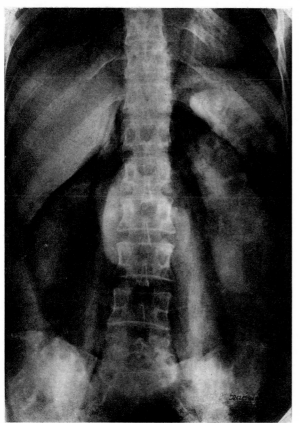

Fig. 1

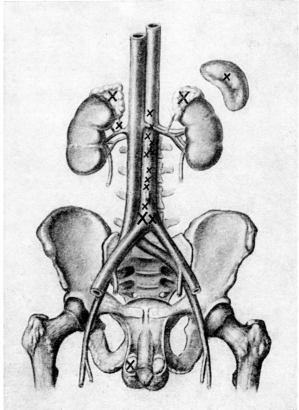

Fig. 2

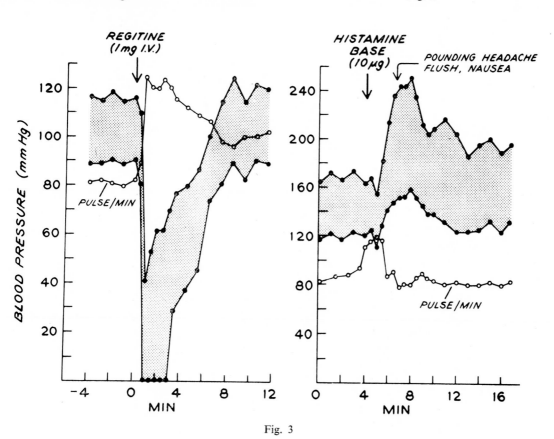

Fig. 3

4. Histamine test: intravenous injection of 0.05 mg histamine induces a typical attack of paroxysmal hypertension with a quick rise in blood pressure of 50 mm or more. All these manifestations disappear after subsequent phentolamine administration.
5. Neutrophilia.
6. Hyperglycemia.
7. High free-fatty-acid level in plasma after meals.
8. Adrenopneumography may reveal an adrenal tumor.
9. Adrenal arteriography and venography usually enable localization of the tumor.
10. Increased basal metabolic rate.

Chapter 4

THE TESTES

ANORCHIDISM

(BILATERAL ANORCHIA)

Anorchidism, the absence of both testes, is characterized by a small penis, underdeveloped "empty" scrotum and some postpubertal eunuchoid features. A careful survey of the inguinal canals and pelvic cavity confirms the absence of the gonads. In some patients the vas deferens is found to end blindly, or there is a rudimentary epididymis on one or both sides of the pelvis. A small nodule consisting of fibrous tissue may be seen on occasion.

The presence of the penis and fused scrotal folds indicates that functioning testes must have been present in fetal life but subsequently have atrophied between the seventh and fourteenth week of fetal life. There is no sexual development during or after the pubertal period, and patients develop childlike fat deposits in the abdomen as well as eunuchoid body proportions, i.e., excessively long extremities in proportion to the trunk. No other abnormalities are present.

There are negative chromatin patterns in buccal mucosa smears and XY sex chromosomes. Urinary and plasma testosterone is low and does not increase after FSH and HCG administration as in normal male subjects. Only in exceedingly rare cases some Leydig cells may be present in the pelvic area and respond to HCG stimulation. After the age of puberty, serum and urinary LH and FSH increase.

The disease is often mistaken for bilateral cryptorchidism but surgical exploration of inguinal canals and pelvis enables differentiation as no testes are found to be present in anorchidism.

Fig. 1A. A 21-year-old patient with anorchidism. Exploratory laparotomy confirmed the absence of gonads in the abdomen and inguinal canals. Infantile face, lack of sexual maturation, slight genu valgum are seen. The XY sex chromosomes are normal. Serum LH 88 mIU/ml, FSH 58 mIU/ml. Serum testosterone 0.6 ng/ml.

Fig. 1B. Extreme underdevelopment of the genitals, fat accumulation on the abdomen and above the hips in the patient shown in Fig. 1A are evident.

Fig. 1C. Closeup view of the genitals of the patient shown in Fig. 1A. The penis is small; the scrotum empty, constituting only a small area of folded skin; very scanty sexual hair.

Fig. 2. Closeup view of the genitals of a 28-year-old anorchid patient following several years therapy with testosterone. Small penis and empty scrotum are evident.

PLATE 1

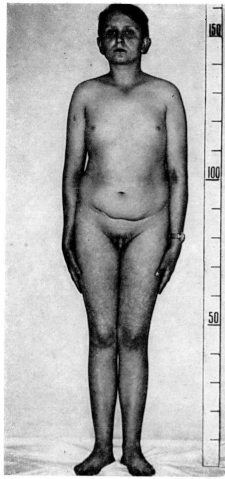

Fig. 1A

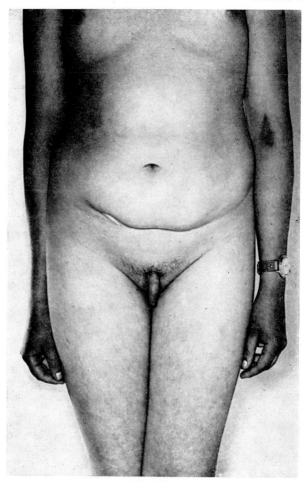

Fig. 1B

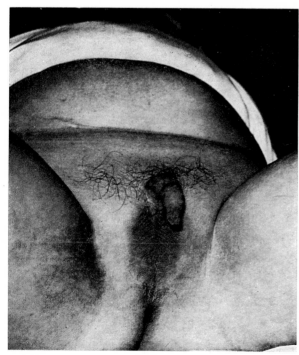

Fig. 1C

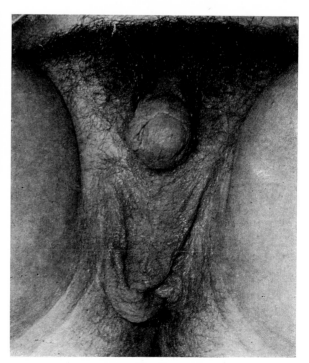

Fig. 2

TESTICULAR DYSGENESIS

(RUDIMENTARY TESTES; DYSGENETIC TESTES)

Testicular dysgenesis is faulty development of the testes originating in the fetus. The testes are small and located in the pelvis or inguinal canals. Histologically the testes show scanty, small seminiferous tubules lined with undifferentiated Sertoli cells and a few spermatogonia. After puberty interstitial tissue may contain sparse Leydig cells. Occasionally a large tubule contains a round intratubular body composed of a core with concentric rings (which stain lightly with eosin) surrounded by sustentacular cells arranged in two layers — the inner against the round body, outer against the basement membrane.

Dysgenetic testes may appear in the following syndromes: male pseudohermaphroditism, male Turner's syndrome, mixed gonadal dysgenesis, and in cryptorchidism in an undescended testis, sometimes associated with polydactylia on the same side.

MALE TURNER'S SYNDROME

A rare congenital disease, resembling Turner's syndrome in females, male Turner's syndrome is characterized by short stature, webbed neck, various congenital anomalies and testicular dysgenesis. Chromatin patterns are negative, and normal XY chromosomes are found.

The disease resembles mixed gonadal dysgenesis in that the same clinical features may be present, but there are no sex chromosome anomalies and no roentgen manifestations as are found in gonadal dysgenesis.

Fig. 1. Laparotomy findings in a patient with anorchidism. No evidence of internal genitals is seen except for a small nodule on the right side wall of the pelvis. Histopathology proved the nodule to be a dysgenetic testis.

Fig. 2. Histopathology of a dysgenic testis from a 6-year-old boy with perineoscrotal hypospadias. Small, densely packed tubules ined with undifferentiated cells are shown; the outlines of the tubules are indistinct. In the middle, an intratubular body consisting of a calcified, laminated core surrounded by 3 concentric layers of granulosa-Sertoli cells is seen (Courtesy J Teter, MD, Warsaw).

Fig. 3. Photomicrograph of another intratubular body in the same patient. The large core, composed of concentric layers of calcified tissue, is surrounded by 2 wreaths of granulosa-Sertoli cells.

PLATE 2

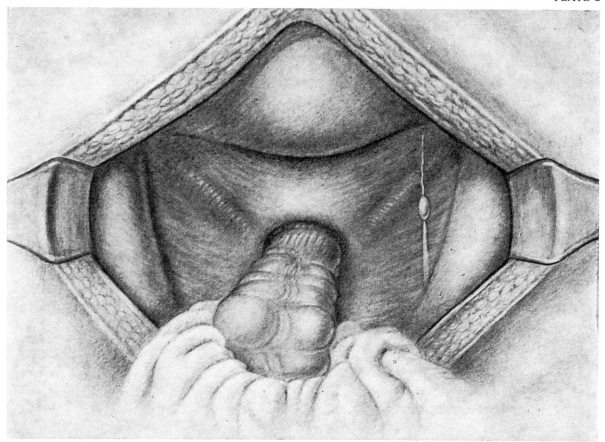

Fig. 1

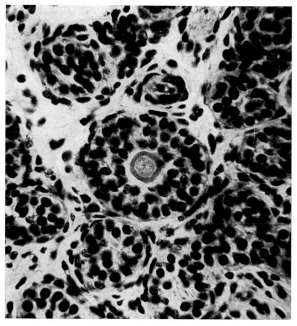

Fig. 2

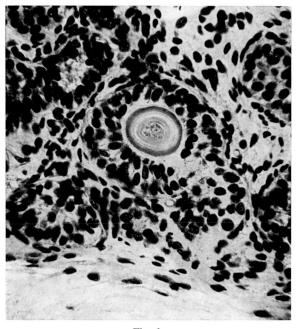

Fig. 3

EUNUCHOIDISM

(HYPOGONADISM)

Eunuchoidism (hypogonadism) is the result of hormonal insufficiency of the testes, i.e., a lack of androgens emanating from Leydig cells. Primary hypogonadism may be caused by mumps during adolescence, trauma or castration, and rarely by hemochromatosis or other diseases affecting the testes. The clinical picture depends on the age of patients at the onset of disease. In adult patients there is a slow regression of secondary sex characteristics, the testes diminish in size and are soft. There are oligospermia or azoospermia, increase in serum FSH when germinal epithelium sclerosis and hyalinization occur. Usually Leydig cell function remains intact and serum testosterone and LH levels are normal.

Secondary hypogonadism results from destruction of the pituitary by craniopharyngioma, chromophobe adenoma or other lesions. The most common form of hypogonadotropic eunuchoidism is isolated gonadotropin deficiency which is sometimes familial. In all forms of hypogonadism with prepubertal onset the clinical manifestations are similar.

HYPOGONADOTROPIC EUNUCHOIDISM

(ISOLATED GONADOTROPIN DEFICIENCY)

Isolated LH and FSH deficiency is caused either by deficient secretion of LH releasing hormone or decreased responsiveness of pituitary gonadotropes to this neurohormone. Hypoosmia or anosmia are frequently associated with hypogonadotropic hypogonadism and can be detected in childhood. Other manifestations such as lack of sexual maturation are evident only at or after puberty, and eunuchoid body proportions are pronounced in later years.

Symptoms

1. Decrease or absence of libido; deficient potency; disinterest in opposite sex.
2. Lack of sexual development at and past the age of puberty.
3. Muscular weakness.
4. Diminished activity; lack of energy.
5. Dizziness.

Fig. 1A. A 30-year-old patient with primary hypogonadism as a result of mumps orchitis. Eunuchoidal body proportions (long extremities compared to the trunk); the hands reach almost to the knees. Lack of sexual development; fat deposits above the hips. Genu valgum. Serum LH 64 mIU/ml. Chromatin pattern negative.

Fig. 1B. Eunuchoidal body proportions of the patient shown in Fig. 1A. The span of the arms exceeds the height by 12 cm (5 in.); the lower dimension from os pubis to sole exceeds the distance from os pubis to vertex by 8 cm (3 in.).

Fig. 2A. A 42-year-old patient with hypogonadotropic eunuchoidism exhibiting poor muscle development, infantile genitals, scanty pubic hair, immature face.

Fig. 2B. Face of the patient shown in Fig. 2A exhibiting infantile features, swollen upper lids, low hairline, complete lack of hair growth on the face, lack of masculine characteristics. The face is soft with rounded contours.

PLATE 3

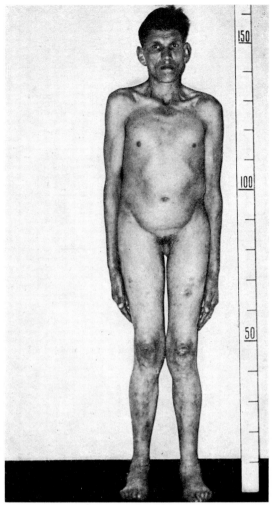

Fig. 1A

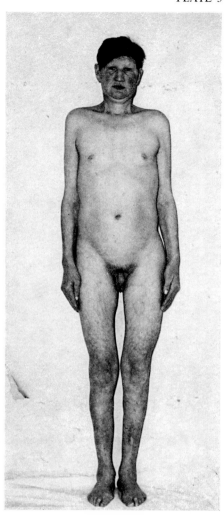

Fig. 2A

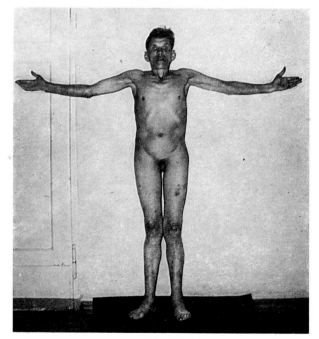

Fig. 1B

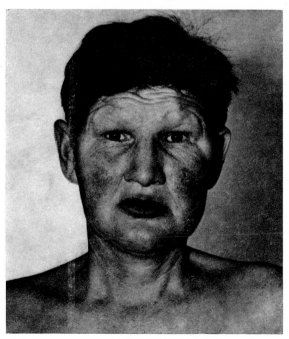

Fig. 2B

Signs

1. Eunuchoid body: disproportionately long extremities compared to the trunk.
2. Height above the average due to continued growth past the age of puberty.
3. Youthful, immature facial features.
4. Noticeable lack of genital development.
5. No beard growth, no facial hair, scanty or absent sexual hair.
6. High-pitched voice.
7. Delicate skin; premature pronounced wrinkles in patients over age 35.
8. Knock-knees (genu valgum).
9. Kyphosis of the spine in older patients.
10. Fat accumulation on the abdomen.
11. Poor muscle development; reduced strength.

The Face

The face has a youthful, immature expression, oval contour and delicate chin. There is a lack of beard. The upper eyelids are sometimes puffed, giving a somnolent look; the skin is pale with a sallow hue. These findings somewhat resemble the face of patients with myxedema. In some patients the supraorbital ridges are prominent. In older patients numerous deep wrinkles and folds develop on the face. The hairline is semicircular with no recession at the temples. The hair is thick, and even in older patients there is no tendency to baldness.

Fig. 1. Face of a 27-year-old patient with hypogonadotropic eunuchoidism and anosmia shows immature features, low hairine on the forehead, recessed chin and complete lack of facial hair. Serum FSH and LH are undetectable, plasma testosterone is 0.6 ng/ml.

Fig. 2. Face of a 50-year-old patient with hypogonadotropic eunuchoidism. The scalp hair extends low on the forehead; numerous wrinkles have appeared around the eyes and mouth, on the cheeks and at the base of the nose; loose skin folds on the neck; complete lack of beard growth.

Figs. 3A and 3B. Many deep folds and wrinkles on the face of a 54-year-old patient with hypogonadotropic hypogonadism. There is no baldness and no recession of the hair at the temples. The chin is recessed and poorly developed; the neck is shortened due to marked osteoporosis of the spine.

PLATE 4

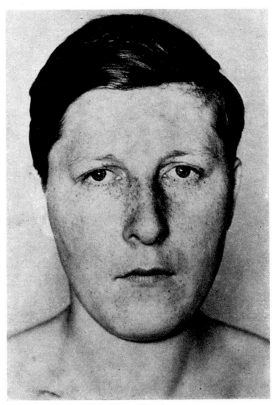

Fig. 1

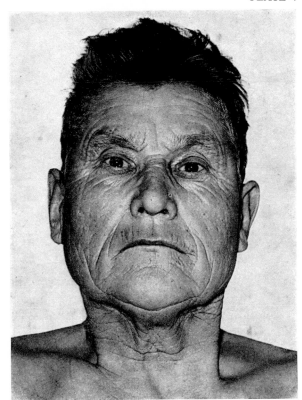

Fig. 2

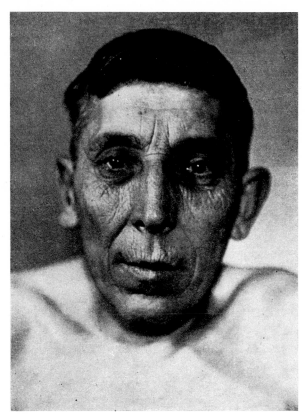

Fig. 3A

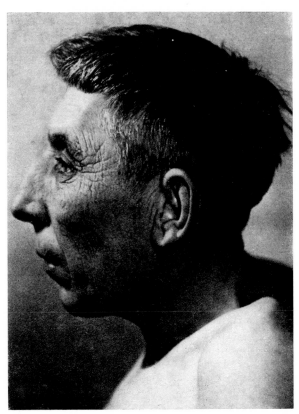

Fig. 3B

Body Proportions

In patients with prepubertal onset of hypogonadism the extremities are greatly elongated in contrast to the trunk, identified as eunuchoid body proportions. The arm span exceeds the height by 7.5 cm or more (3 in. or more); the distance from the os pubis to the sole of the foot is 7.5 cm or more (3 in. or more) greater than the distance from vertex to os pubis. These abnormal proportions evolve after the age of puberty due to the continued growth of the long bones. A deficiency of sex hormones results in lack of fusion of the epiphyses with the shafts of these bones in patients aged 19 to 26 years. By the third decade the patients ultimately have achieved above average height and frequently an arm span of over 195 cm.

The wrists are narrow and delicate; the fingers are unusually elongated, but do not taper; the upper limbs excessively long. Genu valgum is common, and some patients require surgical correction.

Skin, Subcutaneous Fat and Muscles

The skin is pale, smooth and delicate as that of an infant. The body hair is sparse. By the fourth decade of life, many wrinkles have appeared on the dorsa of the hands due to reduced elasticity of the skin. The subcutaneous fat accumulates on the trunk, especially the abdomen, while the extremities remain slender. Peculiar, protruding fat pads appear above the hips, so that the waist line is convex instead of straight. The muscles are poorly developed.

The Genitals

The genitals remain infantile or even at best are markedly underdeveloped. The penis is small; the testes small and soft; the scrotum nonpendulous and pale, without physiologic hyperpigmentation. The pubic hair is scarce and of female escutcheon.

Fig. 1. Extreme atrophy of the genitals of a 50-year-old patient with hypogonadotropic eunuchoidism. The penis is tiny, embedded in fat folds; the scrotum is pale and minute. There is no sexual hair and no physiologic hyperpigmentation. The skin of the abdomen is conspicuously pale and flaccid, with subcutaneous fat accumulations.

Fig. 2. External genitals of a 19-year-old patient with hypogonadotropic eunuchoidism. Note small, soft testes, shrunken scrotum, small penis, very scanty pubic hair.

Fig. 3. Genitals of a 25-year-old patient with craniopharyngioma and gonadotropic deficiency. There is no pubic hair and no physiologic hyperpigmentation; the genitals are atrophic.

Fig. 4. Genitals of a 21-year-old patient with hypogonadism. Underdeveloped penis and scrotum, soft and tiny testes, very scarce pubic hair.

PLATE 5

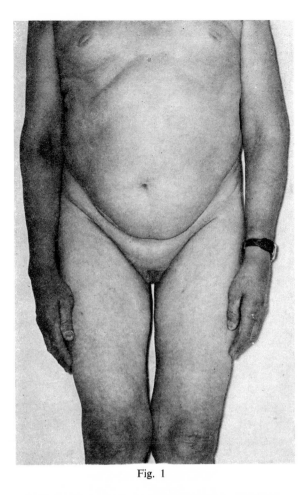

Fig. 1

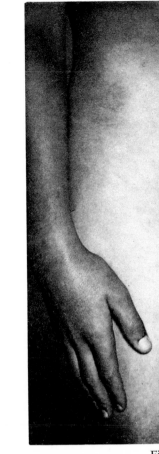

Fig. 2

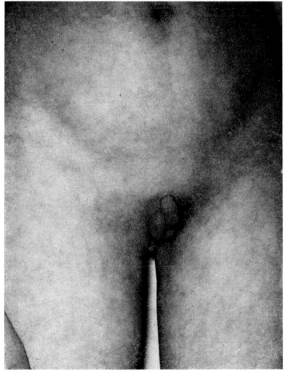

Fig. 3

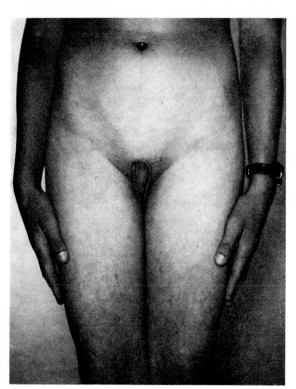

Fig. 4

Roentgen Findings

1. Delayed epiphyseal fusion.
2. Elongated and thickened metacarpals and phalanges.
3. Excessive pneumatization of paranasal sinuses; clubbing of the clinoid processes.
4. Delicate mandible.
5. Osteoporosis, especially of the spine; flattening of the vertebral bodies in patients over 35.

Testicular Histology

Testicular biopsy specimens reveal, in microscopic examination, small, densely packed, immature seminiferous tubules without lumen. The tubules contain mainly undifferentiated epithelial cells but Sertoli cells are not seen. In the interstitial tissue there are no Leydig cells; only fibroblasts are occasionally found. This histologic picture is the same as in prepubertal males.

Figs. 1A to 1D. Roentgenograms of the sella turcica in 4 cases of hypogonadotropic hypogonadism. A small-sized sella (*B*, *C*, and *D*), thickened and clubbed clinoid processes (*A–D*), bridged sella (*C* and *D*), and excessive pneumatization of sphenoidal sinuses are seen.

Fig. 2. Roentgenogram of the finger of a 23-year-old patient with isolated gonadotropin deficiency shows a marked delay in epiphyseal fusion and small spicules of the epiphyses of the medial phalanges pointing distally.

Fig. 3. Roentgenogram of the spine of a 36-year-old untreated patient with hypogonadotropic hypogonadism. Marked flattening and decreased density (osteoporosis) of the vertebral bodies, and irregular, intensively calcified terminal plates are seen.

PLATE 6

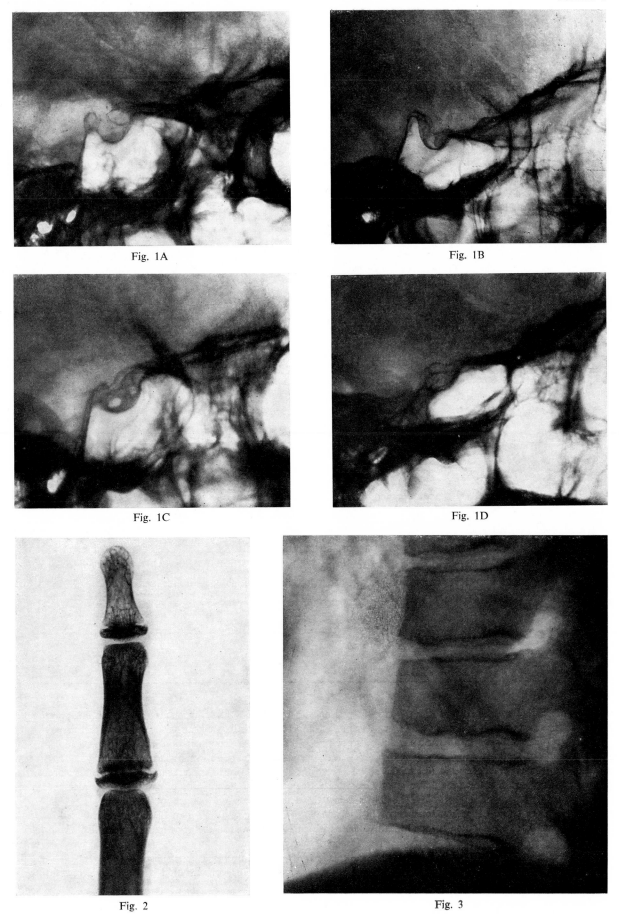

Fig. 1A

Fig. 1B

Fig. 1C

Fig. 1D

Fig. 2

Fig. 3

Laboratory Findings

1. Undetectable or very low serum and urinary LH and FSH.
2. Lowered plasma and urinary testosterone.
3. Negative chromatin findings.
4. Normal XY sex chromosomes.
5. Deficient response of serum LH and FSH to intravenous LH-RH administration.
6. Urinary 17-ketosteroids low-normal.
7. Anosmia or hypoosmia.

KALLMANN'S SYNDROME

(OLFACTORY-GENITAL DYSPLASIA)

Kallmann's syndrome, a subgroup of hypogonadotropic eunuchoidism, is a genetic disorder found only in male subjects. The primary characteristics include eunuchoidism, anosmia, occasional synkinesia, low or absent serum and urinary gonadotropins. Apart from familial occurrence there are no differences between Kallmann's syndrome and isolated gonadotropin deficiency. In both diseases a decrease in smell sensitivity or anosmia is found. The disease is probably caused by deficiency in gonadotropin-releasing hormones due to maldevelopment of neural centers in median eminence, while anosmia results from agenesis of the olfactory lobes of the brain.

Fig. 1. Histopathology of the testis of a 28-year-old patient with hypogonadotropic hypogonadism. Small, infantile tubules lined with immature Sertoli cells and single spermatogonia (clear cells with distinct nucleus) are seen. Interstitial tissue slightly fibrotic and deficient in cells; no Leydig cells are present. The tunica propria is thin and barely perceptible.

Fig. 2. Results of serum testosterone radioimmunoassay in hypogonadal patients. In hypogonadotropic hypogonadism, serum testosterone is considerably lowered (0.1 to 0.8 ng/ml), much the same as in hypopituitarism. In Klinefelter's syndrome the concentration of serum testosterone differs greatly from patient to patient; in the majority of patients testosterone concentration is below the normal range.

Fig. 3. Results of serum LH radioimmunoassay. In hypogonadotropic hypogonadism serum LH is very low, 0 to 4 mIU/ml. Elevated serum LH concentration is found in all patients with anorchidism and in the great majority of patients with Klinefelter's syndrome.

Fig. 4. Results of serum FSH radioimmunoassay. Patients with hypogonadotropic hypogonadism have low or undetectable serum FSH. In anorchidism and in Klinefelter's syndrome serum FSH concentration is markedly increased.

PLATE 7

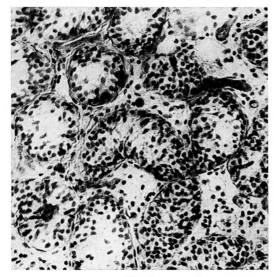

Fig. 1

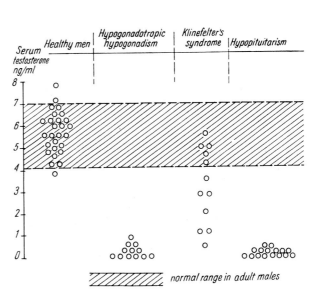

Fig. 2

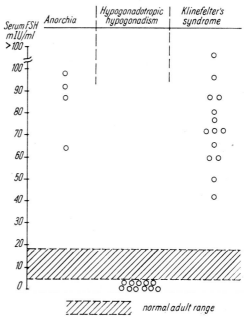

Fig. 3

Fig. 4

KLINEFELTER'S SYNDROME

(SEMINIFEROUS TUBULE DYSGENESIS; SCLEROSING TUBULAR DEGENERATION)

Klinefelter's syndrome is a not uncommon congenital disease associated with abnormalities in sex chromosomes. The principal clinical manifestations include small, firm testes, sterility, positive chromatin findings, increased plasma and urinary gonadotropins, and varying degrees of eunuchoidism. Gynecomastia is found in over half the patients. Chromosome analysis reveals the presence of XXY sex chromosomes in the majority of cases. Prior to puberty there are usually no symptoms, but occasionally mental deficiency is noted; at this time the disease may be diagnosed by detection of a chromatin-positive pattern in buccal mucosa smears.

Patients exhibiting Klinefelter's syndrome variants with mosaicism, most frequently 46,XY/47,XXY, are less severely affected than those with the classic XXY form. Testicular function in these patients may be nearly normal; chromatin findings are negative or borderline (a low percentage of sex chromatin bodies), and some patients are fertile during young adult life.

Symptoms

1. Gynecomastia.
2. Sterility.
3. Anomalous sexual development, sometimes associated with diminished libido and potency.

Fig. 1. An 18-year-old patient with Klinefelter's syndrome. Note narrow shoulders, broad hips, poor sexual development.

Fig. 2. A 19-year-old patient with chromatin-positive Klinefelter's syndrome. Slim build, excessively long extremities, eunuchoid body proportions, scanty pubic hair, underdeveloped genitals are seen.

Fig. 3. An 18-year-old patient with chromatin-positive Klinefelter's syndrome. Gynecomastia, pubic hair of a female escutcheon and pronounced genu valgum are evident.

Fig. 4. A 38-year-old patient with Klinefelter's syndrome. Body proportions are normal. Note lack of beard growth, gynecomastia, female escutcheon of the pubic hair, small and firm testes but otherwise normal genitals. Serum LH elevated 54 mIU/ml.

Fig. 5. A 14-year-old patient with chromatin-positive Klinefelter's syndrome. Slim build, thin extremities with poor muscle development, infantile genitals, congenital heart defect and chest deformity are present.

Fig. 6. An 18-year-old patient with Klinefelter's syndrome. Tall thin habitus, small head, elongated neck, excessively long extremities, poor muscle development, broad hips and small nipples are seen. The genitals are of nearly normal size but the testes are small and firm.

PLATE 8

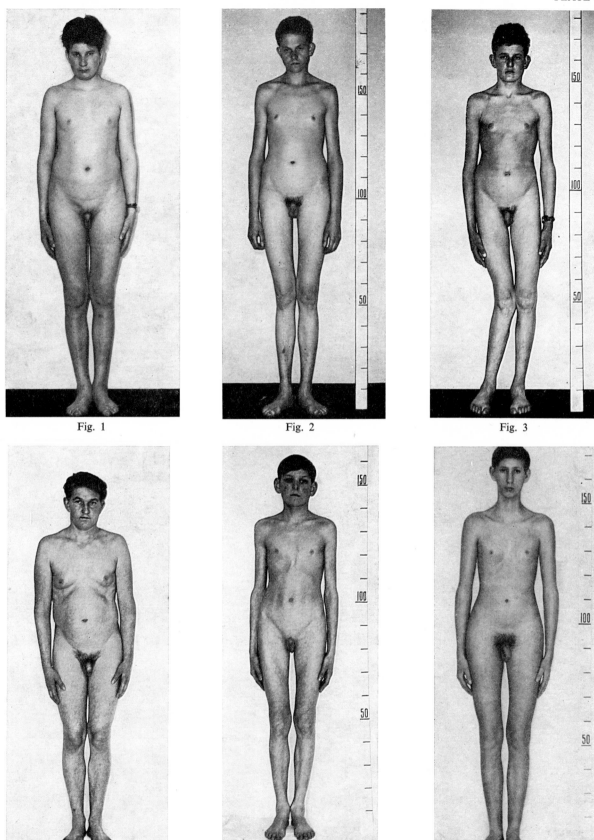

Fig. 1

Fig. 2

Fig. 3

Fig. 4

Fig. 5

Fig. 6

Signs

1. Tallness.
2. Abnormally long legs.
3. Small, firm testes.
4. Genitalia poorly developed.
5. Gynecomastia, in more than half the cases.
6. Paucity of body hair; pubic hair of female escutcheon.
7. Narrow shoulders, broad hips.
8. Mental deficiency, subnormal intelligence; character or personality disorders.

The Head

In some patients the circumference of the cranium is reduced due principally to smaller width of the vault. The face does not differ greatly from that of normal males. The mandible is broad and muscles are heavy; the supraorbital ridges may be protruding. The facial hair, however, is scanty or completely absent, and occasional pallor may be seen. The hairline on the forehead is semicircular without recessions at the temples.

Fig. 1. A 24-year-old patient with chromatin-positive Klinefelter's syndrome and eunuchoid habitus. The face is juvenile with no facial hair.

Fig. 2. A 33-year-old patient with chromatin-positive Klinefelter's syndrome exhibiting immature facial features and complete lack of beard growth. There is no temporal recession of the hairline.

Fig. 3. Face of a 37-year-old patient with Klinefelter's syndrome. Slight puffiness of the upper eyelids, low hairline on the forehead and complete lack of facial hair.

Fig. 4. Face of a 22-year-old patient with Klinefelter's syndrome. The scalp hair extends low on the forehead, no beard growth. Prominent supraorbital ridges give a determined look.

PLATE 9

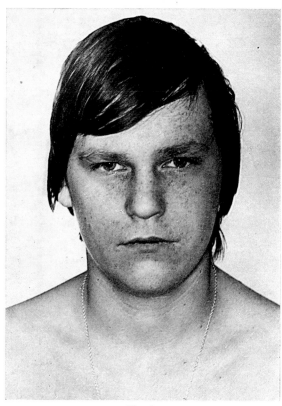

Fig. 1

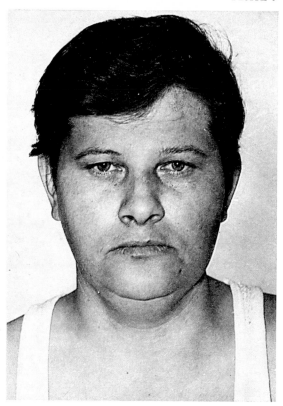

Fig. 2

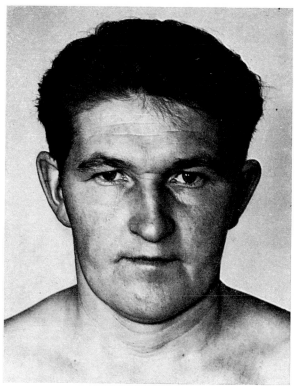

Fig. 3

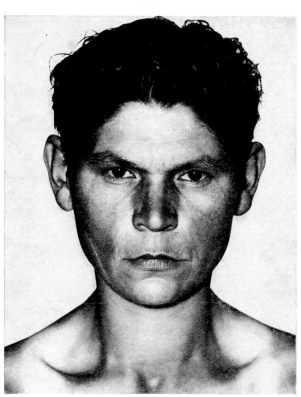

Fig. 4

Body Proportions

The most frequent deviations noted are excessively long legs in contrast to the trunk; the distance from the os pubis to the sole is from 7 to 17 cm greater than the distance from the os pubis to the vertex. The span usually exceeds the height by 5 to 15 cm. Additionally, over half the patients exhibit feminine characteristics such as narrow shoulders and broad hips. In normal males the bihumeral distance exceeds the bitrochanteric distance by 8 to 12 cm, whereas in cases of Klinefelter's syndrome where the shoulders are narrow the difference is only from 3 to 5 cm — as in women.

Fig. 1. Long extremities, deficient muscle mass and pronounced genu valgum in a 22-year-old patient with Klinefelter's syndrome.

Fig. 2. Fat deposits above the hips, typical of eunuchoidism, are frequently seen even in patients of normal weight.

Fig. 3. Sex chromatin in nucleus of buccal mucosal cells obtained from a patient with Klinefelter's syndrome.

Fig. 4. Typical chromosomal analysis from a chromatin-positive Klinefelter's syndrome showing 47, XXY constitution.

PLATE 10

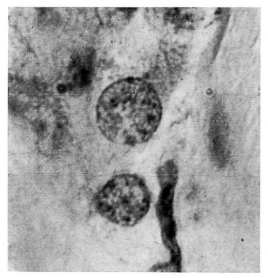

Fig. 1

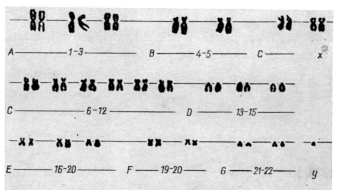

Fig. 2

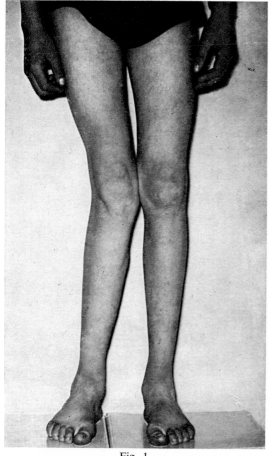

Fig. 3

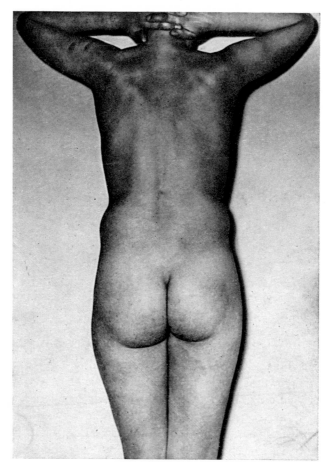

Fig. 4

Sexual Characteristics

The chief complaint of many adult patients is infertility. In other patients anomalous sexual development, scarcity of beard, progressive decrease of libido and of potency are other reasons for seeking medical help.

Physical examination reveals the testes to be firm and small; their diameter does not exceed 1 cm. The size of the penis varies from normal to undersized; the scrotum is small; the prostate normal in size. Axillary hair growth is usually normal, while pubic hair shows a female escutcheon. The beard is scanty, requiring shaving only once a week, and the body hair is markedly reduced.

Other sexual characteristics develop to varying degrees. Some patients with mosaicism differ insignificantly from normal males. In others typical eunuchoid characteristics develop and include poorly developed genitalia, eunuchoid habitus, i.e., elongated extremities and genu valgum, scanty sexual hair, smooth and soft skin resembling that of infants, fat deposits above the hips, semicircular hairline on the forehead without temporal recession, high-pitched voice and poor muscle development.

Chromatin Findings

Buccal smears facilitate sex chromatin examination. Normal female subjects are chromatin-positive, i.e., 20% to 50% of nuclei of their cells have a large chromatin condensation (termed sex chromatin or Barr's body) just beneath the nuclear membrane. Male subjects are chromatin-negative; there is no sex chromatin in the nuclei of their cells. Patients with Klinefelter's syndrome are chromatin-positive as they have an extra X chromosome in their body cells.

Fig. 1. Genitals of a 21-year-old patient exhibiting scanty pubic hair, nearly normal-sized penis, small scrotum and firm, small testes.

Fig. 2. Underdeveloped genitals in a 24-year-old patient. Small testes and nonpendulous scrotum are seen.

Fig. 3. Rounded hips, female escutcheon of the pubic hair, normal penis, small testes in a 22-year-old patient with Klinefelter's syndrome and 47, XXY chromosome constitution.

Fig. 4. Abundant sexual and body hair seen in a 20-year-old patient with nearly normal genitals (only the testes are small and firm). Buccal smears showed chromatin-positive pattern. Mosaicism 46,XY/47,XXY in blood cultures.

PLATE 11

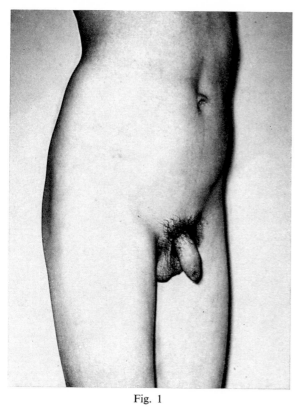

Fig. 1

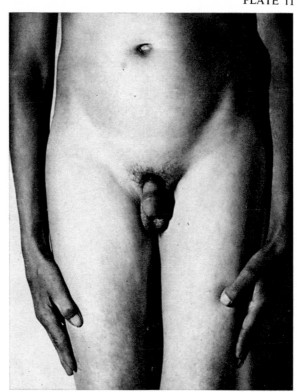

Fig. 2

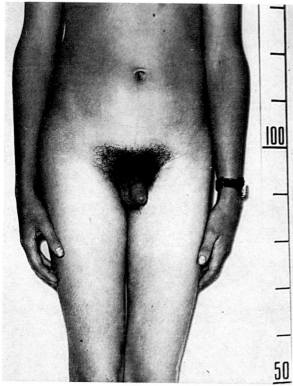

Fig. 3

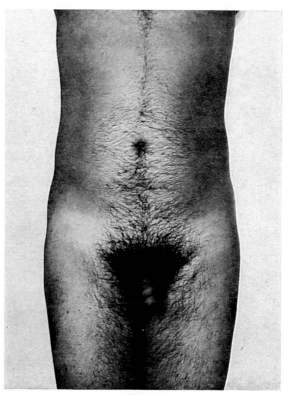

Fig. 4

Roentgen Findings

Roentgenograms of the hand in half the cases reveal shortened distal phalanges and occasional coarse trabecular structure of the wrist (osteoporosis). Skull roentgenograms frequently reveal: flattening of the temporal regions and decreased width of the vault; shortening of the anterior fossa cranii; decreased angle of the base, below 130° (N = 132–135°); small size of the mandibular rami; thinning of the vault at the coronal suture; premature fusion and excessive calcification of this suture.

Figs. 1A to 1D. Lateral roentgenograms of the skull in 4 cases of Klinefelter's syndrome illustrate frequent abnormalities: precocious and excessive calcification of the coronal suture in a 16-year-old patient (A) and 21-year-old patient (B), and irregular thinning of the lamina interna at the major fontanel region (C and D).

Figs. 2A to 2C. Frontal roentgenograms of the skull in a normal subject (B) and 2 cases of Klinefelter's syndrome (A and C). There is a flattening at the temporal regions of the outer contour of the vault in patients with Klinefelter's syndrome.

Figs. 3A and 3B. Basal angle of the skull of a control subject (A) and of a patient with Klinefelter's syndrome (B) which shows a markedly reduced angle of 124° instead of the normal 133 to 135°.

PLATE 12

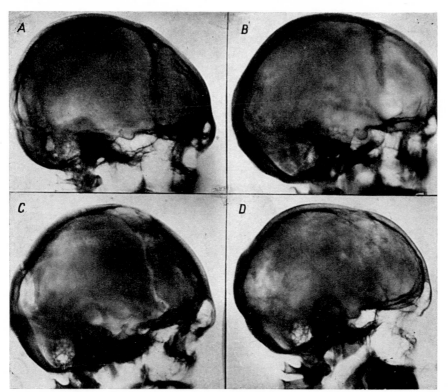

Figs. 1A to 1D

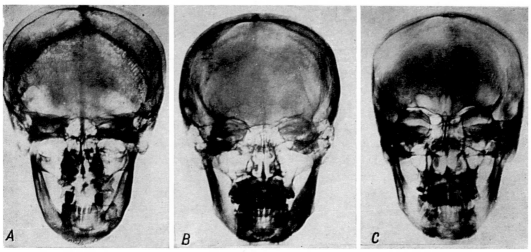

Figs. 2A to 2C

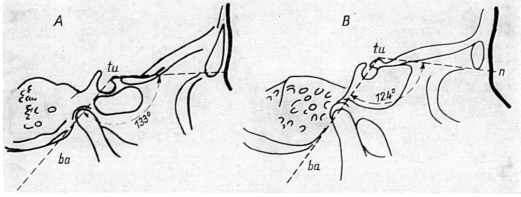

Figs. 3A and 3B

Laboratory Findings

1. Azoospermia.
2. High serum and urinary FSH; high serum LH in the majority of patients.
3. Chromatin positive findings in buccal mucosa smears.
4. Chromosome counts: XXY sex chromosomes or mosaic pattern XY/XXY.
5. Plasma testosterone low or low-normal.
6. Decrease in serum zinc concentration in half the cases.
7. Ability to locate sound impaired.
8. Abnormal EEG: basic rhythm irregular with bursts of high voltage spikes over middle temporal regions.
9. Dactyloscopic findings: short, horizontally oriented loops and central pocket whorls often with a low ridge count.

Figs. 1A to 1D. Fingerprints showing loop patterns in a normal subject (*A*) and 3 patients with Klinefelter's syndrome (*B–D*). Short, horizontally oriented loops with a low ridge count are seen in the latter.

Figs. 2A to 2D. Fingerprints illustrating whorl patterns in 2 control subjects (*A* and *B*) and 2 patients with Klinefelter's syndrome (*C* and *D*). Racket-type whorls with a low ridge count are frequent in this disease.

Figs. 3A and 3B. Fingerprints of the thumbs of patients with Klinefelter's syndrome (*A*) and Turner's syndrome (*B*), illustrating opposite findings: a small horizontal loop with a low ridge count in the patient with Klinefelter's syndrome (*A*) and elongated perpendicular loop with a high ridge count in the patient with Turner's syndrome (*B*).

Figs. 4A to 4C. Fingerprints showing arch pattern: a usual arch pattern in a control subject (*A*) and low arches in 2 patients with Klinefelter's syndrome (*B* and *C*).

Figs. 5A to 5D. Palm of a normal subject (*A*) shows the 3 principal creases: transverse distal, transverse proximal and thenar. In some cases of Klinefelter's syndrome the palm creases are abnormal, e.g., there is a simian crease (*B*), shortened thenar crease (*C*) and rudimentary transverse proximal crease (*D*).

210

PLATE 13

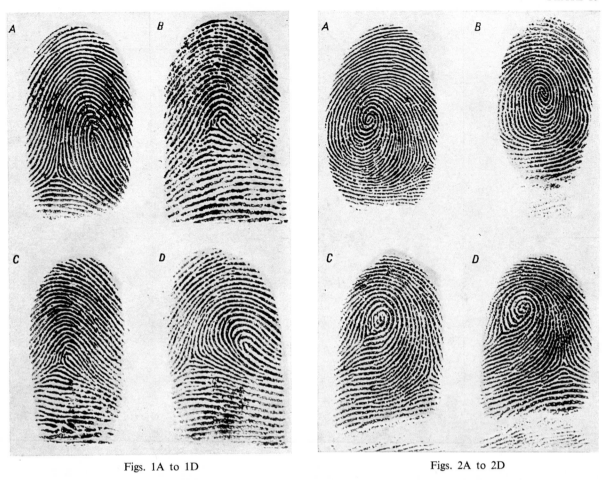

Figs. 1A to 1D

Figs. 2A to 2D

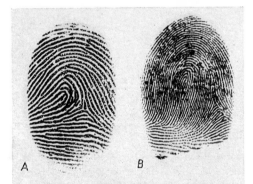

Figs. 3A and 3B

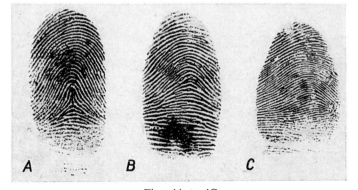

Figs. 4A to 4C

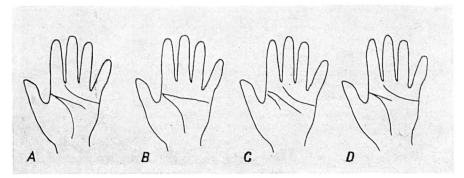

Figs. 5A to 5D

Testicular Histology

In adult patients, the biopsy specimen of the testes shows the seminiferous tubules to differ in size and to be affected to various degrees. Early changes consist of thickening of the basal membrane and degenerative changes in the germ cells. In other tubules the germ cells are absent; only Sertoli cells persist. In later stages there is a complete hyalinization, or fibrosis, of the tubules that have shrunk and are sometimes without lumen; spermatogenesis is absent. The Leydig cells are in excess, forming large clumps; Barr bodies may be seen in the nuclei of these cells.

Prepubertal histologic findings are less characteristic since the hyaline degeneration of the tubules is not yet evident, and Leydig cells are not present at this stage of development.

KLINEFELTER'S SYNDROME WITH MULTIPLE X CHROMOSOMES

The most common chromosome abnormality in Klinefelter's syndrome is the presence of 47, XXY. In some cases there are three or more X chromosomes, e.g., XXXY, XXXXY or mosaicism XXY/XY, XXY/XX or XXXY/XY. In patients with Klinefelter's syndrome, associated with XXXY or XXXXY sex chromosome patterns, two and three Barr bodies respectively are shown to be in the nuclei of some cells by means of buccal mucosa smears.

Patients with XXXY or XXXXY Klinefelter's syndrome are more severely affected than those with the XXY pattern; mental retardation and other congenital anomalies always occur. In the skeletal system, cubitus valgus with the limitation of movements at the elbow joints is common; roentgenograms show fusion (synostosis) of the proximal ends of the ulna and radius. Other changes noted in some patients include microcephaly, short stature, kyphosis, scoliosis, deformed nose or ears, sternum defects, pectus exavatum, coxa vara, abnormalities of the fingers, hyperostosis frontalis interna, strabismus, hypertelorism, cleft palate, cardiac anomalies, cryptorchidism and genital malformations.

ARGONZ DEL CASTILLO SYNDROME

(SERTOLI CELL ONLY SYNDROME; GERMINAL APLASIA)

The cardinal manifestations of the syndrome are infertility, azoospermia and elevated urinary gonadotropins. The etiology is unknown. The patients are of normal height and body proportions; the sex characteristics appear at onset of puberty, and the disease is recognizable in patients who complain of infertility. The buccal smears are chromatin-negative; in blood cultures XY sex chromosomes are found. The testes are of reduced size but of normal consistency. Testicular biopsy specimens show slightly smaller-than-normal seminiferous tubules lined with Sertoli cells but completely devoid of germinal epithelium. The Leydig cells are normal in number and appearance. A similar histologic picture of the testes, i.e., the seminiferous tubules lined with Sertoli cells only, is sometimes seen in cryptorchidism, Klinefelter's syndrome, after orchitis or exposure to irradiation.

Fig. 1. Photomicrograph of the testis from a 20-year-old patient with Klinefelter's syndrome and 47,XXY chromosome constitution. Abundant Leydig cells form large clumps. Various degrees of seminiferous tubular damage; some of the tubules (*center*) show disorganization of the germ cell maturation and sloughing of the epithelium into the lumen of the tubules. Other tubules are fibrotic with haylinized tunica propria (*upper left*).

Fig. 2. Photomicrographic enlargement of the testis of a 24-year-old patient with Klinefelter's syndrome. The tubules are fibrotic with thickened and hyalinized tunica propria and are lined only with Sertoli cells. No germinal epithelium is evident. In the interstitial tissue abundant immature Leydig cells are seen (Courtesy J Teter, MD, Warsaw).

Fig. 3A. Genitals of a 31-year-old patient with Sertoli cell only syndrome. Note male habitus, normal body proportions, sterility, increased serum FSH. The penis, scrotum and pubic hair are normally developed; only the testes are slightly reduced in size.

Fig. 3B. Photomicrograph of the testicular biopsy specimen of the same patient shows large tubules devoid of germ cells, and lined only with Sertoli cells. There is no thickening of the tunica propria and no excess of Leydig cells (Courtesy J Teter, MD, Warsaw).

PLATE 14

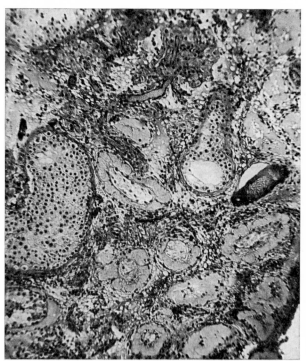

Fig. 1

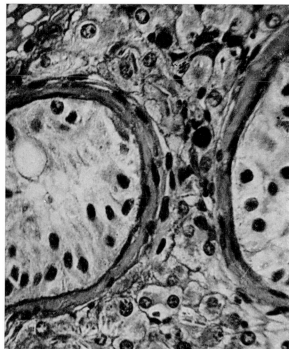

Fig. 2

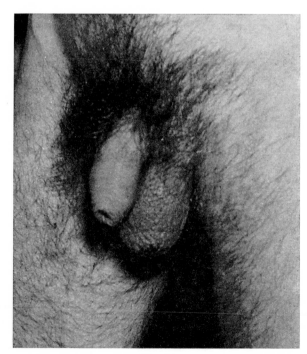

Fig. 3A

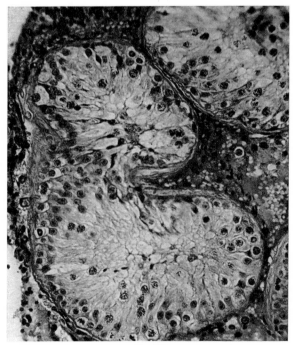

Fig. 3B

47,XYY SYNDROME

Male patients with 47,XYY chromosomes are abnormally tall, usually between 183 and 202 cm. Excessive growth begins in childhood. There are no other important physical abnormalities, sexual development is usually normal. The patients are prone to behavioral disorders and frequently have a criminal record, so the incidence of this syndrome is higher in males in prisons and security hospitals than in the general population. In some patients the ECG shows either a prolongation of the QT period or a right bundle branch block. Roentgenograms of the hand reveal elongated long bones with conspicuously shortened distal phalanges giving rise to a disproportion between the metacarpals and distal phalanges ("metacarpal preponderance"). On skull roentgenograms diminished angle of the base, shortening of anterior fossa cranii and occasional progenia, are seen. The ribs are thin, elongated and slop downward more than is normal. In buccal smears two Y bodies may be detected.

ADULT LEYDIG CELL FAILURE
(MALE CLIMACTERIC)

Idiopathic Leydig cell failure, i.e., male climacteric, is a rare disease characterized by hot flushes, easy fatigability, increased irritability and decrease in libido and sexual potency. Plasma and urinary testosterone is decreased, while plasma and urinary FSH and LH are elevated.

Much more common than male climacteric is the psychogenic impotency seen in neurotic patients. Hormonal studies do not show definite abnormalities.

Deficient Leydig cell function is seen in Klinefelter's syndrome, in post irradiation testicular atrophy, mumps orchitis, advanced vascular changes, hemochromatosis, liver cirrhosis, diabetes and other neuropathies. Diagnosis and treatment depend on the nature of the disease.

ADULT SEMINIFEROUS TUBULE FAILURE

Mumps orchitis, acute orchitis in the course of gonorrheal infection, irradiation, dystrophia myotonica or trauma in adult life may lead to testicular atrophy. The testes are small and soft; there is oligospermia or azoospermia with resultant infertility. Testicular biopsy specimens show disorganization and sloughing of the germinal epithelium; in later stages fibrosis and hyalinization of the seminiferous tubules develop. Leydig cells are usually intact. Serum and urinary FSH are elevated.

Fig. 1A. A 19-year-old patient with 47,XYY chromosomes is excessively tall (height 201 cm, 79 in.), with thin, elongated extremities.

Fig. 1B. Hand of the same patient shows narrow wrist, elongated metacarpals and fingers, and webbing between the second and third digits.

Fig. 2. Normal male genitals but a female escutcheon of the pubic hair in a case of 47,XYY syndrome.

Fig. 3. Roentgenogram of the skull (lateral view) of a patient with 47,XYY syndrome shows diminished angle of the base and shortening of the anterior fossa cranii.

Fig. 4. Roentgenogram of the hand in a patient with 47,XYY syndrome demonstrates metacarpal preponderance over phalanges. The metacarpals are elongated, whereas the distal phalanges are conspicuously shortened — giving rise to a definite disproportion between metacarpal and phalangeal size.

PLATE 15

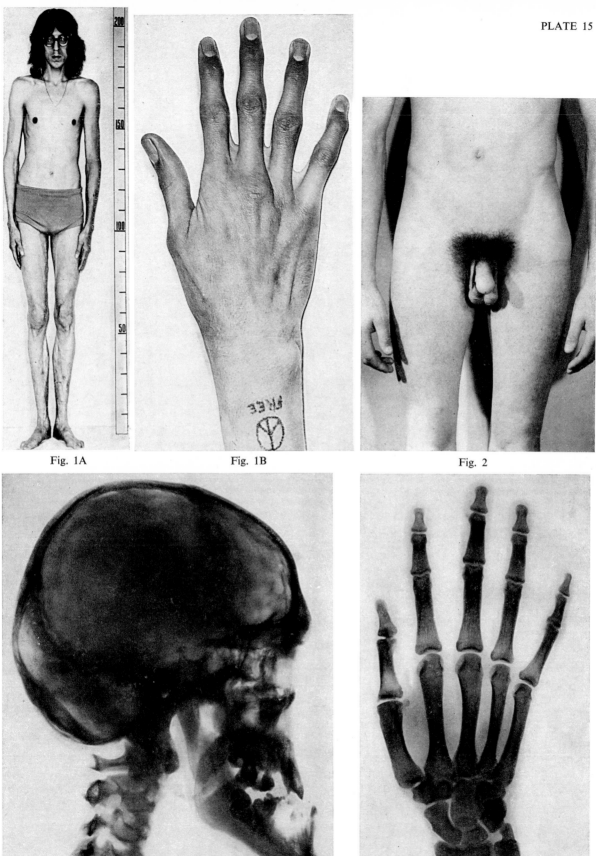

Fig. 1A

Fig. 1B

Fig. 2

Fig. 3

Fig. 4

CRYPTORCHIDISM

(UNDESCENDED TESTIS)

The most common type of cryptorchidism is migratory, or retractile, testis (pseudocryptorchidism), when the testis migrates periodically between the scrotum and inguinal canal. The scrotum is usually well developed. At puberty the testis often descends spontaneously.

True cryptorchidism is the failure of the testes to descend into the scrotum; rather they are located either in the abdomen or inguinal canal. Physical examination shows absence of one or both testes in the scrotum; some cryptorchid testes are palpable in the inguinal canals. Cryptorchidism may be complicated by inguinal hernia. Sterility and prepubertal eunuchoidism may result from bilateral cryptorchidism. In addition, the cryptorchid testes are prone to trauma and torsion. In some cases the intraabdominal testes are dysgenetic and may be the source of malignant changes in postpubertal period.

Ectopic testes are those which, having been diverted before entering the scrotum, are located perineally, femorally or in the superficial inguinal pouch and are usually easily palpable.

GYNECOMASTIA

Gynecomastia or breast enlargement is frequent in adolescent males between the ages of 14 to 16. This may vary from a small, palpable, sometimes painful, tender mass, of about 2 cm in diameter, in the subareolar area to marked enlargement of embarassing size resembling an adult female breast. The changes are usually bilateral, but unilateral gynecomastia also occurs. The etiology is not known, however, estrogens secreted by the pubertal testes are suspected as being the causal factors. The condition may be temporary, regressing in subsequent years, or persistent.

Adolescent gynecomastia should be differentiated from that which appears in Klinefelter's syndrome and is accompanied by small, firm testes, other clinical manifestations and increased serum FSH concentration. In other forms of hypogonadism gynecomastia is found only infrequently.

Gynecomastia associated with hyperprolactinemia is seen in pituitary and suprasellar tumors. In feminizing adrenal cortical carcinoma and interstitial cell tumors gynecomastia is caused by increased estradiol secretion and regresses after removal of the tumor. Ingestion of estrogens or estrogen therapy for prostatic carcinoma frequently cause gynecomastia; it may also follow administration of certain drugs such as phenotiazine and reserpine, probably by stimulation of prolactin secretion.

Liver cirrhosis, combined with testicular atrophy, frequently leads to gynecomastia. The same occurs during recovery from chronic protein malnutrition when the testes resume their hormonal function ("second puberty"). In rare cases gynecomastia may be present in bronchogenic carcinoma or choriccarcinoma of the testis and is then associated with very high chorionic gonadotropin secretion.

Pseudogynecomastia, accumulation of subcutaneous fat without glandular tissue in the areolar area, is frequent in obese adolescent males and regresses when weight is reduced. Unilateral gynecomastia caused by carcinoma of the male breast is of infrequent occurrence in patients above the age of 40.

Fig. 1. Poorly developed external genitals of a 9-year-old male with bilateral cryptorchidism. The testes were palpable high in the inguinal canals. Complete cure, testicular descent and normal sexual development was achieved, following therapy with chorionic gonadotropin.

Fig. 2. Ectopia of the testis. The testis is displaced to the perineum; the scrotum is empty.

Fig. 3. A 13-year-old male with obesity and pubertal gynecomastia. Chromatin findings in buccal smears negative; serum LH and FSH within the normal range. Gynecomastia gradually regressed over a period of 3 years after the patient was put on a low-calorie diet. He attained normal sexual maturation.

Fig. 4. Advanced gynecomastia in a 44-year-old patient with chromatin-positive Klinefelter's syndrome. Plasma testosterone 1.6 ng/ml, serum LH 59 mIU/ml.

PLATE 16

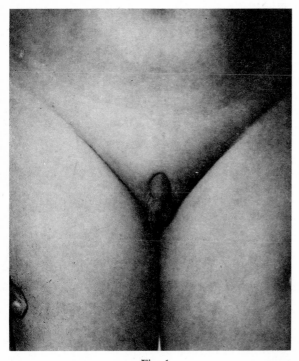

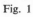

Fig. 1

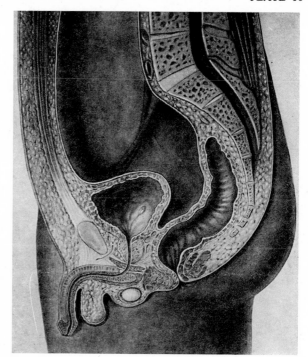

Fig. 2

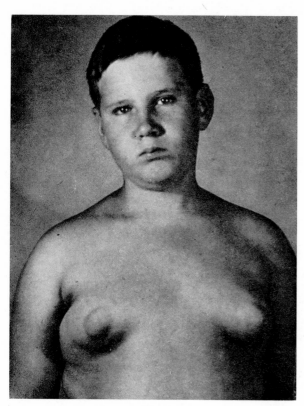

Fig. 3

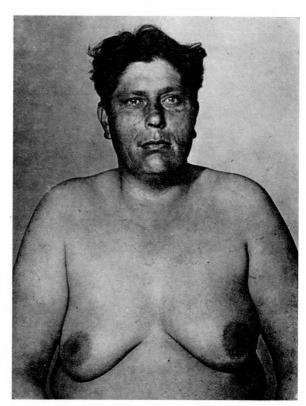

Fig. 4

WERNER'S SYNDROME

(PROGERIA)

Werner's syndrome, found predominantly in males, is a very rare disease which leads to precocious senility in young males. The signs and symptoms of the disease may be present in youth, but become more pronounced in adult life. There is progressive atrophy of the muscles, fat, skin and bones of the upper and lower extremities. Typical clinical manifestations include slim extremities, truncal obesity, precocious graying, partial loss of sexual hair, atrophic changes of the genitalia, impotency, sterility, high-pitched voice, bilateral cataracts, generalized arteriosclerosis and osteitis. The hands and feet gradually diminish in size and become sensitive to pressure.

The testes are of diminished size. Histologic studies reveal various degrees of fibrosis, atrophy of seminiferous tubules and scanty Leydig cells.

LAURENCE-MOON-BIEDL SYNDROME

This is a rare syndrome characterized by a combination of congenital anomalies: polydactylia, mental deficiency, atypical retinitis pigmentosa, obesity and hypogonadism. Males are more often affected than females; familial occurrence has been reported. Chromosomal studies do not show any abnormalities. Supernumerary digits of the hands or feet are noted at birth. In later years mental deficiency becomes more evident, and there is progressive loss of vision. The patients are of short stature, obese and stocky. Genu valgum is common. The hands are broad and short; the distal phalanges are especially reduced in length.

Hypogonadism due to gonadotropin deficiency is frequently present. Histologic examination of testicular biopsy specimens may show hyalinization of the seminiferous tubules similar to that in Klinefelter's syndrome.

Fig. 1A. A 32-year-old patient with Werner's syndrome (premature senility). Short stature (152 cm, 60 in.), thin extremities, truncal obesity, bilateral cataracts (removed at the age 18), early graying of the hair, high-pitched voice, arteriosclerosis, and atrophy of the testes are present.

Fig. 1B. Foot of the same patient showing atrophy of plantar fat tissue and thinning of the skin. Soles painful; the patient cannot walk without the support of microplastic insole.

Fig. 1C. Ulcerations of the toe and fourth digit due to chronic recurrent osteitis.

Fig. 2. Foot of a 5-year-old patient with Laurence-Moon-Biedl syndrome (obesity, mental deficiency), showing polydactylia and webbing between the second and third toe.

Figs. 3A and 3B. Roentgenograms of the hand and foot of a 2-year-old male with Laurence-Moon-Biedl syndrome, mental retardation and polydactylia.

218

PLATE 17

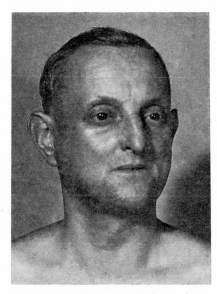

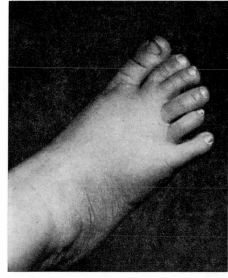

Fig. 1A   Fig. 2

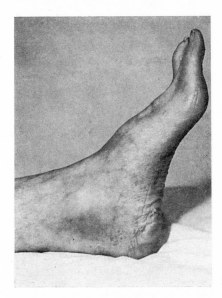

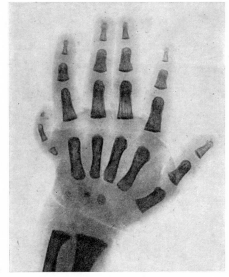

Fig. 1B   Fig. 3A

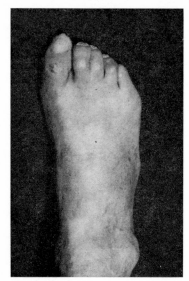

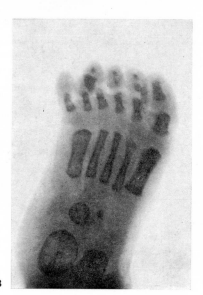

Fig. 1C   Fig. 3B

Chapter 5

THE OVARIES

TURNER'S SYNDROME

(GONADAL DYSGENESIS WITH SHORT STATURE; OVARIAN DYSGENESIS; RUDIMENTARY OVARY SYNDROME)

Turner's syndrome is a congenital disease associated with abnormalities of the sex chromosomes and female phenotype. The cardinal signs are stunted growth, lack of sexual development and numerous congenital anomalies of which the most frequent are changes in the skeleton. A small uterus with Fallopian tubes and whitish fibrous streaks in place of ovaries can be seen on laparotomy.

Signs and Symptoms

In neonates

1. Excessive folds of skin in the neck.
2. Lymphedema cf hands and feet.

In children

1. Stunted growth.
2. Congenital anomalies such as palpebral ptosis, lymphedema, webbing of the neck, congenital heart disease.

In postpuberty

1. Primary amenorrhea.
2. Short stature, usually 125 to 145 cm (49 to 57 in.).
3. Stocky build.
4. Broad, shield-like chest.
5. Sexual infantilism: underdeveloped breasts, hypoplastic areolae and nipples, infantile genitalia.
6. Tendency to obesity.
7. Facial deformities; eye anomalies.
8. Short, broad and sometimes webbed neck.
9. Cubitus valgus; Madelung's deformity.
10. Abnormal palm creases; lymphedema of the back of hands, brachyphalangia; narrowed nails.
11. Thick legs, lymphedema.

Fig. 1. A 16-year-old chromatin-negative patient showing short stature (height 140 cm, 55 in.), stocky build, shield-like chest, webbed neck, broad shoulders, excess weight (52 kg) and lymphedema of the hands and feet. Sexual development absent. Atrophic vaginal smears, serum LH 78 mIU/ml, chromosome constitution 45,X.

Fig. 2. A 21-year-old patient with short stature (height 137 cm, 54 in.), deformed facies, webbed neck, broad chest, small, pale nipples, no breast development, lack of pubic hair, fat accumulation above the hips. Sex chromatin absent in buccal smears; chromosome constitution 45,X; vaginal smears atrophic. Serum FSH 56 mIU/ml, LH 92 mIU/ml.

Fig. 3. A 13-year-old chromatin-negative patient showing dwarfism (height 127 cm, 50 in.), stocky build, broad shoulders and sexual infantilism. The face is slightly deformed; the extremities are shortened; the legs are thick. Serum LH 51 mIU/ml.

Fig. 4. A 16-year-old chromatin-negative patient with dwarfism (height 125 cm, 49 in.) and slightly webbed neck. There is complete absence of sexual development; the areolae are small and pale. Vaginal smears reveal only parabasal cells (89%) and scanty intermediate cells (11%). Serum LH 62 mIU/ml.

Fig. 5. A 17-year-old patient with stunted growth (height 138 cm, 54 in.), broad shoulders, narrow hips. There is complete lack of breast development and scanty pubic hair. Chromosome constitution 45,X/46,XX. Serum LH 69 mIU/ml, FSH 55 mIU/ml.

Fig. 6. A 13-year-old chromatin-positive patient, undersized (height 123 cm, 48 in.). Serum LH 46 mIU/ml. Mosaicism 45,X/46,XX.

PLATE 1

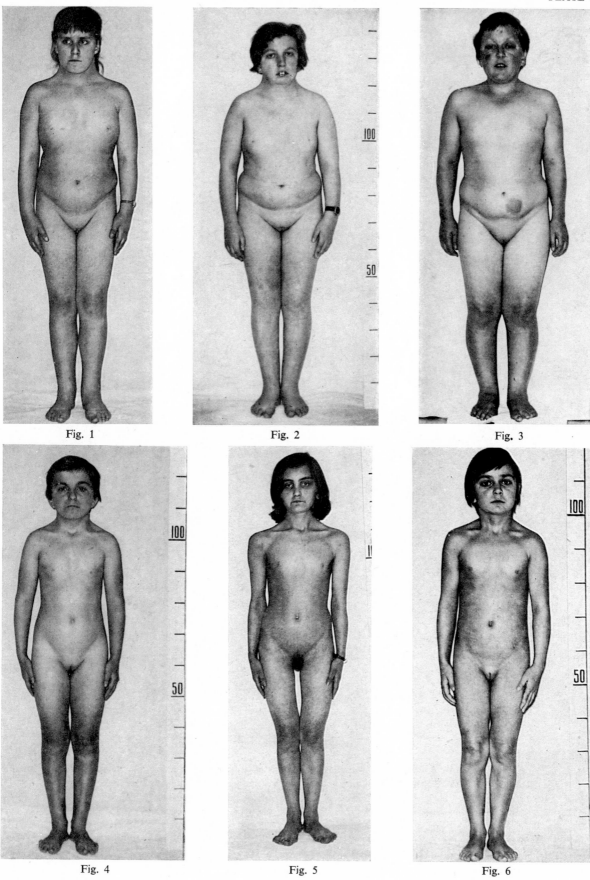

Fig. 1   Fig. 2   Fig. 3

Fig. 4   Fig. 5   Fig. 6

General Appearance

Retarded growth and some congenital anomalies are already noted in the first years of life. On examination of both children and adults with Turner's syndrome a conspicuous finding is stunted growth ranging from dwarfism to small stature. Patients with XO sex chromosomes who are short in childhood, only exceptionally manage to attain a low-normal height after age 20. Patients with Turner's syndrome are usually stocky with wide shoulders, broad chest, narrow hips and thick legs. The chest is frequently expanded with widely spaced nipples — the so-called shield-like chest.

Fig. 1. Face of an 18-year-old chromatin-negative patient. Note the thick hair on the scalp and eyebrows, broad mandible, drooping eyelids, antimongoloid slant to the eyes, pigmented moles.

Fig. 2. Face of a 16-year-old chromatin-positive patient with Turner's syndrome. The face is round with broad mandible.

Fig. 3. Face of a 16-year-old patient with Turner's syndrome. The signs of pretty eyes are present: wing shape, thick, dark eyebrows, long eyelashes.

Figs. 4A and 4B. A 16-year-old patient with Turner's syndrome compared to her 13-year-old healthy sister. Differences are easily seen: the face of the patient is characterized by low set ears, broad mandible, drooping palpebral fissures, wing-shaped eyebrows and drooping corners of the mouth.

PLATE 2

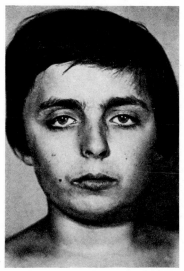

Fig. 1

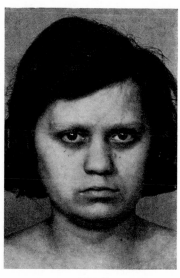

Fig. 2

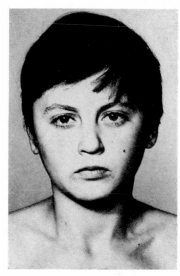

Fig. 3

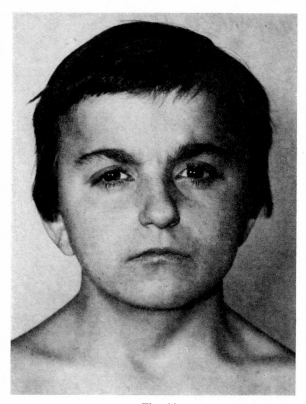

Fig. 4A

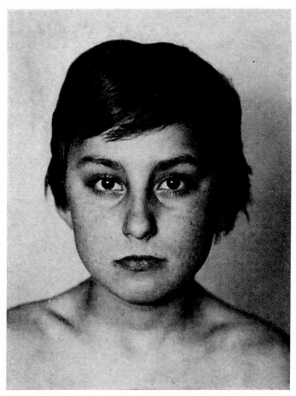

Fig. 4B

The Face

The features are as mature as one could expect for that age. In chromatin-positive patients with mosaicism or structural abnormalities of the X chromosome, facial changes are usually insignificant, i.e., eye changes or pigmented moles may be the only findings.

In chromatin-negative patients the face is often deformed. There are various eye defects, and the ears set low and malformed. The nose is frequently narrow and slender in contrast to pituitary and hypothyroid dwarfs in whom the nose is shortened. The face often has a square appearance due to the broad mandible. In some cases the oral fissure is smaller than normal, in others the corners of the mouth droop, giving it a fishlike appearance. All these deformities cause the faces of the patients to resemble one another, while there is a striking dissimilarity of the patients to other members of their families.

After age 30, seldom earlier, many facial wrinkles appear in untreated patients, probably due to the long standing deficiency of sex hormones. The teeth are sometimes narrow and hypoplastic.

Fig. 1. A 22-year-old patient with Turner's syndrome showing asymmetry, deformed and low set ears, epicantal folds. The neck is short and webbed.

Fig. 2. Face of a 13-year-old chromatin-positive patient with Turner's syndrome. Low set ears, drooping corners of the mouth, antimongoloid slant to the eyes, dark, thick eyelashes and eyebrows.

Fig. 3. Face of a 32-year-old chromatin negative patient with Turner's syndrome. The mandible is heavy and broad, the ears are low set; there is marked blepharoptosis.

Fig. 4. Face of a 43-year-old patient with Turner's syndrome exhibiting premature wrinkles, drooping eyelids, pigmented moles and low set ears.

PLATE 3

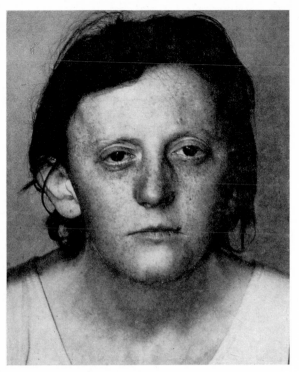

Fig. 1

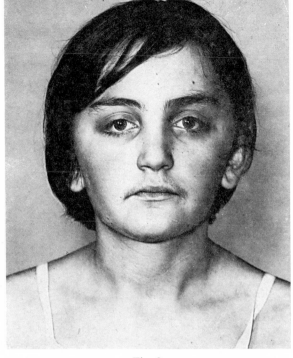

Fig. 2

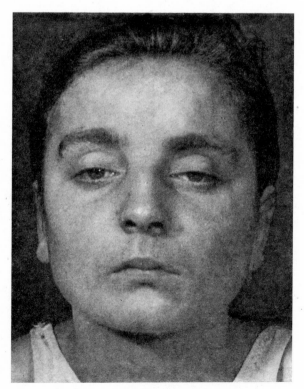

Fig. 3

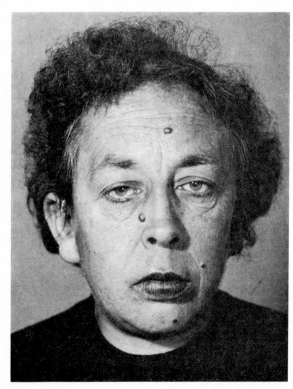

Fig. 4

The Eyes

Changes of the eyes are frequently seen. One third of the patients have very attractive, large eyes with wide, black eyebrows and thick eyelashes that are long, shiny and black, as if artificially darkened. This sign of pretty eyes in Turner's syndrome is an exception since, as a rule, most somatic anomalies give patients an unpleasant appearance. This attractive feature is not present in normal members of the family.

In many other patients anomalies of the eyes may be noted, i.e., antimongoloid, palpebral slants to the eyes causing the outer corners to droop downward, epicanthal folds, ptosis of the upper lids, asymmetric positioning and occasional squint or microphthalmia. Sometimes a peculiar change in the skin around the eyebrows is seen; there is permanent edema of light reddish color without epidermal changes. In patients with webbed neck, the eyebrows are lowered at the periphery, giving the face a sad appearance.

Fig. 1. Pretty eyes frequently seen in patients with Turner's syndrome. They are large, and the eyebrows dark and thick; the eyelashes are long, thick and dark as if artificially darkened.

Fig. 2. Eyes of an 18-year-old chromatin-positive patient. Thick, dark eyebrows and eyelashes, drooping upper lids, anti-mongoloid slant and epicantal folds are evident.

Fig. 3. Eyes of a 19-year-old patient. Thick hair on eyebrows and eyelashes, drooping eyelids and epicantal folds (*left*) are seen

PLATE 4

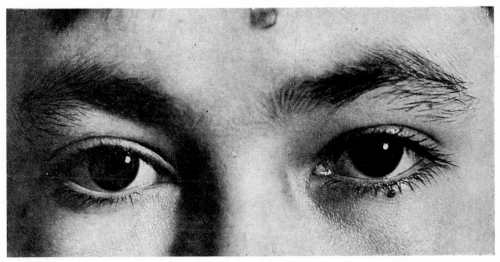

Fig. 1

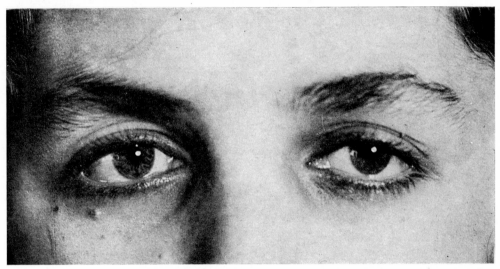

Fig. 2

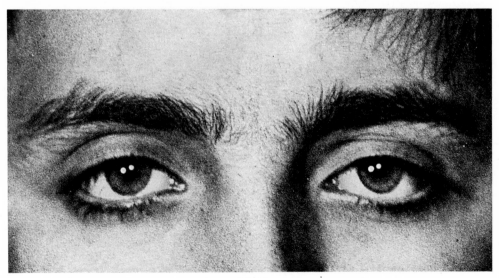

Fig. 3

The Neck

The webbed neck is a conspicuous but infrequent sign found in about 20% of the patients. It is defined as presence of bilateral skin folds extending between the mastoid process of the temporal bone and the acromion. Sometimes a manelike growth of hair extends along these folds. In some cases of Turner's syndrome, especially neonates, redundant skin folds, often arranged longitudinally, are seen at the back of the neck. These folds, characteristic of Bonnevie-Ullrich syndrome later diminish or change into two lateral folds. The webbed neck may also appear associated with a cervical vertebra deformity in Klippel-Feil syndrome, and very rarely in otherwise normal subjects.

In many patients with Turner's syndrome the neck is short and thick. The hair on the back of the neck sometimes grows lower than is normal and the hairline frequently forms two lateral strips as is normally seen in males, instead of three strips (center and both sides) as seen in females.

Figs. 1A and 1B. The webbed neck of an 18-year-old patient with Turner's syndrome. The skin folds extend between the mastoid processes and acromion. The ears are low set.

Fig. 2. A scar from surgical correction of webbed neck in a patient with Turner's syndrome. Long hair is seen growing on the shoulder. The auricle is narrowed, triangular and low set.

Fig. 3. Webbing of the neck and ear deformity in a patient with Turner's syndrome.

230

PLATE 5

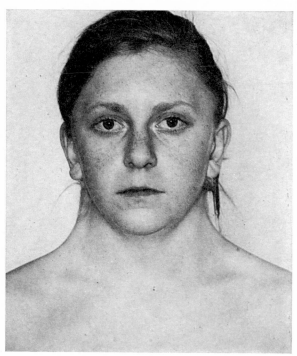

Fig. 1A

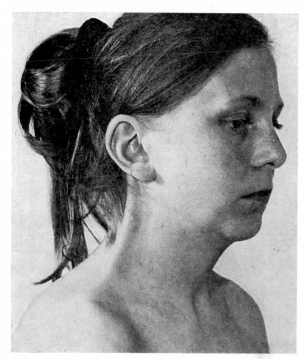

Fig. 1B

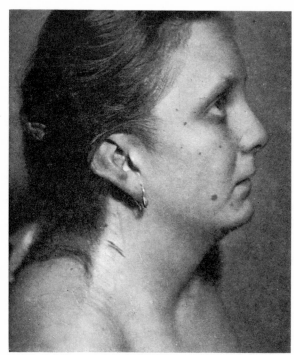
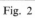

Fig. 2

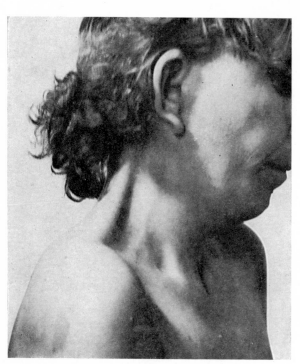

Fig. 3

231

The Elbow

An increase in the carrying angle of the elbow, cubitus valgus, is often found in Turner's syndrome. The angle between the axis of the arm and forearm in normal males is 170 to 180°, in women 160 to 179°; when it is smaller it is termed cubitus valgus. Identification of this anomaly is obtained by having patients extend their arms with the palms pressed together sidewards; the extremities form the letter Y instead of the V found in normal females. In some cases of Turner's syndrome the extension at the elbow is limited, resulting in a spurious increase in the carrying angle.

Madelung's deformity is present in some cases of Turner's syndrome. This deformity is characterized by a "bayonet-like" configuration of the forearm and wrist as well as dorsal subluxation of the ulna. In some other patients the distal end of the ulna protrudes distally more than is normal.

Fig. 1. Hand of a 21-year-old patient showing slender, elongated fingers. The creases at the proximal interphalangeal joints run straight instead of semicircularly.

Fig. 2. Hand of a 14-year-old patient with shortened thumb, fourth and fifth fingers; dimples at the proximal interphalangeal joints and edema of the backs of the fingers.

Fig. 3. Hand of a 12-year-old patient. Brachyphalangia of all fingers; pseudoedema and dimpling on the back of the fourth and fifth fingers are evident. Such a brachyphalangia may also be seen in pseudohypoparathyroidism.

Fig. 4. Slim fingers and narrowed nails, showing lateral hyperconvexity, are deeply set into the nailbeds (frequently found in Turner's syndrome).

232

PLATE 6

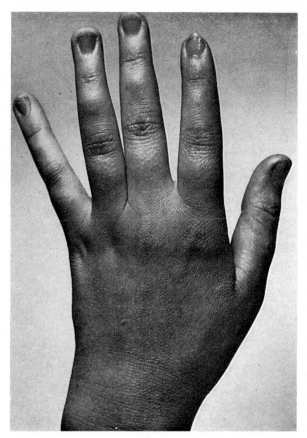

Fig. 1

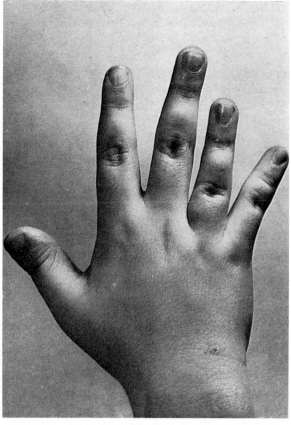

Fig. 2

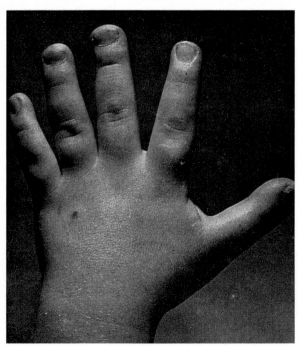

Fig. 3

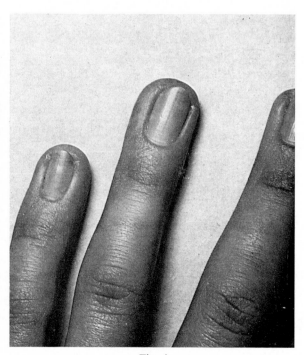

Fig. 4

The Hands

Numerous changes in the hand that are characteristic of the disease can be found in gonadal dysgenesis.

Fingernails. In some patients the nails are narrowed, deeply set into the nailbed and with increased lateral convexity. In others they are shallow and shortened, especially when the distal phalanges are also shortened.

Fingers. In the majority of patients, especially at postpuberty, all the fingers are abnormally long in proportion to the overall stunted growth of the patients and to the stunted metacarpals. Such elongated fingers are not found in other growth disturbances. Lymphedema (edema which does not pit) is occasionally present on the dorsa of the hand and fingers. This finding is most conspicuous in the first two years of life and, less frequently, persists in later years. The creases at the proximal interphalangeal joints sometimes run straight instead of semicircularly as is normally found, or dimples appear in these areas. There is sometimes a shortening of phalanges or metacarpals involving one or more fingers; when all 5 digits are affected the hand is markedly shortened and resembles that seen in pseudohypoparathyroidism.

The metacarpal sign. This finding is positive when a ruler, placed on the metacarpal heads of the clenched fist, simultaneously touches the fifth, fourth and third metacarpals, indicating a relative shortness of the fourth metacarpal bone. It is negative when the ruler runs over the head of the third metacarpal bone. The incidence of a positive metacarpal sign is 60% in gonadal dysgenesis, while in normal population it is only 10%.

The palm. In about 95% of normal subjects three flexion creases can be clearly distinguished on the palm: the transverse distal crease, the transverse proximal crease and the thenar crease. Abnormalities of the flexion creases are found in one third of the patients with gonadal dysgenesis. The presence of a simian line (a transverse crease running horizontally from the radial to the ulnar border of the palm) is most frequent; in these instances the transverse distal crease is lacking or only rudimentary. Other abnormalities of the flexion creases involve a rudimentary transverse proximal crease, an absence of thenar crease or a complete irregularity of the principal flexion creases.

Dermatoglyphics. In one fourth of the patients a high axial triradius is seen in the hypothenar, i.e., the triradius is near the center of the palm. The incidence of this finding in normal subjects is 10%. Dactyloscopic studies of patients with Turner's syndrome show a definite predominance of ulnar loop patterns with reduction of whorls. In addition, the loops are frequently elongated, perpendicularly oriented and have a higher ridge count than the loops in control subjects.

Figs. 1A and 1B. Abnormal palmar creases in two patients with Turner's syndrome. *A.* Completely abnormal palm creases with partial simian crease. *B.* The simian crease running horizontally across the palm from the ulnar to radial border.

Figs. 2A and 2B. *A.* Clenched fist of a patient with Turner's syndrome demonstrating a positive metacarpal sign. *B.* A negative metacarpal sign. In *A,* the ruler does not touch the third metacarpal, while in *B,* it lies simultaneously on the heads of the fifth, fourth and third metacarpals.

Figs. 3A to 3C. Fingerprints of a normal subject (*A*) and of two patients with Turner's syndrome (*B* and *C*) showing differences in the ulnar loop patterns. *B.* The loops are elongated with a high ridge count. *C.* The perpendicularly oriented, elongated loops with a high ridge count typical of Turner's syndrome.

234

PLATE 7

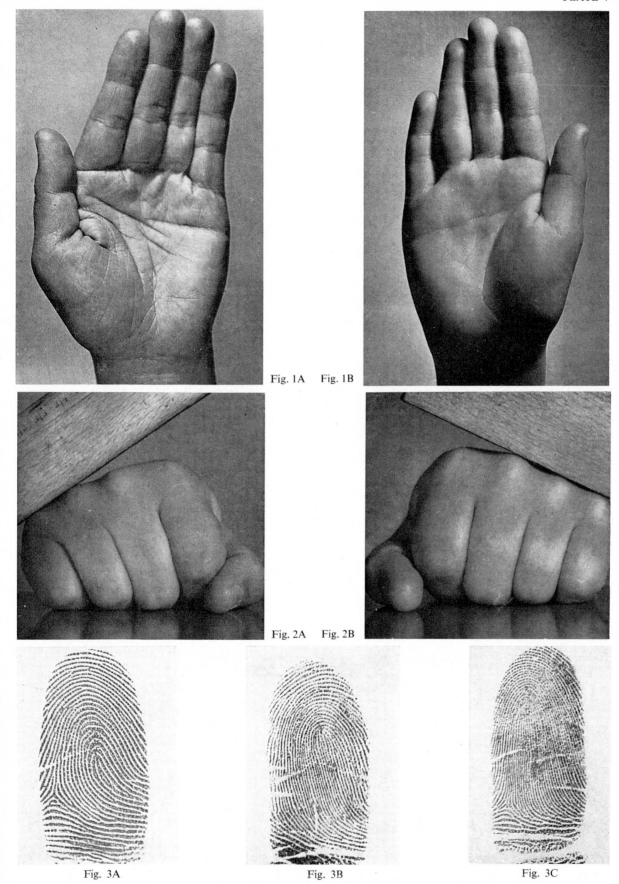

Fig. 1A   Fig. 1B

Fig. 2A   Fig. 2B

Fig. 3A   Fig. 3B   Fig. 3C

The Legs

In half the patients the legs are thick, shapeless, pseudoedematous. Occasionally genu varum may be seen. Talipes equinovarus, lymphedema of the feet — especially in the first years of life — syndactylism, shortened toes and nail anomalies are sometimes seen.

Cardiovascular Anomalies

The most frequent sign is hypertension of a benign nonprogressive course. Congenital heart disease is found in about 10% of the cases of which coarctation of the aorta is the most common. Other cardiovascular anomalies noted are subaortic stenosis and ventricular septal defect. In some patients multiple intestinal telangiectases are seen at laparotomy; these may occasionally cause severe intestinal hemorrhages.

Renal Anomalies

There is a high incidence (about 50%) of renal anomalies in patients with Turner's syndrome. The most common anomalies are horseshoe kidney, double pelvis, double kidney and rotational malformation. The function of the kidneys is not disturbed. In nearly all the patients angiography reveals the presence of multiple renal arteries, i.e., two or three arteries instead of one on each side.

Fig. 1. Cubitus valgus in a patient with Turner's syndrome. The carrying angle of the elbow is decreased, and the extended upper extremities take the shape of the letter Y.

Fig. 2. Palm print of a case of Turner's syndrome showing the simian crease — a transverse line running from the radial to the ulnar border of the palm.

Fig. 3. Thickened legs of a patient with Turner's syndrome showing lymphedema that does not pit on pressure.

Fig. 4. Lymphedema of the foot in a 10-year-old patient with Turner's syndrome with shortening of the third and fourth toes. The nails are short, hyperconvex, deeply set in the beds.

Fig. 5. Madelung's deformity in a case of Turner's syndrome. The styloid process of the ulna protrudes dorsally.

PLATE 8

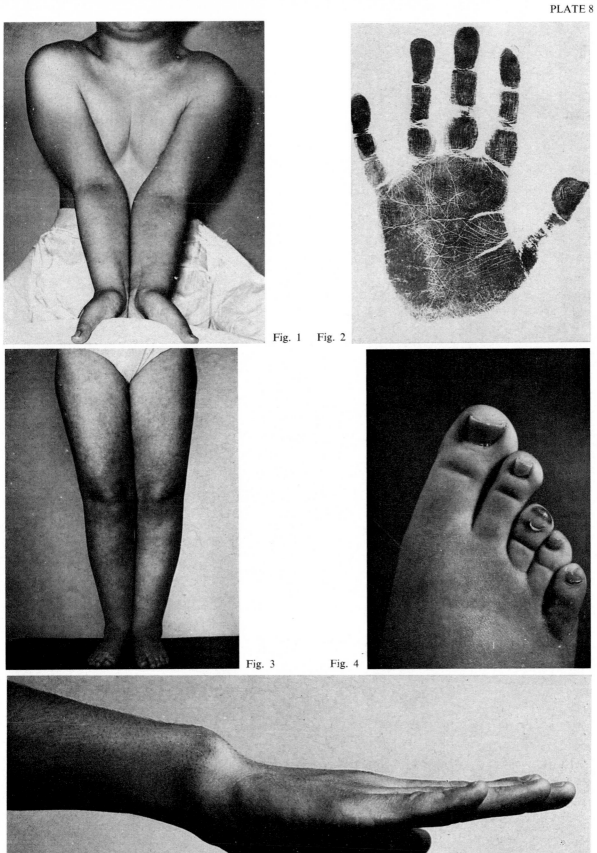

Fig. 1   Fig. 2

Fig. 3   Fig. 4

Fig. 5

Methods Used to Diagnose the Disease

Pelvic Pneumography

After peritoneal gas insufflation pelvic roentgenograms show a small, flattened uterus and long thin Fallopian tubes. No gonads are seen on the roentgenograms. Linear shading of the streaks is rarely evident, as they are usually overlapped by the tubes.

Laparotomy

Laparotomy in Turner's syndrome reveals internal female genitalia and bilateral absence of the ovaries. In the broad ligaments, at the place normally occupied by the ovaries, there are elongated whitish streaks of connective tissue. The fibrous streaks are 3–6 cm long and only 2–3 mm thick. They are nearly always thin and smooth, but in rare instances a slight nodular thickening is seen. The uterus is small and flattened, of fetal or childlike size, exceptionally bicornuate. The tubes are thin, elongated and undulated as in pre-pubertal females.

Fig. 1. Internal genitals of a sexually mature female contrast markedly with those seen in Fig. 2.

Fig. 2. Internal genitals typical of Turner's syndrome. The uterus is small and flattened, the tubes are thin, elongated and undulated. In the broad ligaments whitish streaks are seen instead of ovaries.

Fig. 3. Roentgen pelvic pneumography of a normal female reveals uterus, tubes and ovaries of normal dimensions.

Fig. 4. Roentgen pelvic penumography in a patient with Turner's syndrome shows a flattened uterus and thin tubes and the complete absence of gonads. At laparotomy only whitish streaks, underdeveloped uterus and thin tubes were found.

Figs. 5 and 6. Results of serum FSH and LH radioimmunoassay in control adult subjects and in patients between ages of 12 and 41 years with Turner's syndrome and gonadal dysgenesis. Markedly elevated serum FSH and LH concentration is almost constantly found in patients with gonadal dysgenesis.

238

PLATE 9

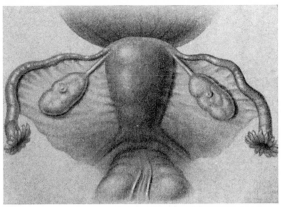

Fig. 1

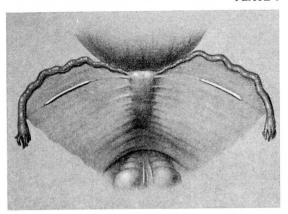

Fig. 2

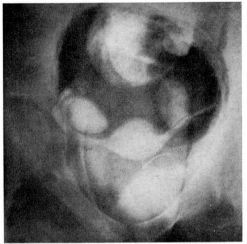

Fig. 3

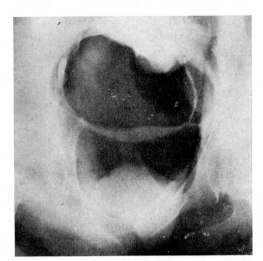

Fig. 4

Fig. 5

Fig. 6

Histologic Examinations

Histologic examination reveals the cortical part of the streak to be composed of connective tissue with numerous fibroblasts arranged in whorls as in the ovarian stroma, but no follicles are seen. In the medullary part, loose connective tissue, numerous vessels, and remnants of the mesonephric tubules are present. In addition, half the patients exhibit large, polygonal Leydig-like cells.

Fig. 1. Infantile external female genitals and absence of the pubic hair in a 17-year-old patient with Turner's syndrome.

Fig. 2. External genitals of a 16-year-old patient with Turner's syndrome. Pubic hair very sparse; labia minora are small, developed only in the upper part.

Fig. 3A. White, elongated streak gonad approximately $6 \times 0.3 \times 0.2$ cm removed at laparotomy from a patient with Turner's syndrome. The streak is bulged at one pole.

Fig. 3B. Photomicrograph of the bulged end of the streak shows a nest of Leydig-like cells (*center*). The whole streak was composed of fibrous tissue devoid of germ cells.

Fig. 4. Photomicrograph of a streak gonad in a patient with Turner's syndrome shows fibrous tissue arranged in whorls and resembling the ovarian stroma. Complete absence of the germinal cells is noted.

PLATE 10

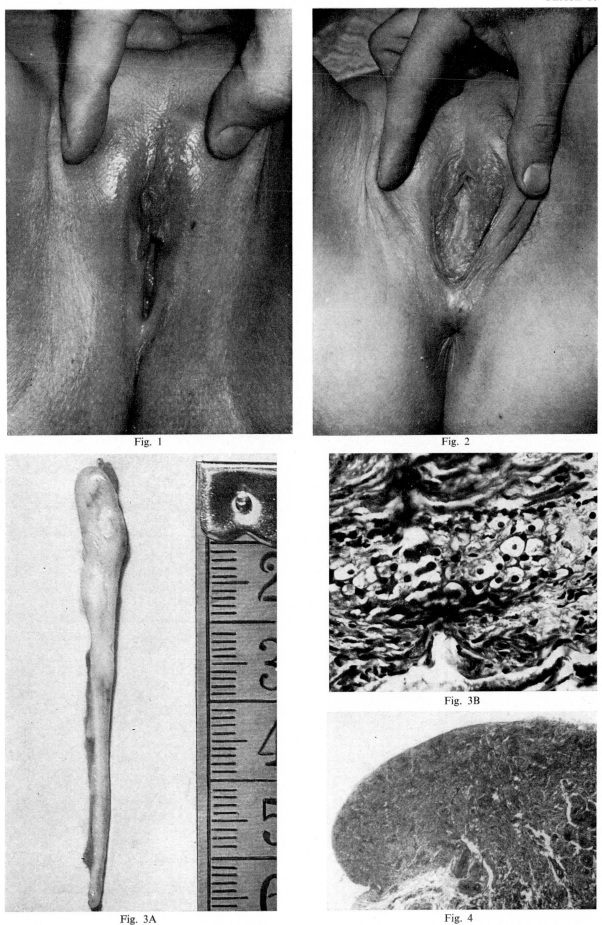

Fig. 1

Fig. 2

Fig. 3A

Fig. 3B

Fig. 4

Vaginal Smears

Smears taken from the vagina reveal definite estrogen deficiency and show a predominance of parabasal cells (small, round, darkly stained cells with large nuclei); they amount to between 85% and 95% of the cells, the remaining being small intermediate cells. Thus the maturation index is usually 90–10–0. After several days of estrogen administration superficial cells appear in the smears.

Chromatin and Chromosomal Findings

Buccal smears show that 60% of the patients are chromatin-negative due to absence of one chromosome X in the cells.

Turner's syndrome is associated with sex chromosome aberrations. The most common anomaly found in two thirds of the cases is the absence of a sex chromosome, so that the patients have a single X and a total of 45 chromosomes. A rare form of chromatin-negative Turner's syndrome is the XO/XY mosaic, a condition which cannot be indentified without chromosomal analysis. The chromatin-positive cases can be divided into two groups, those with mosaicism and those with structural abnormality. The common forms of mosaic are the XO/XX, XO/XX/XXX and, less commonly, the XO/XXX as well as those cases wherein one cell line is an XO and the others contain X chromosomes with structural abnormalities. The second group of chromatin-positive cases contains structural abnormalities of the X chromosome wherein all the cells in the body contain an abnormal X, i.e., isochromosome for the long arm of X, and a ring chromosome or deletion of part of an X chromosome.

Figs. 1A and 1B. Karyotypes in Turner's syndrome showing mosaicism 45,X/46,XX. *A*. Normal female chromosome constitution 46,XX. *B*. Absence of one sex chromosome (45,X constitution).

Figs. 2A and 2B. Photomicrograph of vaginal smears in Turner's syndrome showing small, round parabasal cells (*A*); and larger, oval intermediate cells (*B*).

Figs. 3A and 3B. Urography in 2 patients with Turner's syndrome reveals congenital anomalies of the kidneys, a horseshoe kidney (*A*) and a double kidney (*B*).

242

PLATE 11

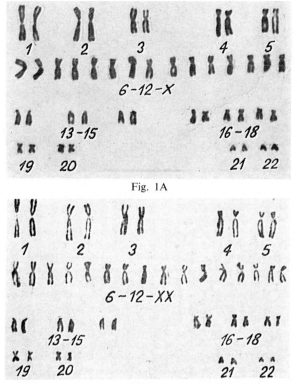

Fig. 1A

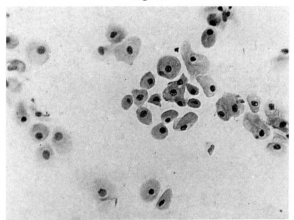

Fig. 1B

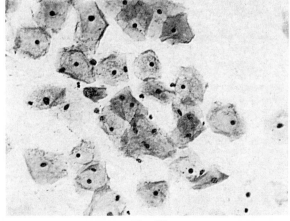

Fig. 2A

Fig. 2B

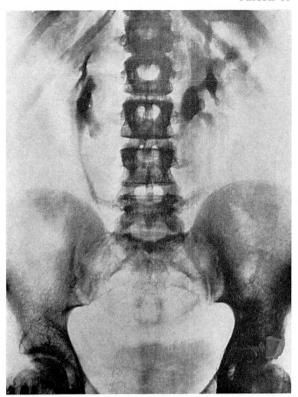

Fig. 3A

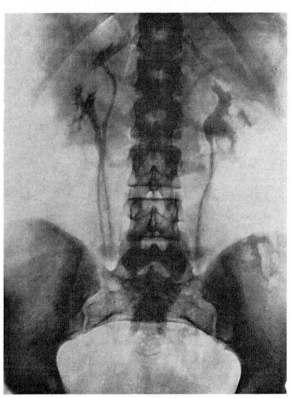

Fig. 3B

Roentgen Findings

The hand. Nearly all patients with gonadal dysgenesis exhibit typical changes in the skeleton. Roentgenograms of the hand and wrist show the bone age to be normal up to age 13 years. After age 13 there is a delay in epiphyseal fusion, with the result that bone age is delayed in patients 15–25 years old. The following findings may also be seen: 1) The distal phalanges are of a peculiar shape, with round and enlarged tufts, and elongated and constricted shafts termed the "drumstick phalanges." 2) A coarse trabecular structure (osteoporosis) is seen in about two thirds of the cases; it is most clearly evident in the carpal bones and the heads and bases of the metacarpals and phalanges. 3) The shafts of the metacarpals and phalanges are slender and narrow across the middle. 4) A shortness of the fourth metacarpal, the so-called metacarpal sign, is frequent. It is present when a tangent drawn to the heads of fourth and fifth metacarpals goes through or touches the head of the third metacarpal. 5) Another finding, called the "preponderance of the phalanges over metacarpals," means a relative lengthening of the phalanges as compared to the stunted metacarpals. 6) In the wrist the notching of the bones of the proximal carpal row is common: it is called the carpal sign.

Fig. 1. Roentgenogram of the hand and wrist of an 18-year-old patient with Turner's syndrome illustrates the common signs: delayed epiphyseal fusion, coarse trabecular structure of the wrist and ends of the long bones, elongated distal phalanges constricted in the middle, marginal projections of epiphyses of the middle phalanges, shortening of the fifth metacarpal, positive carpal sign and convex radial metaphysis with corresponding narrowing of the epiphysis.

PLATE 12

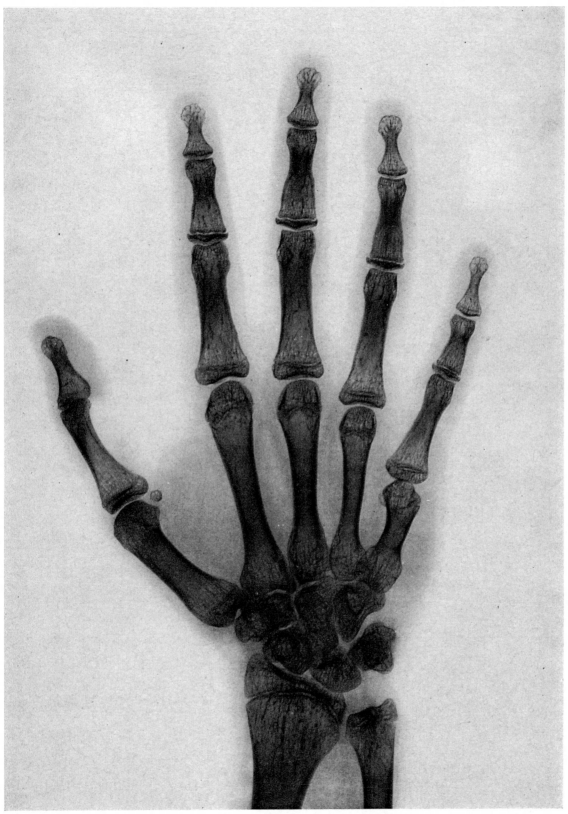

Fig. 1

The distal end of the radius frequently displays a distally convex metaphysis with adaptive narrowing of the epiphysis. The epiphyses of the proximal phalanges of patients between the ages of 15 and 22 years are usually slightly broader than the corresponding metaphyses, and show tiny marginal projections toward the shafts. Madelung's deformity, or distal protrusion of the end of the ulna, may sometimes be seen. A shortening of some phalanges or metacarpals preceded by bulging of epiphyses toward their metaphyses is found in one third of the cases. The metacarpal heads may be flattened and the styloid process of the ulna absent.

The skull. The mastoid processes are very small, the mandible broad and heavy ("male mandible"). The basal angle is increased above 139° in half the patients, and frequently, the petroclinoid processes are calcified.

Fig. 1A. Roentgenogram of the wrist of a patient with Turner's syndrome showing a positive carpal sign: the bones of the proximal carpal row are angularly arranged, forming an angle of 112°.

Fig. 1B. Roentgenogram of the wrist of a normal subject shows the usual arrangement of the bones of the proximal carpal row, which form a slight arch. Two lines drawn tangentially to the contours of these bones form a normal carpal angle of 134°.

Fig. 2A. Distal end of the radius in a 13-year-old patient with Turner's syndrome. The radial metaphysis is convex and the epiphysis is flattened, narrowed in the middle portion. The epiphyseal plate is curved distally.

Fig. 2B. Radius of a healthy 13-year-old female is shown for comparison. The epiphyseal plate runs straight.

Fig. 3. Metacarpal sign. In the majority of patients with Turner's syndrome, a tangent touching the outlines of the fifth and fourth metacarpal heads runs through or touches the head of the third metacarpal. In 90% of normal subjects this tangent runs above the head of the third metacarpal.

Figs. 4A to 4F. "Drumstick" distal phalanges typical of Turner's syndrome (*A–D*) as compared to normal bones (*E* and *F*). The distal phalanges in Turner's syndrome have a round, enlarged tuft, constricted, elongated shaft and a narrow base.

246

PLATE 13

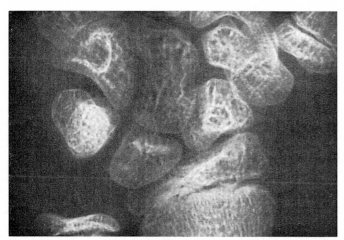

Fig. 1A

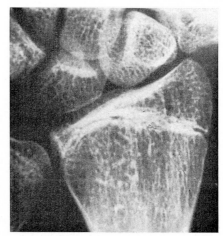

Fig. 2A

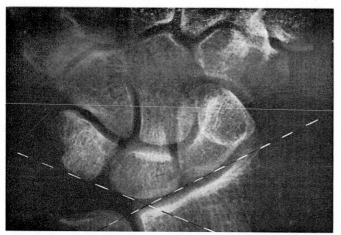

Fig. 1B

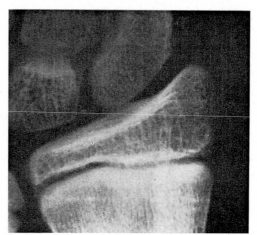

Fig. 2B

METACARPAL SIGN

NEGATIVE   POSITIVE

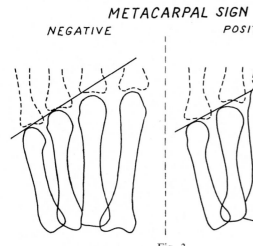

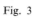

Fig. 3

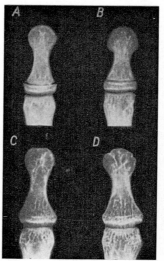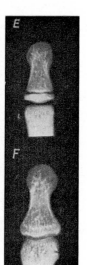

Figs. 4A to 4F

247

The Knee Sign

(Deformity of Medial Condyle of the Tibia; Tibia Vara-Like Deformity)

Frequent changes in the knee, seen roentgenographically, are encountered in 80% of the cases of Turner's syndrome. Three stages of the deformity may be distinguished: in childhood the metaphysis protrudes medially and is sometimes depressed. Adaptive changes occur in femoral epiphyses consisting of flattened lateral condyle and rounded, depressed medial condyle. The tibial epiphyseal plate is extensively curved inferiorly on its medial side.

In teenagers, deformity of the medial tibial metaphysis is associated with corresponding alterations of the tibial epiphysis, which spreads inferiorly to form a pointed projection that covers the protruding part of the metaphysis.

In older patients, after fusion of the epiphysis to its shaft, either a beaklike exostosis or a blunt projection of the medial tibial condyle is evident.

Changes less commonly found in knee roentgenograms include depression of the medial tibial plateau, flattening of the lateral femoral condyle, higher positioning and flattening of the fibular head, beaklike projection of the fibular metaphysis on its medial side. Bone atrophy is found in the majority of cases.

When present, the knee sign is of definite value in the diagnosis of Turner's syndrome since it is not found in growth disturbances other than Turner's syndrome and dyschondroosteosis.

Fig. 1. Medial tibial condyle of 16-year-old patient shows a mushroom enlargement of the metaphysis and a pointed projection of the medial portion of the epiphysis, which overlaps the deformed metaphysis.

Fig. 2. A mushroom enlargement of the tibial metaphysis with slight protrusion of the tibial epiphysis on its medial side is evident in a 15-year-old patient. Coarse trabecular structure (osteoporosis) of the epiphyses.

Fig. 3. A large beaklike projection of the medial tibial condyle is seen in a 26-year-old patient. The medial tibial plateau is depressed, with subsequent lower position of the medial femoral condyle. The fibular head lies higher than normal.

Fig. 4. The type of deformity of the medial tibial condyle commonly seen in adult patients with Turner's syndrome. The medial tibial condyle shows a blunt projection medially and a depressed plateau. The femoral epiphysis reveals coordinate changes: lower position of the medial condyle and higher position and flattening of the lateral condyle. The fibular head is flattened and lies high, close to the joint space.

248

PLATE 14

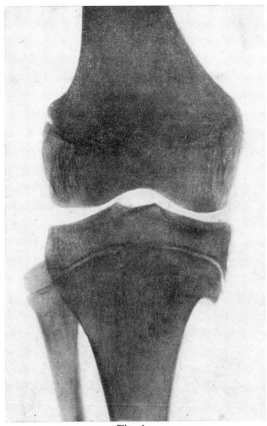

Fig. 1

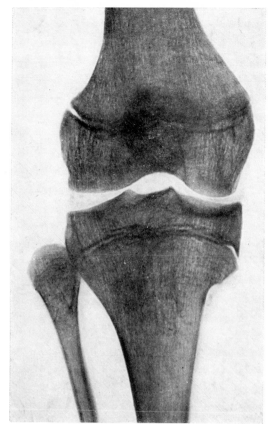

Fig. 2

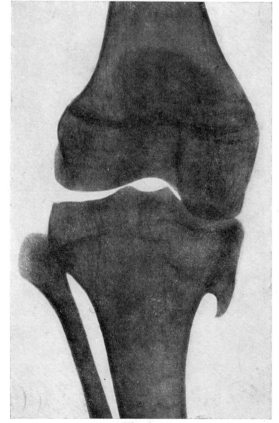

Fig. 3

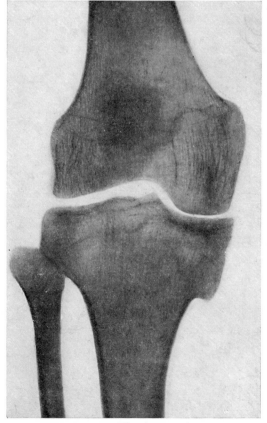

Fig. 4

Laboratory Findings

1. Negative chromatin patterns in two thirds of cases.
2. Chromosome counts showing 45,X or other anomalies.
3. Serum FSH and LH elevated in pubertal and postpubertal period.
4. Plasma and urinary estrogens very low.
5. Atrophic vaginal smears.
6. Pelvic pneumography shows absence of gonads.
7. Roentgen findings: a normal bone age up to age 13; delayed epiphyseal fusion in older patients; osteoporosis; deformity of the medial tibial condyle; positive metacarpal and carpal signs.
8. Palm and fingerprints: a high axial triradius; elongated, perpendicularly oriented loops with an increased ridge count.

Figs. 1A and 1B. Effects of 10-months estrogen treatment (cyclic administration of stilbestrol, 1 mg/day) in a 17-year-old patient with Turner's syndrome. Vaginal bleedings occurred in fourth month of treatment. *A*. Before treatment. There is lack of breast development and very sparse pubic hair. *B*. After therapy. There is definite breast development and growth of pubic hair.

Figs. 2A and 2B. Roentgen pelvic pneumography of the same patient. *A*. Before treatment. Striking underdevelopment of the uterus, which is flattened and small; no gonads are present. *B*. After estrogen therapy. There is evident enlargement of the uterus to nearly normal size.

PLATE 15

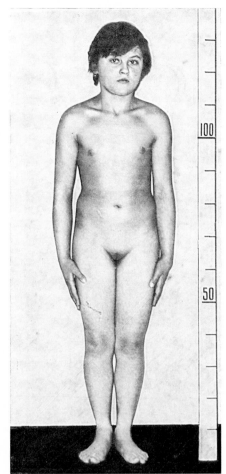 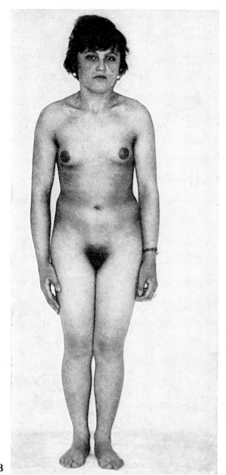

Fig. 1A   Fig. 1B

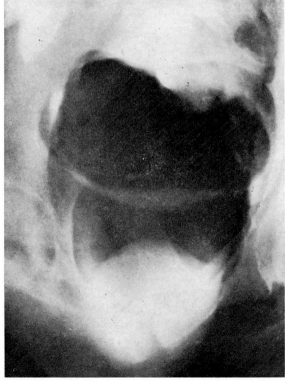 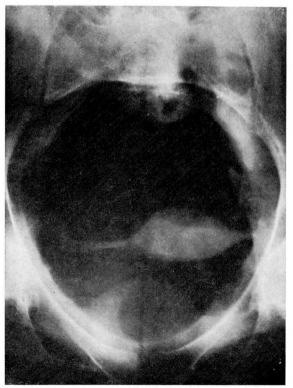

Fig. 2A   Fig. 2B

17*

PURE GONADAL DYSGENESIS

(GONADAL DYSGENESIS WITH NORMAL STATURE)

Pure gonadal dysgenesis appears in phenotypic females. Its cardinal manifestation, evident after the age of puberty, is lack of sexual development, i.e., primary amenorrhea and lack of breast development. The patients are of normal height, but occasionally the extremities are excessively long compared to the trunk due to continued growth of long bones. Thus, the patients assume eunuchoidal body proportions. In the majority of patients their ultimate height exceeds that of other female siblings.

In some cases axillary and pubic hair are poorly developed. There are usually no other anomalies and the disease remains undiagnosed until postpuberty. The external genitalia are feminine, but labia minora are frequently poorly developed. Vaginal smears usually reveal a predominance of intermediate cells and a lack of cyclic changes that indicates a moderate estrogen deficiency. Serum and urinary LH and FSH are markedly elevated.

Fig. 1. A variant of gonadal dysgenesis in an 18-year-old patient. Stunted growth noted in childhood (height 140 cm, 55 in.). Menstrual cycle began at age 14 and appeared regularly for 4 months, then ceased. Female habitus, breasts well developed, normal sexual hair. Chromatin findings positive, karyotype 45,X/46,XX. Laparotomy shows streak gonads. Roentgen signs typical of Turner's syndrome.

Fig. 2. A 20-year-old patient with a variant of gonadal dysgenesis exhibiting short stature (height 142 cm, 56 in.), typically female habitus, normal breast development that started at the age of 13, and primary amenorrhea. Serum LH 68 mIU/ml. Roentgen pelvic pneumography shows absence of gonads and infantile uterus and tubes.

Fig. 3. A variant of gonadal dysgenesis in a 17-year-old patient who gradually attained a low-normal height of 152 cm (60 in.). Presenting manifestations include amenorrhea and complete lack of sexual development. Laparotomy shows streak gonads. Chromatin is positive in buccal smears. Roentgen studies reveal delayed epiphyseal fusion with no other abnormalities.

Fig. 4. A 19-year-old patient with gonadal dysgenesis and low-normal stature (height 154 cm, 61 in.). Note complete lack of breast development, primary amenorrhea, scanty pubic hair. Chromosome constitution 45,X. Pelvic pneumography disclosed the absence of gonads. Serum FSH 68 mIU/ml, LH 93 mIU/ml. Predominance of intermediate cells in the vaginal smears. Roentgen findings typical of Turner's syndrome.

PLATE 16

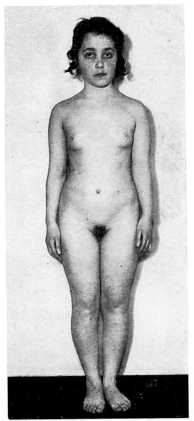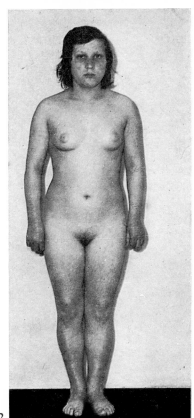

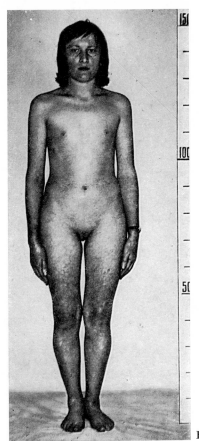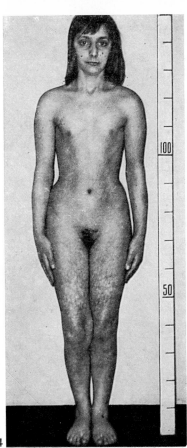

Fig. 1 Fig. 2

Fig. 3 Fig. 4

253

Roentgen pelvic pneumography shows a small uterus and normal tubes, but no ovaries. At laparotomy fibrous streaks, in place of ovaries, are found in the broad ligaments, as in patients with Turner's syndrome. Microscopically, the streaks are composed of connective tissue resembling ovarian stroma; in half the cases nests of Leydig-like cells and mesonephric tubules are seen. Only occasionally are scanty primordial follicles found in the streak gonads.

Two varieties of pure gonadal dysgenesis may be distinguished: 1) chromatin-positive with XX sex chromosomes or mosaicism; and 2) chromatin-negative, in which XY sex chromosomes are usually found.

In patients with XY sex chromosomes, the habitus may show some male characteristics such as wide shoulders and narrow hips. In these cases there is a high incidence of tumors arising from the germ cells (gonocytoma, gonadoblastoma) that are usually associated with signs of masculinization, clitoral hypertrophy, scrotum-like labia majora and excessive sexual hair. Roentgen studies in the XY pure gonadal dysgenesis reveal large cranial dimensions and a large mandible, both characteristic of the male skull.

Fig. 1A. A 19-year-old patient with pure gonadal dysgenesis. Laparotomy disclosed whitish fibrous streaks in place of ovaries. Chromatin-positive findings, normal female chromosome constitution 46,XX, primary amenorrhea, complete lack of breast development and normal pubic hair are found. Vaginal smears reveal predominance of intermediate cells; no cyclic changes of the vaginal epithelium. Height 156 cm (62 in.), normal body proportions. Urinary gonadotropins increased. X ray shows delayed epiphyseal-diaphyseal fusion, no other abnormalities.

Fig. 1B. External genitals of the same patient present normal female appearance, normal sexual hair.

Fig. 2A. Pure gonadal dysgenesis in a 20-year-old patient with chromatin-negative findings and male chromosome constitution 46,XY. Laparotomy reveals streak gonads in the broad ligament, infantile uterus and tubes. Height 174 cm exceeds that of parents and siblings. Broad shoulders, heavy build, primary amenorrhea, no breast development are found. Serum LH 95 mIU/ml. Vaginal smears reveal 90% intermediate cells.

Fig. 2B. External female genitals of the same patient show hypertrophy of the labia minora.

PLATE 17

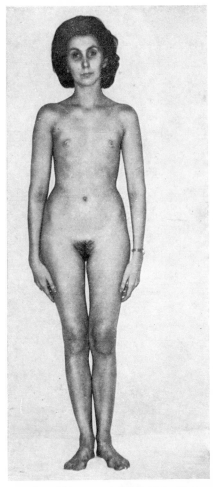

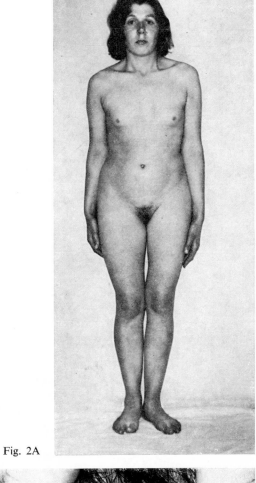

Fig. 1A

Fig. 2A

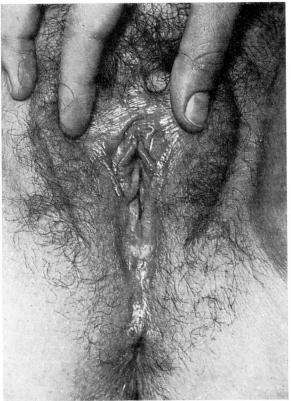

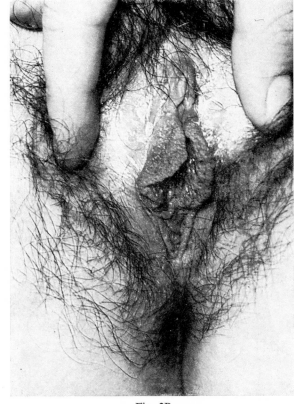

Fig. 1B

Fig. 2B

GONADAL DYSGENESIS WITH FEMINIZATION

In some cases of gonadal dysgenesis there are certain manifestations of Turner's syndrome, e.g., short stature or roentgen changes in the skeleton. At time of puberty, however, sexual characteristics do develop to a certain extent: several spontaneous menses appear, occasionally for several months or even years, and breast development occurs. Despite small stature the habitus is feminine.

Diagnosis of these cases is particularly difficult, and the disease is easily mistaken for primordial dwarfism or familiar short stature. Of diagnostic importance in these patients is the fact that pelvic pneumography reveals the presence of the uterus and tubes, and the absence of the ovaries. At laparotomy typical fibrous streaks are found bilaterally instead of ovaries in the broad ligaments, or exceptionally, a streak gonad is found on one side and a hypoplastic ovary on the other.

Chromatin pattern is usually positive and chromosomal studies demonstrate mosaicism XO/XX or other anomalies.

Roentgenograms of the hand with wrist and of the knee joint frequently show findings typical of those of Turner's syndrome such as normal bone age, osteoporosis, positive carpal and metacarpal signs, knee sign and others.

In contrast to other patients with Turner's syndrome, vaginal smears may reveal some evidence of estrogen effect since not only parabasal cells but also intermediate and superficial cells are seen.

Figs. 1A and 1B. Unilateral gonadal dysgenesis. *A.* At age 10. Typical manifestations of Turner's syndrome are seen: webbed neck, shield-like chest with widely spaced nipples, lymphedema of the legs. Spontaneous menstruations began at age 12, had been regular for 5 years, then ceased at age 18. *B.* The same patient at age 16 shows signs of sexual maturation: normally developed breasts, pubic hair, and feminine fat distribution. Mosaicism 45,X/46,XX.

Figs. 2A to 2C. Internal genitals of the same patient. *A.* Infantile uterus, thin Fallopian tubes, streak gonad, and an ovary are seen. *B.* Histopathology of ovary shows primordial follicles in the cortex. *C.* Histopathology of streak gonad reveals connective tissue arranged in whorls and devoid of germ cells.

PLATE 18

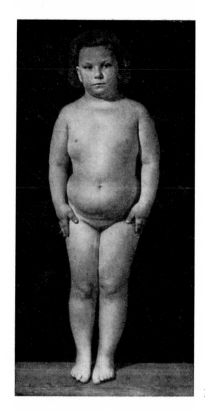

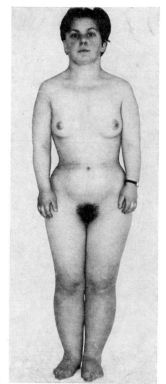

Fig. 1A   Fig. 1B

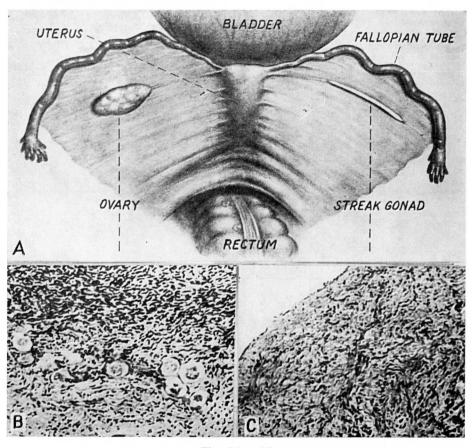

Figs. 2A to 2C

MIXED GONADAL DYSGENESIS

(GONADAL DYSGENESIS WITH HERMAPHRODITISM; ATYPICAL GONADAL DYSGENESIS)

The disease is characterized by ambisexual external genitalia, and the presence of a streak gonad with uterus and tubes on one side, and a testis placed intraabdominally or in the inguinal canal on the other side. The external genitalia are ambisexual; there is an underdeveloped penis (or enlarged clitoris) with hypospadias, and fusion of the labioscrotal folds. Some of the patients are reared as males and others as females. In males, the disease is usually mistaken for bilateral cryptorchidism, but laparotomy confirms a diagnosis of mixed gonadal dysgenesis by revealing a streak gonad on one side and a testis on the other, and internal female genitalia. At puberty, partial masculinization may appear.

Fig. 1A. Mixed gonadal dysgenesis in a 13-year-old patient reared as a male. Short stature (height 139 cm, 55 in.). Roentgen findings are typical of Turner's syndrome: deformity of the medial tibial condyle, osteoporosis; chromatin findings negative; mosaicism 45,X/46,XY.

Fig. 1B. Ambisexual external genitalia of the same patient. Note penis with hypospadias, scrotum-like labia majora, lack of gonads.

Fig. 1C. Findings at laparotomy of the same case: cornuate uterus with only one Fallopian tube; streak gonad (*left*), gonad resembling a testis (*right*) in the inguinal canal.

Fig. 1D. Histopathology of the streak gonad shows fibrous tissue devoid of germ cells.

Fig. 1E. Histopathology of gonad from the inguinal canal presents a picture of a prepubertal testis; densely packed small seminiferous tubules.

258

PLATE 19

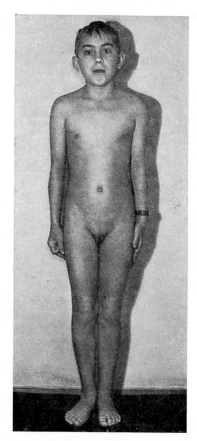

Fig. 1A

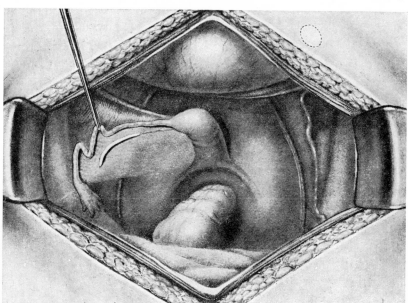

Fig. 1C

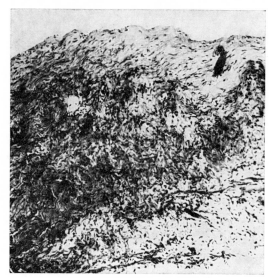

Fig. 1D

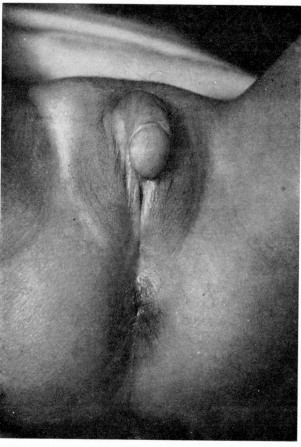

Fig. 1B

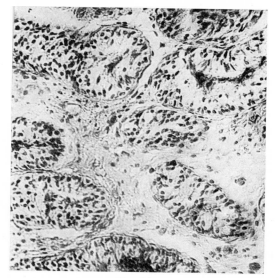

Fig. 1E

In patients reared as females the clinical manifestations are primary amenorrhea, lack of breast development and occasionally some signs of virilization such as a deep voice or facial hair growth.

In mixed gonadal dysgenesis some clinical features of Turner's syndrome such as short stature, roentgen changes in the skeleton, abnormal palmar creases or other somatic anomalies may be present.

The chromatin findings are negative and the sex chromosome constitution is XO or XO/XY in most cases.

Fig. 1A. A 27-year-old patient with pure gonadal dysgenesis and virilization. She had never menstruated, and was taller (height 173 cm, 68 in.) than her parents. Lack of breast development, normal pubic hair can be seen.

Fig. 1B. External genitals of the same patient showing marked hypertrophy of the clitoris and scrotum-like labia majora. The pubic hair was shaved before laparotomy.

Fig. 1C. Internal genitals of the patient as seen at laparotomy: bicornuate uterus, normal Fallopian tubes, and in the broad ligament, yellowish fat nodules on both sides containing minute gonads in the middle. Histopathology revealed bilateral dysgenetic testes with a gonadoblastoma in the right gonad.

Fig. 1D. Karyotype from peripheral blood showing normal male chromosome constitution 46,XY.

Fig. 2. Histopathology of a gonadoblastoma from a case of mixed gonadal dysgenesis with 46,XY chromosomes reveals nests of germ cells scattered among Sertoli-granulosa cells. In the upper portion are seen laminated hyaline-like bodies surrounded by Sertoli-granulosa cells in coronal fashion (Courtesy J Teter, MD, Warsaw).

Fig. 3. Histopathology of a gonocytoma which developed in a dysgenetic gonad. The tumor was removed from a patient with pure gonadal dysgenesis and XY sex chromosomes. Nests of germ cells are separated by connective tissue showing lymphocyte infiltrations. In the upper right corner, psammoma-like calcification is seen (Courtesy J Teter, MD, Warsaw).

260

PLATE 20

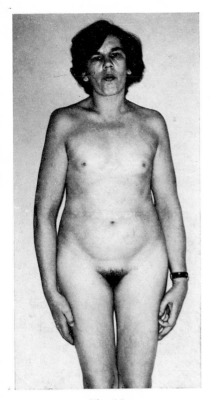

Fig. 1A

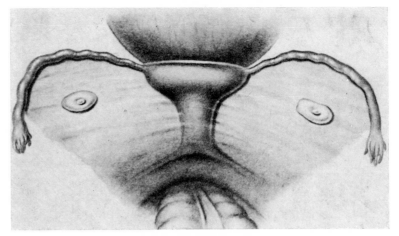

Fig. 1C

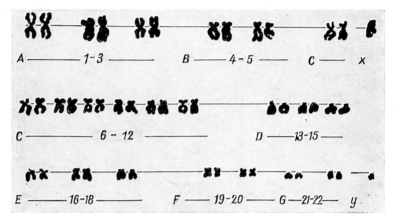

Fig. 1D

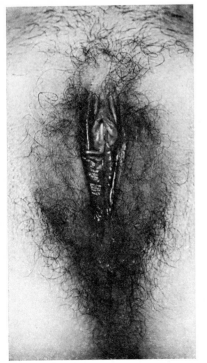

Fig. 1B

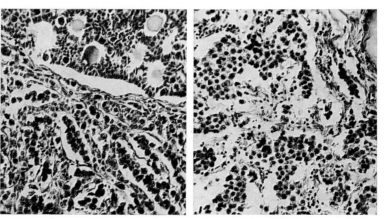

Fig. 2

Fig. 3

HYPOGONADOTROPIC OVARIAN INSUFFICIENCY

(HYPOGONADOTROPIC EUNUCHOIDISM IN FEMALES; ISOLATED GONADOTROPIN DEFICIENCY)

There are two types of hypogonadotropic ovarian insufficiency. The first is idiopathic, of unknown etiology. The second type results from pituitary damage by a chromophobe tumor, craniopharyngeoma or other lesions of the pituitary, giving rise to monotropic pituitary insufficiency.

The cardinal manifestations of idiopathic hypogonadotropic ovarian insufficiency are lack of sexual development during and after the pubertal period, primary amenorrhea, sterility, lack of breast development, scarce or no axillary and pubic hair, underdeveloped genitalia and lack of urinary gonadotropins. The body proportions are usually eunuchoid, the span exceeding the height.

At laparotomy, female internal genitalia of prepubertal size are found; the ovaries are small and oval shaped as in children. On histologic examination they reveal a deficient number of immature follicles. On roentgen pelvic pneumography the uterus and ovaries are of prepubertal dimensions.

Roentgenographic examinations of the skeleton show a delayed fusion of the epiphyses to their shafts. The skull is of the same size and proportion of that found in females, and there are no changes in or around the sella turcica. In some patients osteoporosis develops, first appearing in the spine.

Oral smears are chromatin-positive and there is a normal female XX sex chromosome constitution. Vaginal smears usually show a predominance of the intermediate cells, amounting to about 90%. Serum LH and FSH levels are very low or undetectable.

Despite some similarity in clinical manifestations of hypogonadotropic ovarian insufficiency and pure gonadal dysgenesis, there are certain differences. In hypogonadotropic ovarian insufficiency serum LH and FSH are low; the ovaries, on pelvic pneumography and at laparotomy, are small and ovoid, and there is a response to administration of human FSH. In contrast, in pure gonadal dysgenesis serum LH and FSH are high, no gonads are seen on pelvic pneumography, and instead of ovaries typical fibrous streaks are found at laparotomy; there is no response to human FSH administration. Premature menopause occurs in females who are sexually well developed, have high serum LH and FSH and who have had menstrual cycles — thus differing markedly from hypogonadotropic ovarian insufficiency. The second form of hypogonadotropic ovarian insufficiency, caused by organic pituitary lesions, is described in Chapter 1.

Fig. 1. A 22-year-old patient with isolated gonadotropin deficiency. Height 158 cm (62 in.). Primary amenorrhea and complete lack of sexual development, infantile facial features, slender extremities, fat accumulation on the chin and trunk, especially over the hips. No secondary sex characteristics; infantile genitals are present. Serum LH and FSH are undetectable (below 1 mIU/ml). Atrophic vaginal smears; chromatin findings positive; 46,XX chromosomes. Normal response of serum HGH to insulin-induced hypoglycemia. Normal thyroid and adrenal function. Pelvic pneumography reveals infantile uterus and tubes, small and flattened ovaries.

Fig. 2A. A 21-year-old patient showing isolated gonadotropin deficiency (hypogonadotropic eunuchoidism). Slim build, slender extremities, lack of breast development, scanty pubic hair (the nipples darkened after several estradiol injections) are seen. Primary amenorrhea; vaginal smears show parabasal cells only. Chromosome constitution is 46,XX. Serum LH and FSH below 1 mIU/ml.

Fig. 2B. Hand of the same patient. Note delicate wrist, fine, elongated fingers and narrow nails.

Fig. 2C. Roentgen pelvic pneumography shows small, infantile uterus, tubes and flat ovaries. The left ovary, clearly visible, measures 26 × 6 mm (right ovary, 28 × 6 mm).

Fig. 2D. Effects of FSH stimulation test, which consists of a single intramuscular injection of human FSH 500 units and human LH 50 units in the same patient. Pelvic pneumography taken 12 days after gonadotropin administration shows a marked increase in size of both ovaries and in the uterus. The left ovary now measures 27 × 14 mm, the right ovary, 28 × 15 mm. The vaginal smears revealed definite response to FSH injection, i.e., the appearance of intermediate and superficial cells that persisted for 3 weeks before the smears gradually returned to their previous atrophic state.

PLATE 21

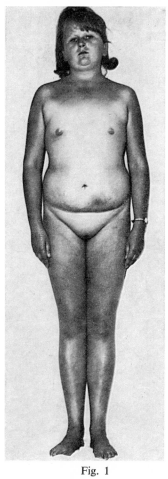

Fig. 1

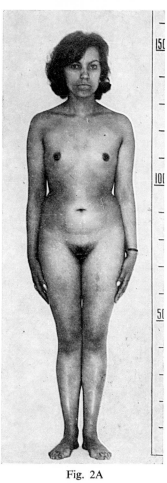

Fig. 2A

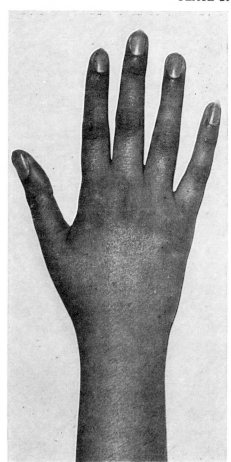

Fig. 2B

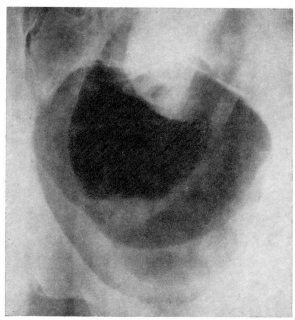

Fig. 2C

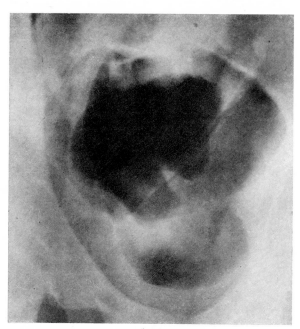

Fig. 2D

The menopause, i.e., cessation of menses, occurs physiologically in females between the ages of 40 and 55 years. It is usually preceded by irregular anovular menses. The duration of menopausal manifestations such as hot flushes and increased irritability lasts from a few months to several years. The symptoms are mild in the majority of cases but are usually more pronounced in those emotionally unbalanced. Artificial menopause is the result of bilateral ovarectomy or irradiation of the ovaries; the younger the castrated women the more acute the symptoms.

Signs and Symptoms

1. Hot flushes.
2. Sweating attacks.
3. Increased nervousness, emotional instability and other psychoneurotic manifestations such as insomnia, palpitation, dyspnea, vertigo, headaches, paresthesias.
4. Weight gain.
5. Gradual atrophy of genitalia.
6. Atrophy of breast tissue.
7. Thinning of sexual hair.

Laboratory Findings

1. High serum FSH and LH.
2. Increased urinary gonadotropins.
3. Vaginal smears show a lack of cyclic changes in the epithelium. The smears are often of a "mixed type," composed of parabasal, intermediate and superficial cells.

Later Complications of Menopause

1. Senile vaginitis causing dyspareunia.
2. Pruritus vulvae.
3. Osteoporosis.

Postmenopausal Osteoporosis

In many females in the postmenopausal period osteoporosis develops; it may also be seen some years after ovarectomy or roentgen castration. The principal symptoms of postmenopausal osteoporosis are pains in the back, ribs and pelvis. On examination kyphosis, scoliosis, limitation of movements and reduction in height (caused by shortening of the vertebral column) may be seen. In advanced stages vertebral collapse or rib fractures may occur. Plasma calcium, phosphate and alkaline phosphatase are normal.

Roentgen examination reveals bone atrophy chiefly localized in spine, ribs and pelvis. In the early stage, there is decreased density of vertebral bodies which have a washed-out structure but thinned and densified terminal plates, sharply outlined as if with a pencil. In other patients vertical striation of the vertebral bodies is seen. When bone atrophy is extensive small herniations of the nucleus pulposus into the vertebral bodies (Schmorl's nodules), flattened or concavoconcave vertebral bodies (fish vertebrae) may appear.

Fig. 1. Results of serum FSH radioimmunoassay in 5 patients with isolated gonadotropin deficiency, in postmenopausal females and in 16 patients with premature menopause. Normal adult range of serum FSH is 4 to 18 mIU/ml. In postmenopausal females and in those with premature menopause serum FSH is definitely elevated, whereas in patients with hypogonadotropic hypogonadism serum FSH is undetectable or very low.

Fig. 2. Roentgenogram of the lumbar spine of a 56-year-old female with advanced postmenopausal osteoporosis. Concavoconcave vertebral bodies of decreased density and marginal condensations of upper and lower surfaces are seen.

Fig. 3. Vaginal smear, stained by Shorr's method, in a 52-year-old postmenopausal female showing marked estrogen deficiency. Parabasal, intermediate and single superficial cells are seen.

PLATE 22

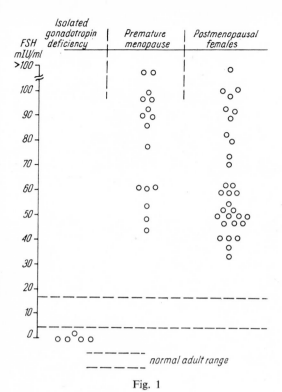

Fig. 1

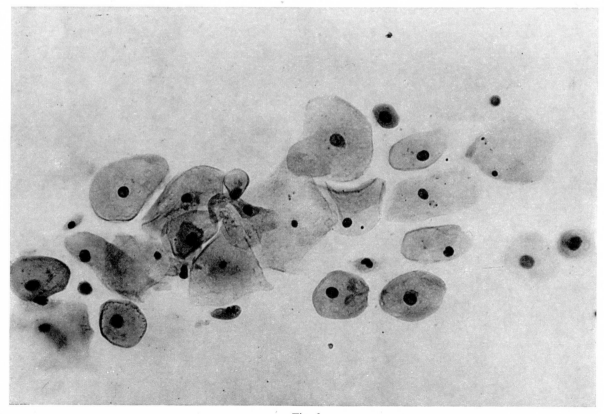

Fig. 2

Fig. 3

The same roentgen picture is found in other diseases such as senile osteoporosis, Cushing's syndrome, prolonged corticosteroid therapy, hypogonadism, primary and secondary hyperparathyroidism and multiple myeloma. In the two last named diseases osteoporosis usually involves the skull, and typical biochemical abnormalities develop which are not found in postmenopausal osteoporosis.

In some patients with Cushing's syndrome and with ectopic ACTH syndrome in which osteoporosis is the predominant manifestation an erroneous diagnosis of postmenopausal osteoporosis is possible. However, hormonal studies reveal an increased plasma cortisol concentration characteristic of these syndromes. In skeletal lesions caused by metastatic cancer small osteolytic areas are usually seen on the roentgenograms and the general condition of the patients is poor.

PREMATURE OVARIAN FAILURE
(PREMATURE MENOPAUSE)

Premature ovarian failure that occurs in women between the ages of 20 and 30 years is characterized by secondary amenorrhea, sterility and climacteric symptoms such as hot flushes, sudden sweats, heart palpitations and increased irritability. Etiology is uncertain; congenital defects of ovarian stroma and autoimmune processes are possible causes. Histopathology of the ovaries shows fibrosis of the stroma and atresia of the follicles. Patients are of normal height and feminine habitus and have normal breast and sexual development. Other congenital anomalies are not evident. Roentgen pelvic pneumography reveals a normal uterus and Fallopian tubes; the ovaries, however, are reduced in size and sometimes shrunken.

Laboratory Findings

1. Low serum and urinary estrogens.
2. Increased plasma and urinary LH and FSH.
3. Vaginal smears are composed of mostly parabasal cells, thus indicating estrogen deficiency.

Fig. 1. Premature ovarian failure (premature menopause) in a 27-year-old patient. Menstruations began at age 14 and were regular until age 26 when they gradually ceased and climacteric symptoms appeared. Female body build; secondary sex characteristics well developed. No changes at gynecologic examination. Serum LH 88 mIU/ml, FSH 71 mIU/ml. Vaginal smears of a mixed type (parabasal, intermediate and superficial cells) show lack of cyclic changes. Urinary 17-ketosteroids 8 mg/24 hr.

Fig. 2. A 33-year-old patient with premature menopause of 2 years duration. Regular menstruations occurred from ages 13 to 30, then secondary amenorrhea and cardiovascular symptoms developed. Serum LH 106 mIU/ml. Vaginal smears indicate estrogen deficiency. Pelvic pneumography shows small uterus, shrunken ovaries. The patient is of normal height (162 cm, 64 in.). Broad hips, typically feminine habitus, normal female external genitalia are present.

Fig. 3. Results of serum LH radioimmunoassay in premature ovarian failure. Serum LH concentration increases to levels found in postmenopausal females in all cases. (*See also* serum FSH results on the Plate 22.)

Fig. 4. Vaginal smear of "mixed type" from a 27-year-old patient with premature menopause composed of cells from all 3 layers of the mucosa.

PLATE 23

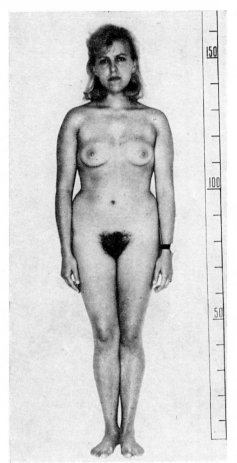

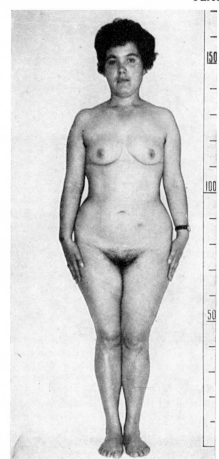

Fig. 1   Fig. 2

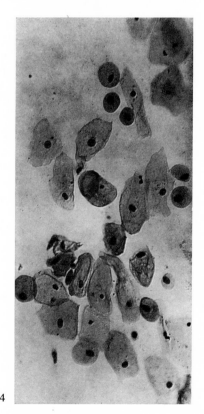

Fig. 3   Fig. 4

THE POLYCYSTIC OVARY

(STEIN-LEVENTHAL SYNDROME; THE ANDROGENIC OVARY)

This is a common disease in women characterized by bilateral enlargement of the ovaries, irregular menstruations, hirsutism and infertility. The signs and symptoms usually commence some years after puberty.

Symptoms

1. Menstrual disturbances, usually oligomenorrhea or secondary amenorrhea; primary amenorrhea in exceptional cases.
2. Hirsutism, sometimes requiring frequent shaving or depilation.
3. Sterility.

Signs

1. Hirsutism: excessive growth of hair on the face, thighs, abdomen and around the areolae — more prominent in brunettes.
2. Enlarged ovaries that are smooth, hard but pain-free may be noted on gynecologic examination. The uterus is sometimes infantile.
3. Monophasic curve of the basal temperature.
4. Tendency to obesity in some patients.
5. Occasional acne.
6. Laparotomy reveals the ovaries to be large and pearly white in color. Cross section of the ovaries displays a hard and thickened albuginea, beneath which are numerous small follicular cysts.

Figs. 1A and 1B. Marked hirsutism in a 26-year-old patient with Stein-Leventhal syndrome accompanied by sterility and secondary amenorrhea. Excessive hair growth on the breasts around the areolae, along the linea alba and on the buttocks and thighs. Vaginal smears showed a maturation index of 5/90/5 with striking predominance of intermediate cells. Serum LH is 32 mIU/ml. Chromatin findings positive. Enlarged ovaries were found on gynecologic examination and on roentgen pelvic pneumography.

Fig. 1C. Laparotomy findings in the same patient: greatly enlarged, billiard-ball-like ovary with pearly white surface. The ovarian membrane was found to be greatly thickened with numerous cysts underneath. Restoration of regular cycles after wedge resection of the ovaries. The patient became pregnant one year later.

PLATE 24

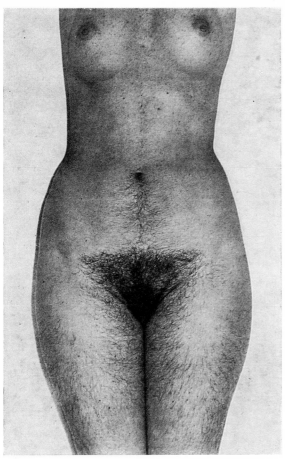

Fig. 1A

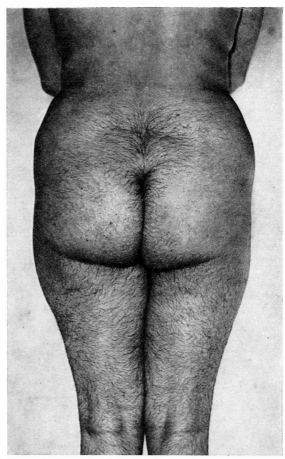

Fig. 1B

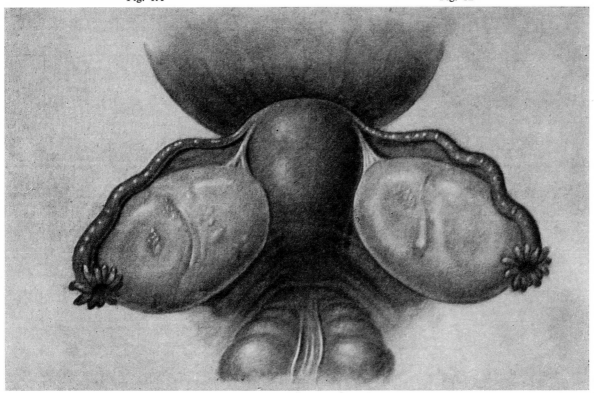

Fig. 1C

Laboratory Findings

1. Increased plasma and urinary testosterone.
2. Abnormal cystic fluid contains increased amounts of androstenedione and only minimal amounts of estradiol, estrone and progesterone.
3. Predominance of intermediate cells in vaginal smears.
4. Pelvic pneumography shows enlargement and increased density of the ovaries, and generally a small uterus.
5. Increase in plasma and urinary LH in some cases.

Fig. 1A. A 19-year-old patient with primary amenorrhea, hirsutism and enlarged ovaries in which the juvenile form of Stein-Leventhal syndrome was diagnosed. Height is normal, as is female habitus. Hair growth found on abdomen and thighs. Vaginal smears show no cyclic changes of vaginal epithelium and 90%-94% intermediate cells. Enlarged ovaries seen on pelvic pneumography.

Fig. 1B. Closeup view of external genitalia of the same patient showing excessive hair growth on the medial aspect of the thigh. Marked hypertrophy of the labia minora which protrude 2 cm beyond the labia majora.

Fig. 1C. Roentgen pelvic pneumography showing small uterus and greatly enlarged ovaries measuring 62 × 41 mm and 60 × 42 mm.

Fig. 1D. Laparotomy in the same patient revealed large, elongated ovaries with multiple cysts located just beneath the membrane.

270

PLATE 25

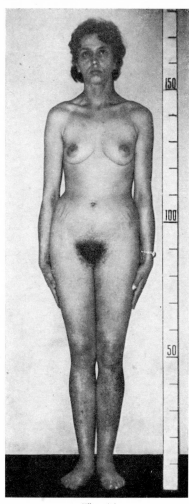

Fig. 1A

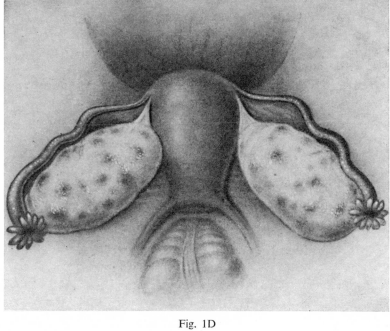

Fig. 1D

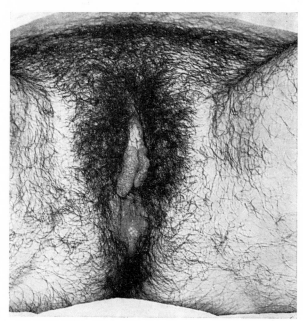

Fig. 1B

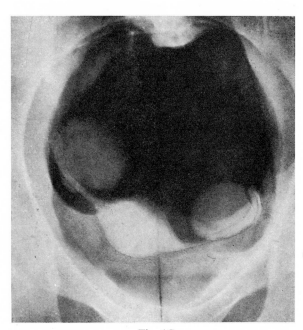

Fig. 1C

Masculinizing tumors of the ovary develop in women during the reproductive years and are manifested by virilization and secondary amenorrhea. Histologically the tumors are usually arrhenoblastomas, and rarely luteomas, hilus cells (Leydig cells) tumors or adrenal rest tumors (masculinovoblastomas).

Signs and Symptoms

1. Cessation of menses; sterility.
2. Hirsutism; hair growth on upper lip, chin, cheeks and breasts; male escutcheon.
3. Deepening of the voice.
4. Hypertrophy of the clitoris.
5. Acne.
6. Thinning of the hair at the temples; baldness.
7. Tumor mass palpable in the abdomen.
8. Masculine distribution of subcutaneous fat.

Laboratory Findings

1. Increased plasma and urinary testosterone.
2. Urinary 17-ketosteroids normal or slightly increased.
3. Negative dexamethasone suppression test.
4. Vaginal smears show estrogen deficiency and lack of cyclic changes.
5. Pelvic pneumography reveals enlargement of the ovary.

Following successful treatment signs of masculinization regress, menses and fertility are restored, but baldness, if present, remains.

HIRSUTISM

Hirsutism accompanies hormonal disturbances of the ovaries and adrenals and is seen in Stein-Leventhal syndrome, masculinizing tumors of the ovary, mixed gonadal dysgenesis, male pseudohermaphroditism, congenital adrenogenital syndrome, virilizing adrenocortical tumors and Cushing's syndrome. These diseases usually evoke virilization, amenorrhea or menstrual disturbances, sterility, vaginal smears of intermediate type, and other characteristic signs and symptoms. After a careful exclusion of all these diseases there remains idiopathic hirsutism, excessive hair growth of a male type not accompanied by other clinical manifestations and found in a large number of females. The exact etiology of idiopathic hirsutism has not yet been determined. In some patients basal plasma testosterone is elevated; others show an exaggerated plasma testosterone response to ACTH administration, indicating hyperresponsiveness of the adrenal cortex. In yet other patients administration of chorionic

---

Fig. 1A. A 48-year-old patient with arrhenoblastoma of the left ovary. The voice deepened and clitoral hypertrophy developed. A large tumor of the ovary was found on pelvic pneumography. Abundant thick hair growth above the upper lip and on the chin is seen.

Fig. 1B. Laparotomy findings in the same patient. A large, lobulated tumor measuring 20 × 16 cm of gray-yellow color was found in the broad ligament on the left side. Histopathology showed an arrhenoblastoma.

Fig. 2. Extensive hirsutism in an 18-year-old patient with the juvenile form of Stein-Leventhal syndrome. Hair growth above the upper lip, on the chin and on the chest is evident. At laparotomy both ovaries were grossly enlarged and contained numerous cysts.

Fig. 3. Face of a 61-year-old patient with an adrenocortical virilizing adenoma associated with signs of Cushing's syndrome (hypertension, osteoporosis, plethoric face, truncal obesity). Marked facial hair growth is found, especially on the chin.

PLATE 26

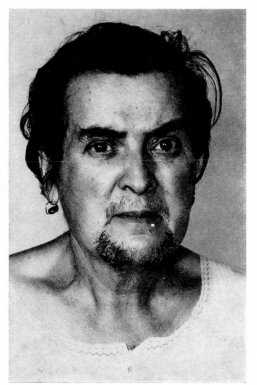

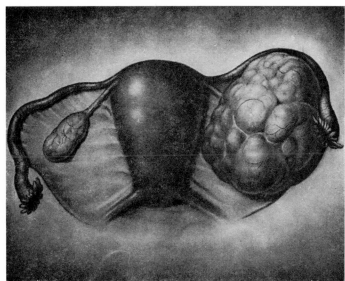

Fig. 1B

Fig. 1A

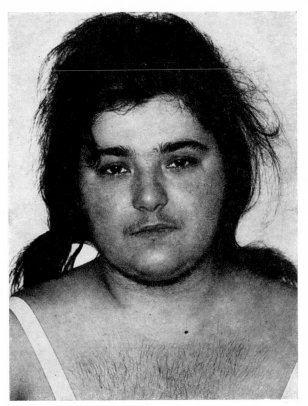

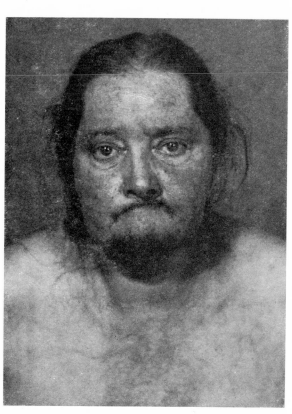

Fig. 2

Fig. 3

gonadotropin together with dexamethasone increases plasma testosterone, pointing to an ovarian defect in steroidogenesis. In hirsute females with normal basal plasma testosterone and normal response to ACTH and HCG stimulation tests, receptor defects such as abnormal androgen metabolism in the skin or increased sensitivity of hair follicles to circulating androgens are suspected. Another possible cause may be a lowered serum concentration or a reduced avidity of testosterone-binding proteins that lead to elevation in free testosterone concentration in the plasma.

Excessive hair growth appears on the chin, cheeks, upper lip, around the areolae, on the chest, on the abdomen along the linea alba, on the thighs and lower limbs. The growth may be thick, the hair coarse, presenting a difficult cosmetic problem. Menstrual cycles are normal; the patients usually possess normal fertility.

FEMINIZING TUMORS OF THE OVARY

These are rare tumors found in females, composed of granulosa cells or theca cells, that secrete estrogens and cause signs and symptoms of feminization. The clinical manifestations depend on the age of the patients: pseudoprecocious puberty develops in prepubertal females, amenorrhea or irregular menstruations during the reproductive age, and vaginal bleedings and swelling of the breasts in postmenopausal females. Ovarian tumor may be palpable in the abdomen or viewed by roentgen pelvic pneumography. Plasma and urinary estrogens are very high. Vaginal smears reveal persistence of high estrogen effect consisting of superficial cells with very high maturation, karyopycnotic and eosinophilic indexes. Surgical removal of the tumor leads to regression of clinical and laboratory abnormalities.

Chapter 6

INTERSEXUALITY

TRUE HERMAPHRODITISM

True hermaphroditism is a rare disease wherein ovarian and testicular structures are present in one individual. One of each gonad, ovary and testis, may be present either separately or joined to form one ovotestis composed of ovarian and testicular tissue. The external genitalia are male, female or ambiguous, and various malformations occur (Figs. 1–6). During puberty male and/or female sex characteristics develop to varying degrees. The internal genitalia usually consist of a uterus and one or two Fallopian tubes. There may also be a prostate. In over half the patients menstrual cycles appear, but the patients nearly always are sterile.

Chromatin findings are predominantly positive and XX sex chromosome constitution is more frequent than is XY or mosaicism.

Fig. 1. Male external genitalia with the urethrovaginal opening behind the scrotum. Ovotestis present in the scrotum on one side, and an ovary on the other. Uterus and a Fallopian tube found at laparotomy.

Fig. 2. Female external genitalia with hypertrophied clitoris; internal genitalia have an ovary. Testis found in the hernial sac.

Fig. 3. Male external genitalia, penis with hypospadias. A testis is seen in the scrotum and an ovotestis intraabdominally in the broad ligament. Uterus and a Fallopian tube are also present; separate vaginal orifice located posteriorly to the scrotum.

Fig. 4. External genitalia are of male appearance, i.e., penis with hypospadias, scrotum with one testis. At laparotomy rudimentary vagina, uterus and an ovary were found.

Fig. 5. External genitalia are feminine: hypertrophied clitoris, separate urethral and vaginal orifices. Laparotomy disclosed uterus, Fallopian tubes and an ovary on one side, and an ovotestis on the other.

Fig. 6. Penile urethra, well developed penis, rudimentary empty scrotum are seen. Internal genitalia consist of bilateral ovotestes, Fallopian tubes and infantile uterus.

PLATE 1

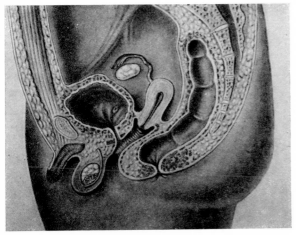

Fig. 1

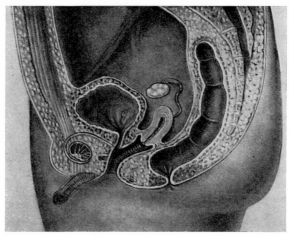

Fig. 2

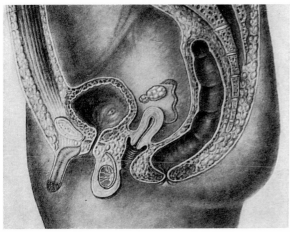

Fig. 3

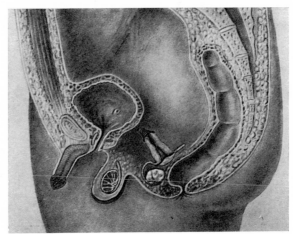

Fig. 4

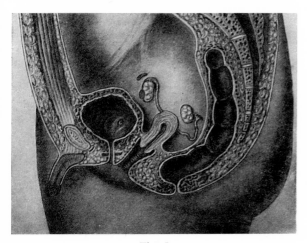

Fig. 5

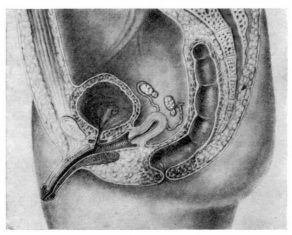

Fig. 6

TESTICULAR FEMINIZATION SYNDROME

(FEMINIZING TESTES; ANDROGEN INSENSITIVITY SYNDROME)

Other synonyms for this syndrome are Goldberg-Maxwell syndrome, Morris syndrome, hereditary male pseudohermaphroditism. The syndrome is an extreme form of male pseudohermaphroditism characterized by a typically female habitus and female external genitals but the presence of testes which lie intra-abdominally or in inguinal canals. There are negative chromatin findings and a male chromosomal pattern. All the clinical manifestations may be attributed to a deficiency or abnormality of the androgen receptors in target tissues. There is a definite familial predisposition to this syndrome, the abnormality being transmitted maternally. The infants are assigned a feminine gender identity.

Symptoms

1. In infants, there may be a bilateral inguinal hernia in which the gonads are often present.
2. Primary amenorrhea; sterility.
3. Lack of sexual hair.
4. Inguinal pains caused by the presence of testes in inguinal canals, or hernia.
5. Infrequent difficulties in sexual relations due to underdevelopment of the vagina.
6. Sometimes symptoms of menopause such as hot flushes, appear in patients as early as the third decade of life.

Fig. 1A. A 19-year-old patient with testicular feminization syndrome. Height 170 cm (67 in.). Slender build, typically feminine habitus, well developed breasts, lack of pubic hair are exhibiting features. Chromatin pattern negative; 46,XY chromosome constitution.

Fig. 1B. Side view of the same patient showing complete lack of axillary and pubic hair, full breasts, the presence of palpable masses (testes) in the inguinal regions.

Fig. 1C. Internal genitalia of the patient shown in Fig. 1. Present are bilateral, normal-sized testes, closely connected with bicornuate uterus (*shaded area*), embedded in the broad ligaments.

PLATE 2

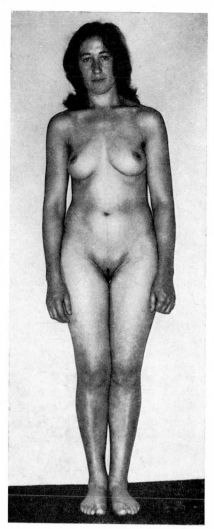

Fig. 1A

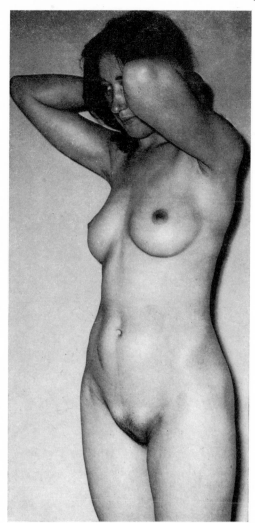

Fig. 1B

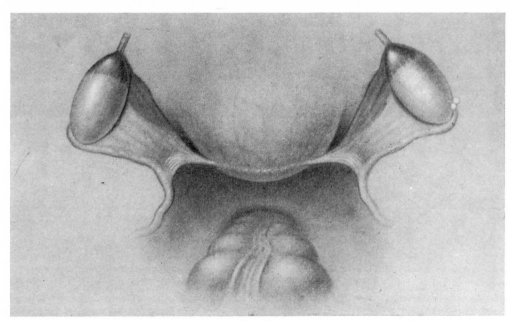

Fig. 1C

279

Signs

1. Typical female external appearance with feminine fat deposition and female proportions of the shoulders and hips.
2. Normal breast development, but the nipples may remain infantile.
3. Lack of pubic and axillary hair; occasional scarce vulval hair.
4. Female external genitalia, but the labia majora, minora and clitoris may be underdeveloped; the vagina is significantly shortened, usually measuring 2 to 5 cm and ending blindly; portio vaginalis of the uterus is lacking; slight or no perineal pigmentation.
5. Height above average.
6. Long limbs; occasionally eunuchoid features, the span of the arms exceeding the height.
7. Bilateral inguinal hernia which frequently contains ovoid bodies representing the testes. In some cases the testes may be palpable in inguinal canals.
8. Thick hair on the head, but body hair is scarce, usually present only on the forearms and calves.
9. The skull is rather large with broad mandible, as in males.
10. Psychosexually the patients are typically female and of normal intelligence.
11. Familial occurrence.

Laboratory Findings

1. Negative chromatin pattern.
2. Presence of Y-fluorescent body in buccal smears.
3. Male chromosome constitution 46,XY.
4. Plasma and urinary testosterone near or in the normal male range.
5. Serum FSH and LH are normal in younger patients, but increase in some older patients.
6. Androgen-sensitive tissues (e.g., sexual hair, voice) unresponsive to administration of testosterone, even in large doses.
7. Roentgen manifestation: typically male skull with broad mandible.

Fig. 1. A 30-year-old patient with testicular feminization is shown with a 26-year-old healthy sister. The patient is taller and of heavier build, has a larger head and broader mandible, and no sexual hair.

Fig. 2. Internal genitalia of the patient shown in Fig. 1. Cornuate uterus and bilateral testes are seen.

Fig. 3. Lateral view of the pelvis in testicular feminization. Normal female external genitalia, the vagina is markedly shortened and with blind end; testis with rudimentary uterus is attached to the lateral wall of the pelvis.

Fig. 4. External genitalia of a 28-year-old patient with testicular feminization syndrome show a normal feminine appearance, only the pubic hair is scarce.

PLATE 3

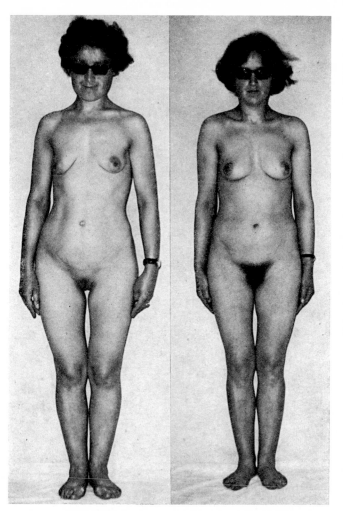

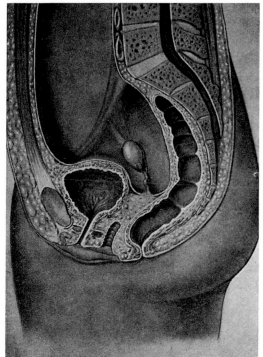

Fig. 3

Fig. 1

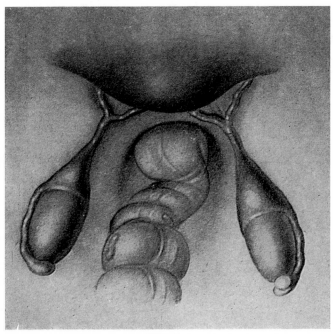

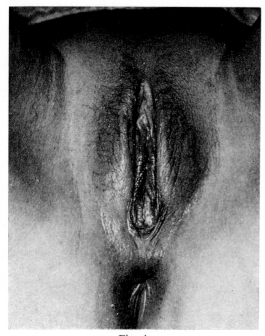

Fig. 2

Fig. 4

INCOMPLETE TESTICULAR FEMINIZATION

(PARTIAL TESTICULAR FEMINIZATION)

Incomplete testicular feminization is a form of familial male pseudohermaphroditism characterized by sign of masculinization, breast development, ambiguous external genitalia with labial testes and XY sex chromosome constitution. A congenital defect in androgen receptor is probably responsible for reduced sensitivity of the target tissues to androgens. The patients are usually reared as females.

Signs and Symptoms

 1. Male habitus, broad shoulders and narrow hips.
 2. Female breast development.
 3. Normal growth of pubic and axillary hair.
 4. Ambisexual external genitalia with clitoral enlargement.
 5. Testes undescended or located in the labia majora.
 6. Internal genitalia absent.
 7. Plasma testosterone and urinary 17-ketosteroid excretion in the male range.
 8. Negative chromatin pattern; presence of Y-fluorescent body.
 9. Normal male chromosome constitution 46,XY.
10. Familial occurrence.

The syndrome is similar to testicular feminization especially in the prepubertal period. In postpubertal patients there are differences. Clitoral enlargement, pubic and axillary hair growth, and increase in 17-ketosteroid excretion are characteristic of incomplete testicular feminization and do not occur in true testicular feminization. The incomplete testicular feminization syndrome differs from other types of male pseudohermaphroditism because of the presence of well developed breasts which do not appear in the latter diseases.

Fig. 1A. A 22-year-old patient with partial feminization syndrome shows height and breast development to be normal, feminine body habitus.

Fig. 1B. External genitals of the same patient show feminine labia majora and minora, and clitoris. A testis is seen in the left labium.

Fig. 1C. Photomicrograph of the testis found on the right side in the inguinal canal at laparotomy. The seminiferous tubules show fibrosis, sloughing of the epithelium and hyalinization. The interstitial Leydig cells are abundant.

Fig. 1D. Karyotype of the same patient shows a normal male 46,XY chromosome constitution.

PLATE 4

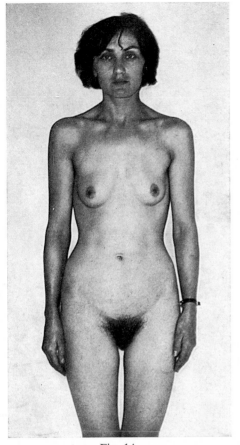

Fig. 1A

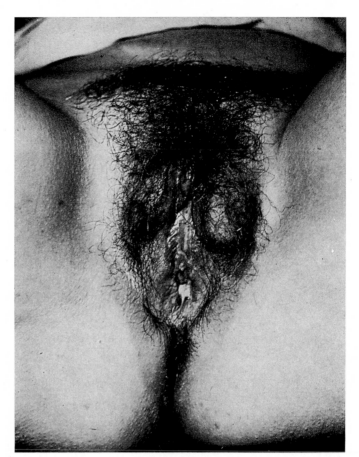

Fig. 1B

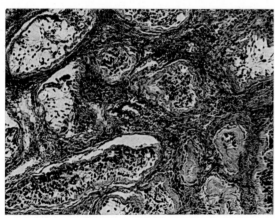

Fig. 1C

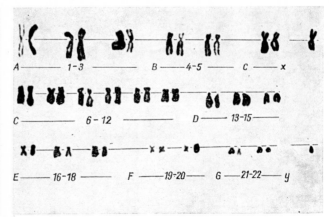

Fig. 1D

REIFENSTEIN'S SYNDROME

Reifenstein's syndrome is a hereditary form of male pseudohermaphroditism characterized by hypospadias, eunuchoidism of varying degree, postpubertal tubular atrophy, azoospermia and gynecomastia. Plasma testosterone is lowered while gonadotropins are usually elevated. Chromatin pattern is negative and there is a normal XY sex chromosome constitution. In histologic studies the testes show various degrees of tubular fibrosis and inconstantly abundant Leydig cells. In contrast to testicular feminization, the patients respond to testosterone administration in an appropriate manner.

DYSGENETIC TESTES IN EUNUCHOID FEMALES

This variant of male pseudohermaphroditism is not recognized until puberty at which time female sexual development fails to occur. There is primary amenorrhea and lack of breast development, whereas axillary and pubic hair does appear. The patients, who are invariably reared as girls, are of normal height and normal or eunuchoid body proportions. They have female external genitalia with some clitoral enlargement. Chromatin findings are negative, and chromosome analysis shows 46,XY. Psychosexual orientation is feminine.

In some patients laparotomy shows a small uterus, Fallopian tubes and tiny testes instead of ovaries. In patients in whom no structures developed from the Müllerian ducts, the testes lie on the lateral pelvic walls. In histologic examination the testes show small, irregularly situated seminiferous tubules lined with Sertoli cells only. Fibrosclerotic degeneration of the seminiferous tubules is frequent, especially after puberty. There is a high incidence of tumors, usually gonadoblastoma, developing from the dysgenetic testes, hence their removal is recommended.

Fig. 1. A 27-year-old patient with male pseudohermaphroditism (Reifenstein's syndrome) exhibiting slight build, long, thin extremities, female breast development and ambisexual genitalia. Negative chromatin pattern, XY sex chromosomes.

Fig. 2. A 22-year-old patient with Reifenstein's syndrome. Height 173 cm (68 in.), broad hips, enormous gynecomastia, ambisexual genitalia.

Fig. 3. Karyotype of peripheral blood cultures of the patient shown in Fig. 2 reveals a normal male chromosome constitution, 46,XY.

Fig. 4. Ambiguous external genitalia of the patient shown in Fig. 2. Bilateral testes of normal size in labioscrotal folds, rudimentary penis resembling clitoris, hypospadias, normal pubic hair.

Fig. 5. Ambiguous external genitalia of the patient shown in Fig. 1. There are two separate scrotal folds, resembling labia majora, with testes inside, a small penis and hypospadias. Scarce pubic hair.

PLATE 5

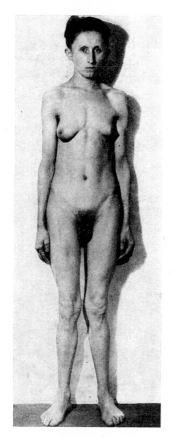

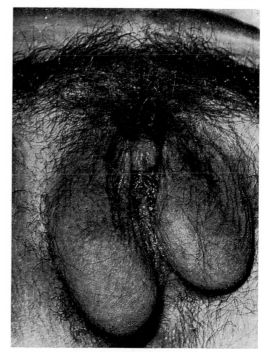

Fig. 4

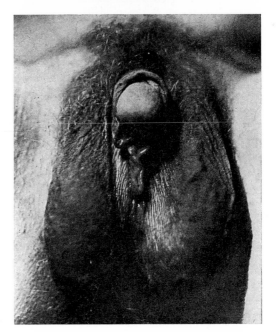

Fig. 5

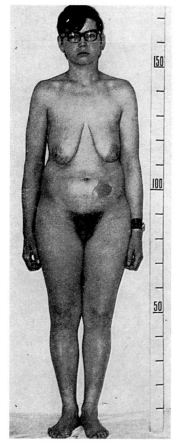

Fig. 1

Fig. 2   Fig. 3

MALE PSEUDOHERMAPHRODITISM

In male pseudohermaphroditism the external genitalia are ambiguous, and the testes may be located intraabdominaly in inguinal canals or labioscrotal folds. Because of ambiguous genitalia the patients may be reared as boys or girls. The disease is caused either by a failure of the fetal testes to produce Müllerian suppressor substance during sex differentiation or by a decreased response of the androgen-sensitive tissue to masculinization. The body build is male or slightly eunuchoid; at puberty male sex characteristics develop to varying degrees, but pubic hair is of a female escutcheon and there is usually no beard growth. The patients are chromatin-negative and have XY sex chromosomes. Before puberty it is not possible to differentiate this form of male pseudohermaphroditism from incomplete testicular feminization in which breast development occurs.

Histologic examination of the testes after puberty reveals small, irregularly situated seminiferous tubules varying in size and development, with tubular sclerosis and peritubular fibrosis.

FEMALE PSEUDOHERMAPHRODITISM

(FEMALE INTERSEXUALITY)

In female pseudohermaphroditism the external genitalia are ambiguous while internal genitalia, i.e., uterus, ovaries and Fallopian tubes, are normally developed. The condition is the result of exposure to androgens during early stages of fetal development, or it may occur spontaneously. The ovaries are fertile. The chromatin pattern is positive and the karyotype is 46,XX. The most common form is congenital virilizing adrenal hyperplasia described in Chapter 3. A similar masculinization of the female external genitalia may be provoked by maternal ingestion of testosterone, methyltestosterone or progesterone derivatives in the first trimester of pregnancy or by a virilizing tumor in the mother. In this form of female pseudohermaphroditism there are no hormonal abnormalities. Specifically, the urinary 17-ketosteroids, 17-ketogenic steroids, and testosterone are normal.

CONGENITAL ABSENCE OF THE VAGINA

(ROKITANSKY'S DISEASE; CHIARI SYNDROME)

In this syndrome there is a congenital absence of the vagina. The uterus is also absent or may be bicornuate, while the ovaries are normal. At the age of puberty secondary sex characteristics normally develop; there is, however, primary amenorrhea. Urinary estrogens are in the female range and urinary smears show cyclic changes in the epithelium indicating appropriate ovarian function. Chromatin pattern is positive, karyotype is 46,XX. The external genitalia are feminine, except that the vaginal opening is represented by only a dimple. The disease is frequently associated with congenital anomalies of the urinary tract; other anomalies are rare.

Fig. 1. An 18-year-old patient with male pseudohermaphroditism reared as a male. Normal height and build, no beard growth, pubic hair of female escutcheon. 46,XY chromosome constitution.

Fig. 2A. A 22-year-old patient with male pseudohermaphroditism, reared as a girl because of ambisexual genitalia. Normal height and build, female escutcheon of pubic hair, no breast development. Negative chromatin pattern.

Fig. 2B. Pelvic pneumography performed on the patient shown in Fig. 2A reveals bilateral gonads at the lateral borders of the pelvis with no other internal genitalia. On laparotomy and in histologic studies the gonads proved to be testes.

Fig. 3. External ambiguous genitalia of the patient in Fig. 1. Note nearly normal-sized penis, hypospadias, shrunken and empty scrotum.

Fig. 4. Karyotype of the patient shown in Fig. 1 shows a normal 46,XY chromosome constitution.

PLATE 6

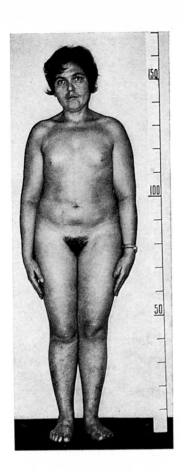

Fig. 2A

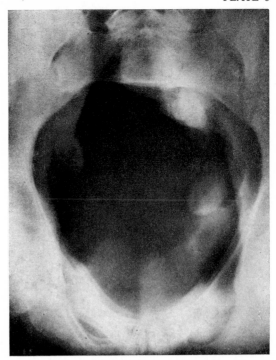

Fig. 2B

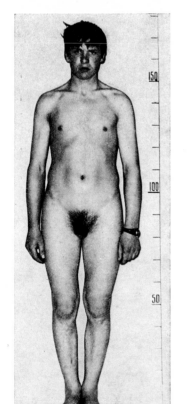

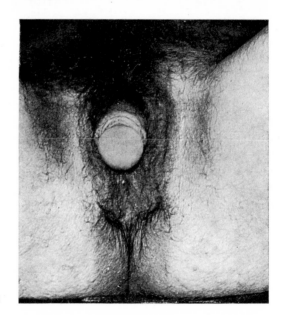

Fig. 3

Fig. 1   Fig. 4

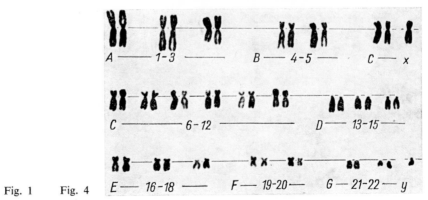

Chapter 7

PRECOCIOUS PUBERTY

PRECOCIOUS PUBERTY

(SEXUAL PRECOCITY)

Precocious puberty, or true precocious puberty, is a condition whereby pituitary and gonadal functions are activated prematurely in females before age 8, and in males before age 10. True precocious puberty in females is characterized by sexual maturation, regular cycles and ovulation. In males, secondary sex characteristics develop, the testes assume adult size and spermatogenesis occurs. True precocious puberty invariably arises from a disturbed function of the brain. On the other hand, pseudoprecocious puberty is due to disorders in gonadal or adrenocortical functions in which secondary sexual characteristics develop while the gonads, testes or ovaries, remain immature.

TYPES OF PRECOCIOUS PUBERTY IN YOUNG FEMALES

Precocious puberty is at least twice as common in females as in males. About 80% of the females show no evidence of organic brain abnormality although many of them have abnormal EEGs. Four main types of precocious puberty may be distinguished: idiopathic, Albright's syndrome, neurogenic and that associated with hypothyroidism.

IDIOPATHIC PRECOCIOUS PUBERTY

In females between the ages of 1 and 7 years, there is breast development, onset of menarche, maturation of genitals and development of pubic and axillary hair. Growth is accelerated, the hips are rounded and the patients attain feminine body contours. Mental development is normal.

Hormonal Findings

1. Serum LH and FSH are in adolescent or adult female range.
2. Serum estrogens are in adolescent or adult female range.
3. Vaginal smears show superficial and intermediate cells.
4. Serum testosterone low, in adolescent range.
5. Urinary 17-ketosteroids low, 2 to 12 mg/day.

Roentgen Findings

1. Bone age accelerated several years in advance of the chronologic age.
2. Premature fusion of the epiphyses from about ages 9 to 11 years.
3. Adult female size and shape of the pelvis.
4. Roentgen pelvic pneumography: uterus and ovaries of the adolescent or adult size, without evidence of ovarian tumor.

Fig. 1. A 7-year-old female with idiopathic precocious puberty. Breast development began at age 5, followed by menarche 8 months later. Height 131 cm (52 in.). Female habitus, well developed breasts, sparse pubic hair are seen. Mental development compatible with chronologic age. Superficial cells are seen in the vaginal smears. No neurologic changes have occurred. Bone age accelerated (14 years).

Fig. 2. An 8-year-old patient with neurogenic precocious puberty following encephalitis at age 7 exhibits mental deficiency. Height 140 cm (55 in.), weight 54 kg. Obesity and full sexual development are seen.

Fig. 3. Roentgenogram of the hand of a 4-year-old female with neurogenic precocious puberty who died from severe cerebral complications. At autopsy it was found that a large tumor (9 cm in diameter), which proved to be astrocytoma, had damaged the hypothalamus. Bone age (8 years) was greatly accelerated.

Fig. 4. EEG of a 7-year-old patient with idiopathic precocious puberty shows gross irregularity in the basic rhythm.

PLATE 1

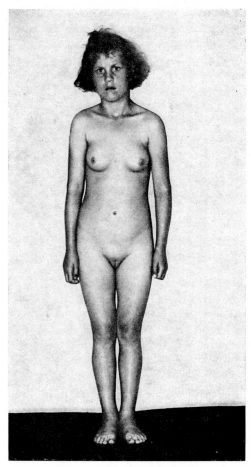

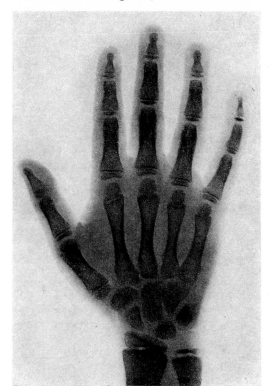

Fig. 1

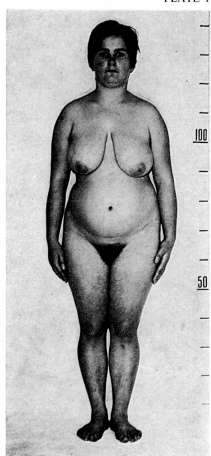

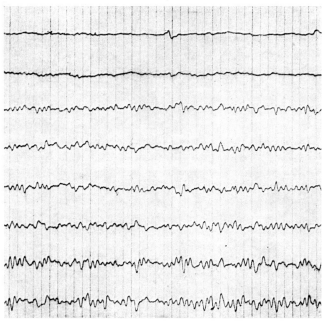

Fig. 2

Fig. 3

Fig. 4

ALBRIGHT'S SYNDROME

(PRECOCIOUS PUBERTY, AREAS OF SKIN PIGMENTATION AND FIBROUS DYSPLASIA OF BONE)

The primary manifestations of the syndrome are sexual precocity, areas of skin hyperpigmentation and fibrous dysplasia of bone. The syndrome is encountered almost exclusively in females. Menarche may begin as early as 3 months of age and usually precedes breast development and the appearance of pubic hair by several months to years. The skin changes, usually present at birth, consist of brown nonelevated areas of pigmentation that are often distributed unilaterally on the trunk and extremities. Bone lesions occasionally lead to pathologic fractures and deformities. Roentgenograms of the skull frequently show sclerotic overgrowth of the base, which may overshadow the sella turcica. In the long bones patchy areas of rarefaction with cystic appearance and loss of trabecular structure are seen. In the majority of patients EEGs reveal abnormalities, slowing of the basic rhythm and paroxysmal activity which includes spikes, sharp wave or spike-wave pattern. Other clinical, hormonal and roentgenographic manifestations are the same as those found in idiopathic precocious puberty.

NEUROGENIC PRECOCIOUS PUBERTY

The condition arises from damage to the hypothalamus by hamartoma; tumors such as craniopharyngioma, glioma, astrocytoma; inflammatory lesions such as encephalitis; granulomatous lesions, i.e., tuberculosis, sarcoidosis, reticuloendotheliosis; and internal hydrocephalus, regardless of cause. Neurogenic precocious puberty is associated with other manifestations of the hypothalamic syndrome.

Clinical Manifestations

1. Headache.
2. Loss of vision: diplopia.
3. Papilledema.
4. Hyperbulimia and obesity.
5. Occasional anorexia; loss of weight.
6. Convulsions.
7. Behavior disturbances.
8. Somnolence or other sleep disturbances.
9. Mental retardation.
10. Hyperthermia; variations in body temperature.
11. Manifestations of diabetes insipidus.

Neurologic examination, roentgenograms of the skull, pneumoencephalography or arteriography are usually helpful in locating the site and in determining the extent of the tumor.

Fig. 1A. A 4-year-old female with Albright's syndrome. Menarche started at the age 18 months; breast development followed 6 months later. Irregular areas of skin pigmentation on the upper limb and back, and breast development are clearly evident. Height 118 cm (47 in.). Normal mental development. Profuse EEG abnormalities.

Fig. 1B. External genitals of the same patient, showing pubertal development and scarcity of pubic hair.

Fig. 1C. Cystic changes in the humerus of the same patient.

Fig. 1D. Fingers of the same patient show markedly expanded ends of the fourth and fifth digits caused by fibrous dysplasia of bone.

Fig. 1E. Roentgenogram of the skull of the same patient at age 7 shows sclerotic overgrowth of the base that overshadows the sphenoidal sinuses and the sella turcica.

Fig. 1F. Roentgenogram of the hand of the same patient at age 6 shows greatly accelerated bone age (10 years), fibrous dysplasia — cystic changes in the ulna — expanded shafts of the phalanges of the fourth digits with loss of trabecular structure.

PLATE 2

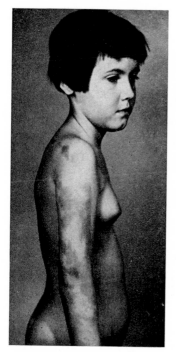

Fig. 1A

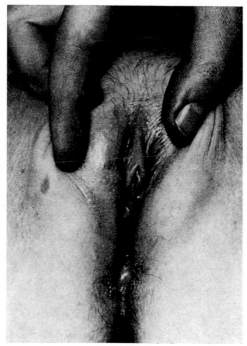

Fig. 1B

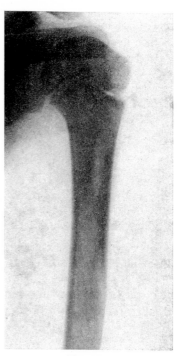

Fig. 1C

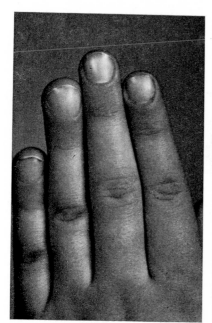

Fig. 1D

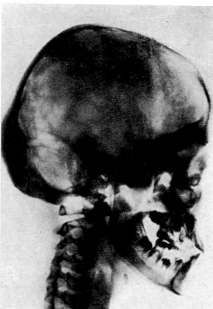

Fig. 1E

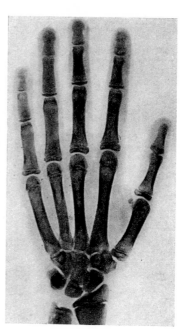

Fig. 1F

HYPOTHYROIDISM ASSOCIATED WITH PRECOCIOUS PUBERTY

Juvenile hypothyroidism is very rarely associated with true precocious puberty. Galactorrhea and hyperpigmentation may be present occasionally. The clinical manifestations include both hypothyroidism and precocious puberty; there is, however, no stimulation of linear growth and acceleration of bone age as seen in other types of sexual precocity. Serum TSH and prolactin are markedly elevated; serum thyroxine is lowered. Manifestations regress on thyroxine replacement therapy.

GONADAL PSEUDOPRECOCIOUS PUBERTY

(OVARIAN PSEUDOPRECOCIOUS PUBERTY)

In females usually between 2 and 7 years of age, some ovarian tumors such as granulosa cell tumor, thecoma or luteoma secrete estrogens that initiate sexual precocity and vaginal bleeding without ovulation. Another cause of gonadal sexual precocity may be ovarian tumors like chorioepithelioma or teratoma that secrete chorionic gonadotropins and stimulate the ovaries. Large ovarian tumors may be palpable on abdominal or rectal examination. On the other hand, small tumors are visualized only by roentgen pelvic pneumography. Plasma estrogens are usually elevated to within the adult female range. Patients with chorio-epithelioma also have very high serum and urinary HCG. Superficial cells are seen in vaginal smears. Surgical removal of the ovarian tumor causes regression of sexual precocity, cessation of vaginal bleedings and disappearance of estrogens and gonadotropins — if they were present — in body fluids.

ADRENAL PSEUDOPRECOCIOUS PUBERTY

In some patients with congenital adrenocortical hyperplasia, sexual precocity, breast enlargement and vaginal bleeding may precede the appearance of virilization by months or even years. Clitoral enlargement and the elevated urinary 17-ketosteroids, which are returned to normal by dexamethasone, indicate the adrenal etiology of sexual precocity in these patients.

TYPES OF PRECOCIOUS PUBERTY IN YOUNG MALES

About 60% of the males with precocious puberty undergo organic changes in the brain that involve the hypothalamus. Other types of sexual precocity: idiopathic, Albright's syndrome or that associated with juvenile hypothyroidism are extremely rare.

Fig. 1. A 2-year-old female with "premature thelarche." Breast enlargement persisted for the next 14 months of observation but nipples and areolae remained pale and undeveloped. No other signs of precocious puberty were noted. Serum LH and FSH are undetectable, serum prolactin is 8 ng/ml.

Fig. 2A. An 8-year-old male with neurogenic precocious puberty caused by a spongioblastoma damaging the floor of the third ventricle exhibits sexual maturation, excessive height (148 cm, 58 in.), gynecomastia, sloping shoulders, short extremities as compared to trunk. Bone age is accelerated (16 years). Serum prolactin markedly elevated, 390 ng/ml, serum LH 98 mIU/ml and FSH 18 mIU/ml (Courtesy S Sobieszczyk, MD, Poznań, Poland).

Fig. 2B. The same patient showing intensive acne on the face, convergent squint, sloping shoulders and enlarged breasts with dark nipples.

Fig. 2C. Genitalia of the same patient. Note penis, testes and scrotum of adult male size and presence of pubic hair.

PLATE 3

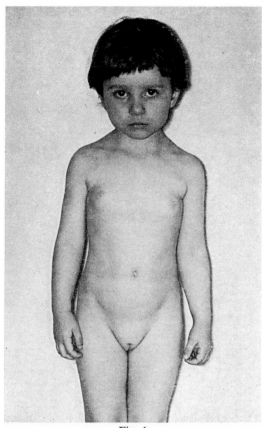

Fig. 1

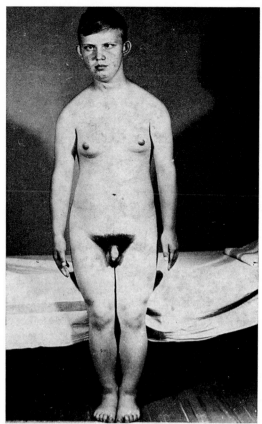

Fig. 2A

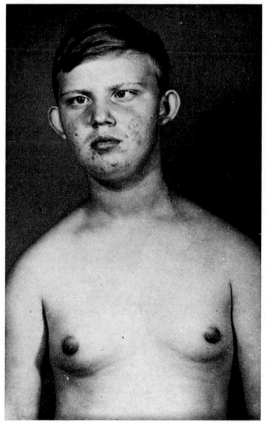

Fig. 2B

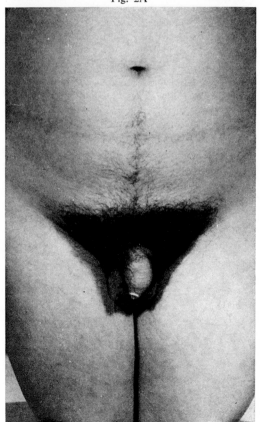

Fig. 2C

NEUROGENIC PRECOCIOUS PUBERTY

Brain tumors such as hamartoma of the hypothalamus or tuber cinereum, glioma, astrocytoma, tumor of the pineal gland or ectopic pinealoma, teratoma, internal hydrocephalus, inflammatory processes (encephalitis, meningoencephalitis) or granulomatous changes are among the causes of neurogenic precocious puberty. Clinical evidence of hypothalamic involvement is noted in the majority of these patients. Pineal tumors may evoke sexual precocity either by altered secretion of biogenic amines or by direct pressure on the hypothalamus. Clinical manifestations usually appear between the ages of 3 and 9 years. The genitals enlarge and the testes gradually assume the size of those of a normal adult male. Spermatogenesis may be identified by seminal fluid examination or by testicular biopsy. Pubic and axillary hair appear; the voice becomes low pitched; there is acceleration of growth and muscular development. Hormonal studies show plasma testosterone has increased to adult male levels and does not respond to dexamethasone suppression. Roentgen studies show advanced bone age, and, frequently, in cases with suprasellar tumors, enlargement of the sella turcica and shortening of the dorsum.

There is a high incidence of EEG abnormalities. Neurologic manifestations of brain tumor or hypothalamic syndrome are common and include headache, visual disturbances, papilledema, extremes in appetite leading to obesity or emaciation, deficient mental development, convulsions, behavioral deviations, temperature elevation, insomnia or somnolence, increased thirst and other signs of diabetes insipidus.

All patients need careful neurologic examination, including cerebral angiography and pneumoencephalography to diagnose the cause of the condition and to determine the site and extension of the lesion.

Idiopathic precocious puberty in young males may be diagnosed only after careful exclusion of organic lesion of the brain; neurologic, ophthalmologic and roentgenographic examinations should be repeated periodically as a small brain tumor may be undetectable in the first stage.

GONADAL PSEUDOPRECOCIOUS PUBERTY IN YOUNG MALES

Endocrine tumors of the testes, especially interstitial cell adenoma and sometimes ectopic testicular tumors, secrete large quantities of androgens and initiate sexual precocity in young males. Testicular tumors vary in diameter from 1 to 10 cm, and are easily palpable on examination. The contralateral testis remains infantile. Urinary 17-ketosteroids are elevated in half the cases. Plasma and urinary testosterone are elevated but revert to normal levels after surgical removal of the tumor.

Fig. 1A. A 3$^1/_2$-year-old male with neurogenic precocious puberty after surgical removal of a hamartoma in the hypothalamus. At the age of 3$^1/_2$ headaches started, followed by unsteady gait, seizures, visual disturbances and vomiting. Height increased to 117 cm (46 in.). Exophthalmos, squint, marked emaciation, and enlargement of the genitals are seen. The testes are of nearly adult size; very scanty pubic hair.

Fig. 1B. Roentgenogram of the hand of the above patient reveals an advanced bone age (7 years).

Fig. 1C. Roentgenogram of the skull of the same patient shows enormous enlargement of the pituitary fossa with destruction of clinoid processes and shortening of the dorsum of the sella.

Fig. 2. Sexual maturation, enlargement of the genitals, especially the testes, and development of pubic and axillary hair in a 7-year-old patient with neurogenic precocious puberty caused by internal hydrocephalus.

PLATE 4

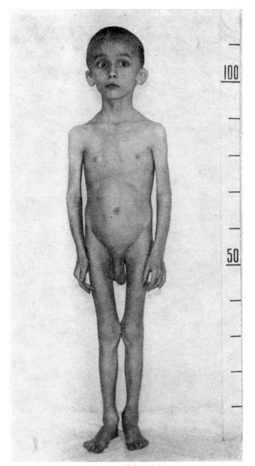

Fig. 1A

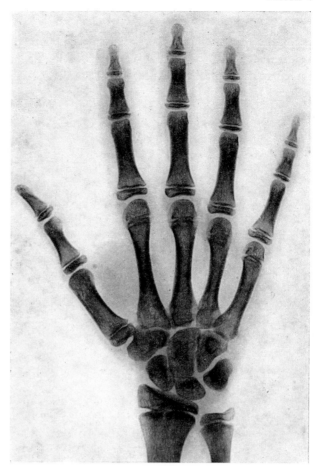

Fig. 1B

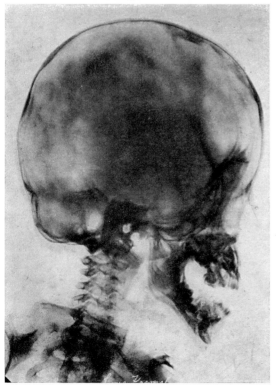

Fig. 1C

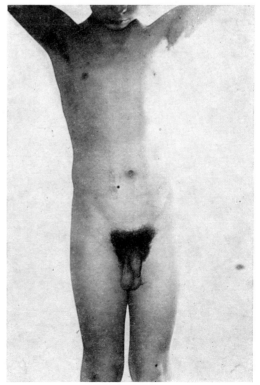

Fig. 2

ADRENAL PSEUDOPRECOCIOUS PUBERTY IN YOUNG MALES

Congenital adrenal hyperplasia precipitates precocious sexual development of a masculine nature in young males. The testes, however, remain infantile, and there is no spermatogenesis. Physical growth and muscular development is grossly accelerated. The urinary 17-ketosteroids are markedly elevated and are reduced to normal levels by administration of cortisol or its derivatives. (Further discussion of adrenal pseudoprecocious puberty is found in Chapter 3.)

ECTOPIC TUMORS ASSOCIATED WITH PSEUDOPRECOCIOUS PUBERTY

There are rare types of precocious sexual development due to excessive secretion of gonadotropins from abnormal sources. Chorioepitheliomas and some teratomas may secrete large amounts of chorionic gonadotropin and stimulate the Leydig cells. It is also probable that the effects of hepatoblastomas are due to secretion by the tumors of substances similar to chorionic gonadotropin or gonadotropin-releasing hormone as the testes in these patients show marked Leydig cell hyperplasia without maturation of the seminiferous tubules or spermatogenesis.

Chapter 8

THE PARATHYROIDS

PRIMARY HYPERPARATHYROIDISM

Primary hyperparathyroidism is a chronic condition in which there is an excess of parathyroid hormone with subsequent hypercalcemia and pathologic changes in the kidneys, and in the gastrointestinal and the skeletal systems. The most common cause is a single adenoma located in one of the parathyroids or, infrequently, in the mediastinum. Rare occurrences result from multiple adenomas, hyperplasia or parathyroid cancer. The disease is insidious and may escape diagnosis for several years until recurring kidney stones, bone changes or a laboratory finding of hypercalcemia disclose hyperparathyroidism as being the true cause of these abnormalities.

Symptoms

1. Easy fatigability.
2. Polyuria and polydipsia, resembling diabetes insipidus; nocturia.
3. Lack of appetite; weight loss.
4. Nausea, vomiting; constipation.
5. Pains in legs or spine, sometimes pains in other bones.
6. Apathy.
7. Symptoms of renal calculi.
8. Symptoms of duodenal ulcer.

Signs

1. No signs in some patients.
2. Bone fractures or deformities, genu varum.
3. Local swellings of bones due to osteoclastoma.
4. Tumor of the jaw (epulis).
5. Clubbing of fingers.
6. Hypotonia of muscles (decrease in the muscle tone).
7. Corneal calcifications.

Renal Manifestations

An increase in the daily output of urine and excessive thirst are early symptoms. Patients drink large quantities of liquids, usually from 2 to 5 liters/day, sometimes as much as 10 liters. These symptoms closely resemble those of diabetes insipidus. Polydipsia and polyuria disappear immediately following removal of the parathyroid tumor.

The renal function in hyperparathyroidism is impaired early, the first sign is a loss of concentrating ability. During a concentration test the specific gravity of the urine remains low, ranging from 1.005 to 1.015.

In the majority of cases urolithiasis develops; the stones are often bilateral and recurrent. In some cases calcium deposits accumulate in the renal parenchyma; this nephrocalcinosis can be seen on roentgenograms or stated histologically in renal biopsy specimens. Nephrocalcinosis is not characteristic of hyperparathyroidism, as it occurs occasionally in hypervitaminosis D, tubular acidosis, sarcoidosis, multiple myeloma, chronic pyelonephritis or skeletal metastases of malignant tumors. Long standing hyperparathyroidism may lead to chronic renal insufficiency and death.

Fig. 1A. Roentgenogram of the skull of a 38-year-old female with hyperparathyroidism and advanced osteodystrophy. Numerous small areas of bone resorption, leading to the characteristic salt-and-pepper appearance of the vault — note the "motheaten" contour. Area of increased density above the orbital roof is a giant cell tumor; there is a cyst in the mandibular shaft. Plasma calcium 6.2 mEq/liter, serum parathyroid hormone concentration 5.8 ng/ml.

Fig. 1B. Roentgenogram of the chest of the same patient reveals a decrease in bone density, cystic changes and fractures in several ribs.

Fig. 1C. Roentgenogram of the hand of the same patient shows a general decline in bone density, multiple cysts and expansion of shafts in phalanges and metacarpals.

Fig. 1D. Extensive osteodystrophy of the humerus and ulna in the same patient. There are multiple cystlike lesions in the distal end of the humerus, a huge cyst completely destroying the bone structure and deforming the outline of the ulna, and an area of increased density (osteoclastoma) in the distal portion of the radius.

Fig. 2. Numerous cysts in both tibia in a patient with primary hyperparathyroidism.

PLATE 1

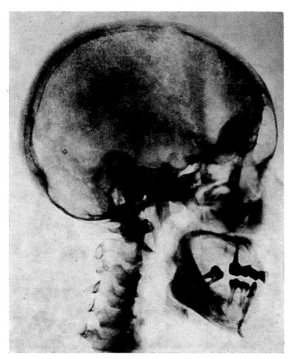

Fig. 1A

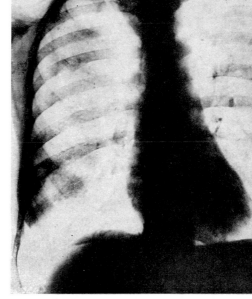

Fig. 1B

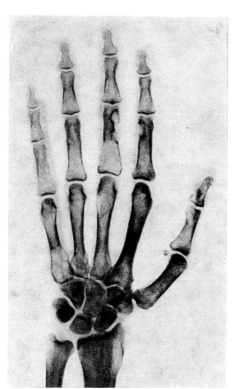

Fig. 1C

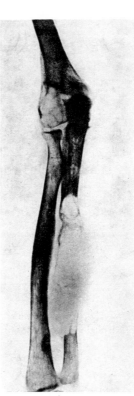

Fig. 1D

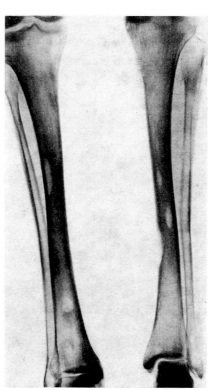

Fig. 2

Gastrointestinal Manifestations

Anorexia with subsequent loss of weight is a frequent occurrence in the majority of patients. Nausea, pernicious vomiting and constipation frequently occur also. The incidence of peptic ulcers, especially duodenal ulcers, is definitely higher than in the general population. The epigastric pains become more severe if large quantities of milk are ingested.

Skeletal and Roentgen Manifestations

Skeletal changes are frequently found in the advanced stages of hyperparathyroidism. The first symptom may be bone deformity, tumor or fracture. In the early stages, about 40% of the cases show skeletal involvement. Roentgen studies show a generalized decrease in bone density, most noticeable in the spine. The cortex of long bones is thinned. In the shafts and metaphyses of long bones, ribs and clavicles multiple cysts of varying sizes develop, leading to bowing, deformities and fractures. A classic sign of parathyroid hormone excess is subperiosteal bone resorption, primarily found radially in the middle phalanges and in the proximal ends of the tibia. Resorption in the distal phalanges may cause dissolution of the phalangeal tufts and clubbing of the fingers.

The skull frequently reveals coarse, meshed trabeculation with granular or miliary areas of bone resorption. Osteoclastomas may appear in the jaw; the lamina dura of the teeth disappear. After surgical removal of the parathyroid adenoma the cysts and bone atrophy gradually regress while the osteoclastomas calcify extensively. In addition to the signs already mentioned, roentgen studies are also of assistance in diagnosing nephrolithiasis and nephrocalcinosis, and calcifications in the pancreas, liver, prostate and in other sites.

Fig. 1A. Hand of a 56-year-old female with primary hyperparathyroidism shows shortened, clubbed distal phalanges, constricted middle phalanges and dry, atrophic skin.

Fig. 1B. Roentgenogram of the hand of the same patient reveals marked thinning of distal phalanges, partial disappearance of tufts, advanced subperiosteal bone resorption in middle and proximal phalanges, typical of hyperparathyroidism.

Fig. 1C. Roentgenogram of the chest of the same patient showing a generalized demineralization of ribs and concave shape of sides of thorax.

Fig. 2. Duodenal ulcer is seen in a 34-year-old female with primary hyperparathyroidism.

PLATE 2

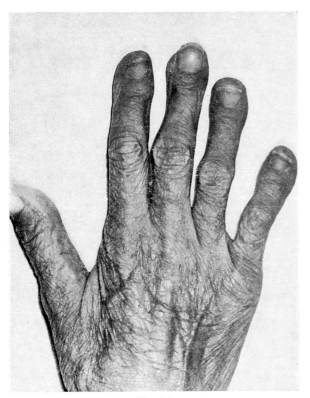

Fig. 1A

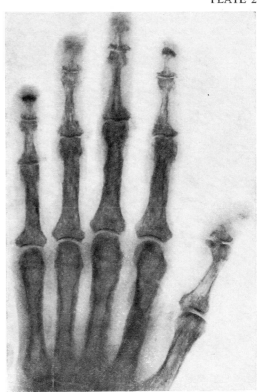

Fig. 1B

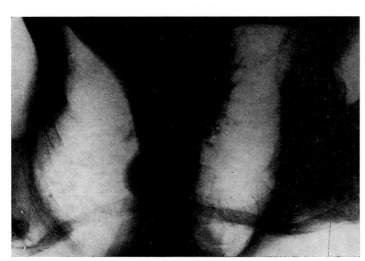

Fig. 1C

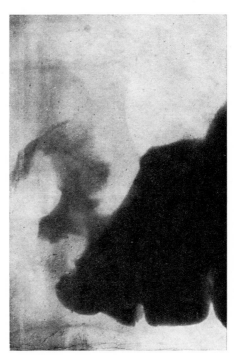

Fig. 2

Laboratory Findings

1. Hypercalcemia — a constant finding. The ionic calcium fraction is especially high.
2. Increased plasma parathyroid hormone concentration.
3. No drop in plasma parathyroid hormone concentration during calcium infusion in the majority of patients.
4. Hypercalciuria found in 60% of cases. However, patients in early stages, as well as those with renal insufficiency, may not have hypercalciuria.
5. Hypophosphatemia found in about 50% of cases.
6. Plasma alkaline phospohatase increased in cases complicated by bone disease.
7. Decrease in tubular reabsorption rate of phosphorus to below 65% after phosphorus load 2.5 g/day for three days.
8. Cortisone suppression test: administration of corticosteroids, e.g., cortisone 150 mg/day for 7 to 10 days, does not reduce hypercalcemia in hyperparathyroidism as it does in sarcoidosis, multiple myeloma and hypervitaminosis D.
9. Increased urinary hydroxyproline.
10. No response to parathyroid hormone in tubular reabsorption rate of phosphorus. Parathyroid hormone administration decreases tubular reabsorption rate in both normal subjects and patients with hypercalcemia, whereas patients with hyperparathyroidism are resistant.
11. Augmentation of hypercalcemia and hypercalciuria during phosphorus and calcium deprivation.
12. Parathyroid adenoma may occasionally be detected by parathyroid scan after ^{75}Se selenomethionine administration.
13. Hyposthenuria; low specific gravity of the urine.
14. ECG: QT interval shorter in patients with marked hypercalcemia.

ACUTE HYPERPARATHYROIDISM

In chronic hyperparathyroidism a sudden deterioration, called hyperparathyroid crisis (or acute hyperparathyroidism), is characterized by rapid progression of renal, gastrointestinal and psychic manifestations along with an abrupt rise in the plasma calcium due to excessive secretion of parathyroid hormone.

The general condition becomes serious; prostration, fever, tachycardia, abdominal pains, persistent vomiting, gastrointestinal hemorrhages with hematemesis and melena develop. Symptoms in the central nervous system include agitation, usually followed by apathy and coma. Renal infarctions, tubular and glomerular necrosis lead to acute renal insufficiency manifested by oliguria, and an increase in creatinine, urea, potassium and inorganic phosphorus in the serum. Acute hyperparythyroidism frequently terminates in death.

SECONDARY HYPERPARATHYROIDISM

Secondary hyperparathyroidism may be encountered in a variety of clinical conditions involved with disturbed calcium homeostasis, including malabsorption, kidney disease, vitamin D deficiency and pseudohypoparathyroidism. Malabsorption syndromes, i.e., pancreatic disease, sprue, celiac disease, et al., severely impair calcium and vitamin D absorption. In chronic

---

Fig. 1. The posterior of the thyroid showing the location of the parathyroid glands and a small adenoma in the right lower gland.

Figs. 2A to 2C. Subperiosteal bone resorption in renal osteodystrophy. *A.* Before treatment. Extensive erosion of the periosteal surfaces and uneven outline of the phalanges are seen. *B.* After therapy. Regression of changes and smooth surface of the phalanges are evident. *C.* Note complete reconstruction of the cortex and normal appearance of the bones after prolonged therapy (Courtesy CE Dent, London).

Fig. 3. Nephrocalcinosis in a 41-year-old patient with hyperparathyroidism. Calcium deposits are primarily located in the medulla of the kidney, around the renal pelvis and calyces.

Fig. 4. Band keratopathy as seen in hyperparathyroidism and other hypercalcemic states. White bands appear on lateral margins of cornea, in contrast to those which develop on superior and inferior margins in arcus juvenilis and senilis (Courtesy IM Braverman, reproduced from Skin Signs of Systemic Disease, WB Saunders, 1970).

Fig. 5. Results of parathyroid hormone (PTH) radioimmunoassay in patients with chronic renal failure, in control subjects and in 4 cases of primary hyperparathyroidism with skeletal involvement. Markedly elevated PTH is found in the majority of patients with chronic uremia indicating a high occurrence of secondary hyperparathyroidism.

PLATE 3

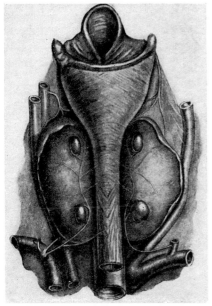

Fig. 1

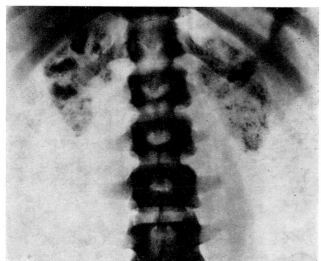

Figs. 2A to 2C

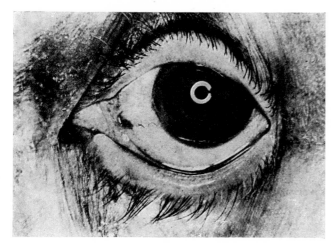

Fig. 3

Fig. 4

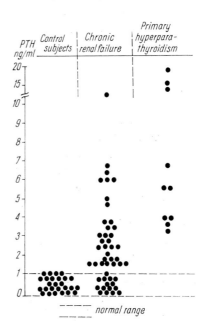

Fig. 5

renal failure, deficient secretion of 1,25-dihydrocholecalciferol leads to reduced calcium and phosphate absorption from the intestine, and lowering of plasma calcium. These changes cause enlargement of parathyroids and excessive secretion of parathyroid hormone. Clinical manifestations consist of apathy, muscular weakness and bone tenderness. Radiologic evidence of rickets is seen in children, and osteomalatia and osteitis fibrosa in adults. Serum parathyroid hormone is greatly elevated, although plasma calcium is low or normal. This is in contrast to primary hyperparathyroidism where the plasma calcium is constantly elevated.

HYPOPARATHYROIDISM

Hypoparathyroidism is a chronic condition characterized by parathyroid hormone deficiency, hypocalcemia and tetany. The most common cause is removal of or damage to the parathyroids during thyroidectomy. Idiopathic hypoparathyroidism, a very rare condition, is probably the result of faulty development of parathyroids; its manifestations appear in childhood.

Signs and Symptoms

1. Painful paresthesia in the limbs; tingling in the extremities.
2. Muscular cramps; carpopedal spasms common; stiffness in hands and feet.
3. Laryngeal stridor.
4. Twitching in face and eyelids.
5. Generalized epileptoid convulsions; incontinence of urine sometimes seen in severe cases.
6. Cataracts.
7. Dry skin; brittle nails; falling hair.
8. Latent tetany: grimacing, awkwardness, tremor, stumbling and muscular rigidity.
9. Trousseau's sign: induction of a typical carpal spasm within 3 min after application of pressure on the arm to stop the blood flow.
10. Chvostek's sign: twitching of the facial muscles on tapping.
11. Idiopathic hypoparathyroidism: mental retardation, sometimes blepharitis and photophobia.

Laboratory Findings

1. Hypocalcemia.
2. Hyperphosphatemia.
3. Low or undetectable serum parathyroid hormone.
4. Absence of signs and symptoms of renal insufficiency, rickets, osteomalacia, chronic diarrhea or alkalosis.
5. EEG: increased diffuse activity resembling *grand mal* epilepsy.
6. ECG: QT period prolonged.
7. Electromyogram (EMG): appearance of periodic electrical discharges lasting several minutes following release of pressure on the arm.
8. Roentgenogram of the skull: calcification of the basal ganglia in idiopathic hypoparathyroidism.

Fig. 1. A positive Trousseau's sign (obstetric hand) that developed following thyroidectomy in a patient with hypoparathyroidism. Extension of fingers in interphalangeal joints, flexion in the metacarpophalangeal joints and wrist, and adduction of the thumb are typical of tetany.

Fig. 2. ECG of a 32-year-old patient with postoperative hypoparathyroidism and tetany. Marked prolongation of the QT period is clearly seen.

Fig. 3. EMG of a 28-year-old patient with hypoparathyroidism, taken 5 min after removal of peripheral circulatory occlusion, shows periodic appearance of spontaneous discharges.

Figs. 4A and 4B. *A*. Results of plasma calcium assays in 12 patients with hypoparathyroidism before and during vitamin D therapy. In all untreated patients plasma total and ionized calcium concentrations are definitely lowered. *B*. In some cases phosphate concentration is elevated. After treatment with large doses of vitamin D 50,000 to 150,000 U/day, plasma calcium reverts to almost normal range.

PLATE 4

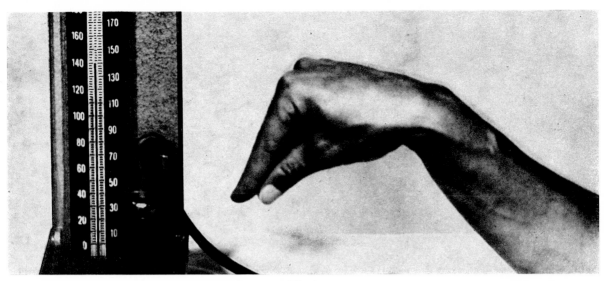

Fig. 1

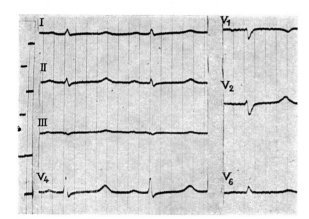

Fig. 2

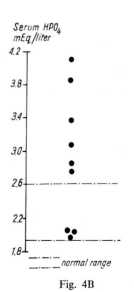

Fig. 3

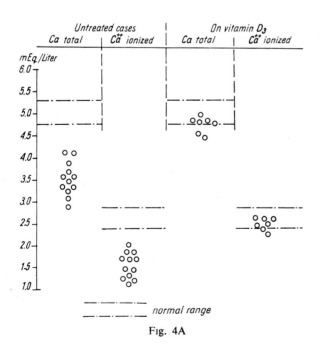

Fig. 4A

Fig. 4B

307

PSEUDOHYPOPARATHYROIDISM

The clinical manifestations of this rare condition are short stature, rounded face, strabismus, fourth and fifth fingers and toes shortened and, usually, mental deficiency. The disease is often familial. Muscular weakness and a latent or manifest tetany are present as well as low plasma calcium and high plasma phosphorus. Plasma parathyroid hormone concentration is elevated. The tetany is resistant to parathyroid hormone administration and there is no response to this hormone in plasma calcium level and urinary cyclic AMP excretion.

Roentgen findings. Roentgenograms of the skull may show intracranial calcifications and increased thickness and density of the calvarial bones. Roentgenograms of the hand reveal shortening of the metacarpals, predominantly the fourth and fifth, less frequently the first or others. The shortened metacarpal usually has a broad shaft and squared head of diminished density. The epiphyses of some phalanges are abnormally triangular in shape and fuse precociously with their shafts, the end result being brachyphalangia. Ectopic calcifications are occasionally noted.

PSEUDO-PSEUDOHYPOPARATHYROIDISM

The condition is characterized by the same clinical and roentgenographic manifestations as pseudo-hypoparathyroidism, but tetany is not present, and plasma calcium and phosphorus are normal.

Fig. 1. A 10-year-old female with pseudohypoparathyroidism and mental retardation. Short stature (height 121 cm, 48 in.), round face and squint are evident.

Fig. 2. The 16-year-old sister of the patient shown in Fig. 1 with pseudohypoparathyroidism. Height 138 cm (54 in.). Rounded face, normal sexual maturation can be seen. No response in urinary cyclic AMP to intravenous PTH administration.

Fig. 3. Roentgenogram of the hand of the patient shown in Fig. 1. Shortening of the 4th and 5th metacarpals and premature fusion of the epiphyses of several phalanges are seen.

Fig. 4. Effects of PTH 300 U on urinary excretion of cyclic 3′,5′-AMP in control subjects and in patients with pseudohypoparathyroidism. There is a brisk rise in cyclic AMP excretion in all control subjects 15 min after PTH infusion. No response is seen in pseudohypoparathyroidism (Courtesy Chase LR, Melson GL, Aurbach GD: J Clin Invest 48:1832, 1969).

PLATE 5

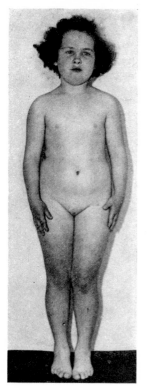

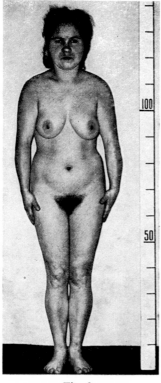

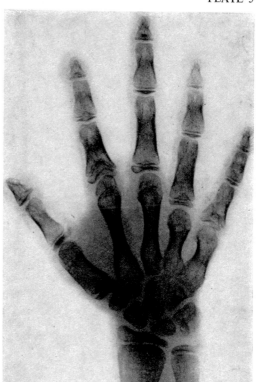

Fig. 1   Fig. 2   Fig. 3

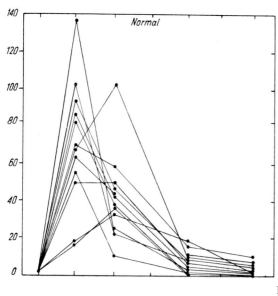

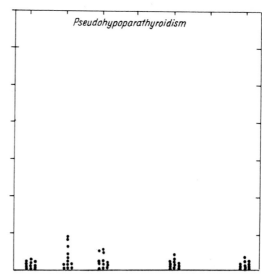

Fig. 4

PANCREATIC TUMORS WITH HORMONAL ACTIVITY

INSULINOMA

(HYPERINSULINISM)

Insulinoma, a tumor composed of beta cells and located in the pancreatic islets, produces excessive amounts of insulin and gives rise to attacks of hypoglycemia. Clinical manifestations of hypoglycemic episodes, which usually follow a prolonged fast, vary greatly from one person to another, but in a given individual the episodes tend to be similar though they differ in severity. The tumor is usually benign, rarely malignant or multiple, and affects adults and children over the age of 4.

All clinical manifestations disappear after successful surgical removal of insulinoma. In untreated patients severe hypoglycemia may cause permanent damage to the brain and irreparable mental disturbances.

Signs and Symptoms

1. Sweating.
2. Heart palpitations.
3. Slurred speech.
4. Fainting.
5. Disorders of gait.
6. Paresthesias.
7. Transient hemiparesis.
8. Dizziness.
9. Confusion; mental disturbances; occasionally aggression.
10. Trembling.
11. Seizures.
12. Deep coma.
    The manifestations disappear rapidly on intravenous administration of glucose.

Laboratory Findings

1. High plasma insulin levels after an overnight fast.
2. Hypoglycemia, ranging from 20 to 50 mg/100 ml, after fasting for 12 to 24 hr.
3. Prolonged fasting is a particularly useful diagnostic procedure; 24 to 48 hr fast with exercise provokes hypoglycemic episodes with clinical manifestations and a marked drop in blood sugar.
4. Intravenous tolbutamide administration induces marked hypoglycemia and excessive insulin response.
5. Glucose tolerance test in some cases shows a low fasting level of blood glucose, a small rise following glucose administration and hypoglycemic values after 2 to 4 hr.
6. Disappearance of hyperinsulinism and hypoglycemia after removal of the tumor.

Fig. 1. Results of repetitive determinations of blood glucose in 6 patients with surgically confirmed pancreatic tumors (4 patients with benign insulinoma and 2 patients with carcinoma). Basal blood glucose is definitely lowered to below 50 mg/100 ml, only sporadically reaching normal levels.

Fig. 2. Basal serum insulin levels by radioimmunoassay in control subjects and in 5 cases of insulinoma. In the majority of healthy subjects basal serum insulin concentration is between undetectable and 20 μU/ml; after 24 hr without food, the patient presents very low serum insulin, 0 to 10 μU/ml. In patients with insulinoma, serum insulin is definitely elevated, both in basal conditions and after food deprivation.

Fig. 3. Effects of tolbutamine test on serum insulin concentration in 2 patients with functional hypoglycemia (5 and 6), in control subjects and in 4 patients with insulinoma (1 to 4). In healthy subjects and in patients with functional hypoglycemia, tolbutamide administration 1 g intravenously produced a moderate rise in serum insulin (maximum level 28 to 125 μU/ml).

In 4 patients with insulinoma there was a striking increase in serum insulin, from 190 to over 1000 μU/ml.

Fig. 4. A small adenoma removed from a patient with severe hypoglycemic attacks that began 10 months before. All manifestations disappeared completely after removal of the tumor. Acid ethanol extracts of the tumor in radioimmunoassay revealed very high content of insulin, 2.5 U/mg.

PLATE 1

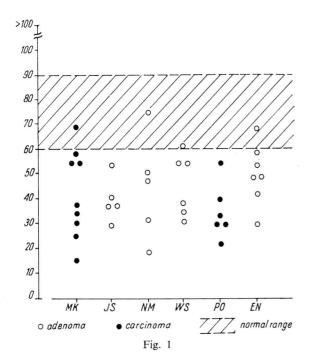

Fig. 1

○ adenoma   ● carcinoma   ▨▨▨ normal range

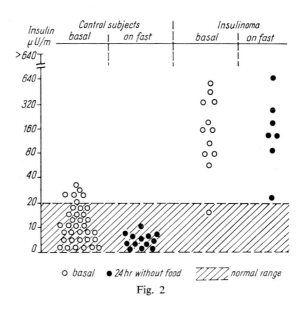

Fig. 2

○ basal   ● 24 hr without food   ▨▨▨ normal range

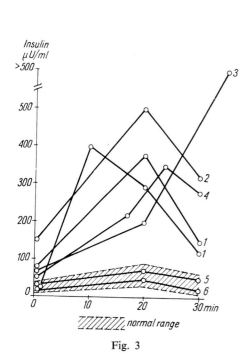

Fig. 3

▨▨▨ normal range

Fig. 4

GLUCAGONOMA

(ALPHA CELL TUMOR)

Alpha cell tumors producing glucagon are very rare and are characterized by weight loss, anemia, dermatitis and stomatitis. The diagnosis can be made on finding a pancreatic tumor associated with diabetes mellitus and excessive amounts of glucagon in plasma. In histopathologic examinations the tumor cells resemble alpha cells of the pancreatic islets. Surgical excision of the tumor leads to disappearance of clinical manifestations and a drop in plasma glucagon concentration to normal.

PANCREATIC TUMOR WITH CUSHING'S SYNDROME

A malignant islet-cell tumor may be an ectopic source of corticotropin that, upon release, may give rise to manifestations of Cushing's syndrome. Obesity and striae, however, are not so frequent as in Cushing's syndrome of adrenal origin. Plasma ACTH is elevated, as are plasma and urinary cortisol. In some patients there is skin hyperpigmentation due to an increase in plasma melanocyte-stimulating hormone. The islet-cell tumor associated with Cushing's syndrome is usually highly malignant, so the survival rate for these patients is not good.

PANCREATIC TUMOR WITH CARCINOID SYNDROME

Carcinoid syndrome in most cases is due to a malignant carcinoid tumor of the ileocecal area. Occasionally pancreatic tumor alone is associated with carcinoid syndrome and is characterized by "flushing," diarrhea and sometimes asthma. Blood serotonin is elevated and urinary 5-hydroxy-indoloacetic acid increased. In some patients the disease is accompanied by hypoglycemia or Cushing's syndrome, as islet-cell tumors can produce a variety of hormones.

ZOLLINGER-ELLISON SYNDROME

Islet-cell tumors that secrete gastrin are associated with hyperacidity and duodenal or jejunal ulcers, forming the Zollinger-Ellison syndrome. The tumors are usually composed of D cells; two thirds of them are malignant. In some cases diarrhea and hypokalemia may develop. Serum gastrin is greatly elevated (above 500 pg/ml) and is not suppressed by HCl administration.

CELLS OF THE APUD SERIES AND ENDOCRINE TUMOR SYNDROMES

(MULTIPLE ENDOCRINE ADENOMATOSIS)

A conception and description of the main characteristics of this group of cells was presented by Pearse in 1969. The term APUD derives from the letters of the 3 most important features of these cells — Amine and Amine Precursor Uptake and Decarboxylation. These characteristics are: the ability of uptake and storage of monoamines and their precursors such as dopa and 5-hydroxytryptamine, and production of polypeptide hormones. The most common methods used in the detection of APUD cells are specific immunofluorescence, argyrophil and argentaphin reaction, masked metachromasia and APUD-formaldehyde induced fluorescence.

Excessive hormone secretion by adenomas or carcinomas composed of the APUD cells may cause several endocrine diseases and involve one or more of the following glands: parathyroids, pituitary, pancreatic islets, thyroid and adrenals. The disease is frequently familial inherited in an autosomal dominant pattern. Simultaneous occurrence of two or more adenomas in various combinations in a patient is termed multiple endocrine adenomatosis; the following variants have been described in literature: type I: adenomas of the anterior pituitary, pancreatic islets, thyroid and adrenal medulla; type II: medullary thyroid carcinoma-pheochromocytoma syndrome; carcinoid syndrome, carcinoid, medullary carcinoma of the thyroid, bronchial adenoma, oat-cell carcinoma, insulinoma; tumors secreting ACTH or ACTH-like substances, neuroblastoma, pheochromocytoma, carcinoid, insulinoma, thyroid medullary carcinoma and bronchial adenoma.

314

Chapter 10

SYNDROMES SIMULATING ENDOCRINE DISORDERS

Primordial dwarfism, or true dwarfism, is characterized by very short stature (3 standard deviations or more below average), but normal mental development and sexual maturation. The condition occurs sporadically in normal families, chiefly affecting the female members. The patients are usually very small at birth, and already in the first years of life growth is markedly stunted and the body build conspicuously delicate. The skin is fine and smooth; the hands and feet are of tiny proportions. The circumference of the head is smaller than normal, amounting in teenagers to between 50 and 52 cm (20 in.). The facial features, however, are mature, corresponding to the chronologic age of the patients. Growth ceases at the normal postpubertal period; the ultimate height attained is usually between 110 and 139 cm (43 to 55 in.).

Laboratory tests do not reveal any abnormalities. Fasting serum HGH is normal and rises in response to hypoglycemia. Serum cholesterol, phosphorus, water loading test, ECGs, reflexograms, ^{131}I uptake, chromatin pattern and chromosomes are also normal.

Postpubertal diagnosis is based on clinical manifestations such as dwarfism and normal sexual development that lacks other abnormalities. In younger female patients the diagnosis is more difficult and the disease is easily mistaken for pituitary dwarfism or Turner's syndrome.

Roentgen studies of the skeletal system are of assistance in early diagnosis. Bone age is normal and the epiphyses fuse to their shafts at the proper time. The dimensions of all bones are proportionally decreased. In females, roentgen pelvic pneumography shows normal-sized internal genitalia. No roentgen manifestations typical of Turner's syndrome are seen. Pituitary dwarfism is characterized by lowered serum HGH concentration which does not rise during hypoglycemia, in contrast to primordial dwarfism in which the levels are normal.

FAMILIAL SHORT STATURE

(FAMILIAL SHORTNESS)

Short stature in otherwise normal subjects is common, especially in young females. The mothers (rarely the fathers), or other female members of the family are also short in stature, the lack of height being more pronounced in the affected patients. Familial short stature is an intermediate stage between normal height and primordial dwarfism.

The patients grow steadily at a rate slightly less than normal and finally attain the height 2 to 3 standard deviations below average [140 to 150 cm (55 to 59 in.) in females and 145 to 155 cm (57 to 61 in.) in males]. Sexual development is normal.

HGH assays and other laboratory studies show normal results. Roentgen examinations of the skeletal system reveal bone age to be normal, but dimensions of the bones are slightly diminished.

During the pubertal period in females it is difficult to differentiate this condition from Turner's syndrome. On roentgen pelvic pneumography normal ovaries are seen; they are absent in Turner's syndrome.

Fig. 1. A 19-year-old patient with primordial dwarfism, undersized and underweight at birth. Regular menstrual cycles began at age 13. Mental development normal. Height 135 cm (53 in.). Feminine body contours, broad hips, female sex characteristics are present. Brisk response of serum HGH to insulin-induced hypoglycemia (3, 31 and 36 ng/ml). Normal serum LH 12 mIU/ml, and FSH 10 mIU/ml.

Fig. 2A. A 16-year-old patient with primordial dwarfism. Stunted growth from birth, delicate build, normal mental and sexual development. Regular menses commenced at age 12. Height 126 cm (50 in.). Typically female habitus; breasts normally developed. A normal HGH response to insulin; serum HGH 2, 29 and 14 ng/ml at 0, 30 and 60 min, respectively.

Fig. 2B. Face of the patient seen in Fig. 2A with no pathologic features present, but with a somewhat childlike appearance.

Fig. 2C. Roentgenogram of the hand and wrist of the same patient shows a proportional diminishing in size of all the bones, which are normal in shape and structure. The epiphyses are already fused to the shafts.

PLATE 1

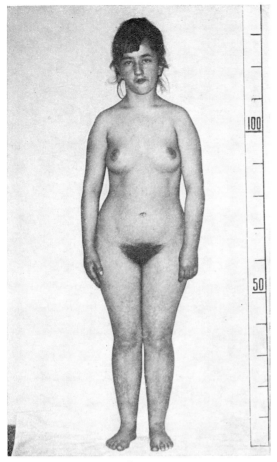

Fig. 1

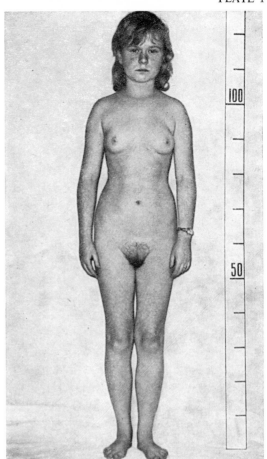

Fig. 2A

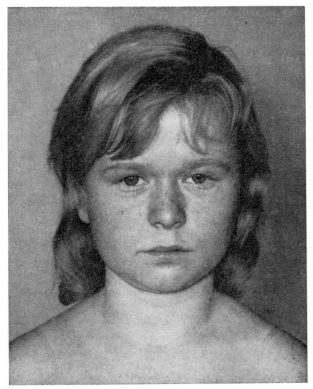

Fig. 2B

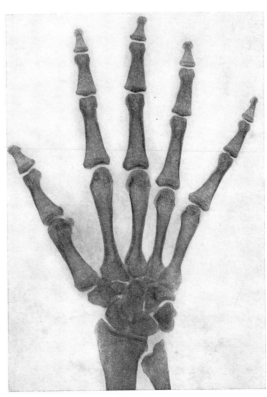

Fig. 2C

PROGERIA

(GILFORD'S PROGERIA; HUTCHINSON-GILFORD SYNDROME)

Progeria is a rare congenital disorder, manifestations of which appear between the first months of life and 3 years. The patients are normal at birth, but their growth subsequently ceases almost completely and they become emaciated and develop a senilitic appearance. The skin becomes wrinkled; there is atrophy of subcutaneous fat and muscles, and baldness; deformities in the joints and early arteriosclerotic changes appear. Typical facial features are prominent scalp vessels, close-set eyes, thin protruding nose and recessed chin. The cause of the disease is entirely unknown. The patients die at an early age from infections or arteriosclerotic complications.

Laboratory findings do not show any definite abnormalities. The bone age is normal.

PROGERIAL DWARFISM

(CACHECTIC DWARFISM; MICROCEPHALIC DWARFISM)

Progerial, cachectic and microcephalic dwarfism are less clearly defined forms of dwarfism in which only some signs and symptoms of Gilford's progeria are present. Marked dwarfism, microcephaly, mental deficiency and cachectic or senile appearance are the cardinal manifestations, but baldness is absent and arteriosclerosis develops later than in progeria. Sexual development is deficient. Death usually occurs between the ages of 15 and 40 years. Roentgen examinations show a normal bone age; on roentgenograms of the skull, calcification of the basal ganglia is common.

Fig. 1A. A 35-year-old female with cachectic dwarfism. Height 119 cm (47 in.), weight 21 kg. Note emaciated and aged appearance; normal sexual hair; poor breast development. Mental retardation present. Menarche commenced at age 19 and ceased several years later.

Fig. 1B. Face of the same patient shows marked progeria, i.e., deep-set eyes with bilateral cataracts, hollow cheeks, thin lips, many wrinkles, suppurating nodule below the left eye (epithelioma on histopathology). Calcification of the basal ganglia is revealed on the roentgenogram of the skull, but no other abnormalities are seen. HGH response to insulin-induced hypoglycemia is normal.

Fig. 2. Gilford's progeria in an 8-year-old male. Height 97 cm (38 in.). Dwarfism, complete baldness, prominent veins on the scalp, thinned extremities, muscular atrophy, protruding abdomen and scleroderma were evident (Courtesy M Walczak, MD, Poznań, Poland).

Figs. 3A and 3B. Face of a 38-year-old female with bird-headed dwarfism. Height 124 cm (49 in.). Note aged appearance, prominent frontal bosses, flattened occiput and beak-like nose. No evidence of hormonal deficiency. Mental retardation present.

PLATE 2

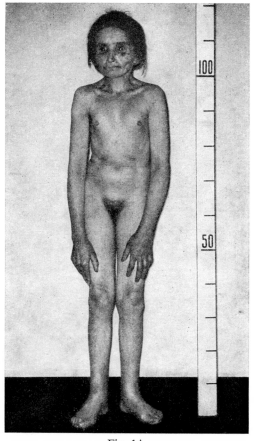

Fig. 1A

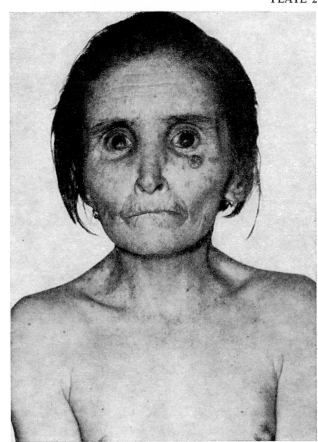

Fig. 1B

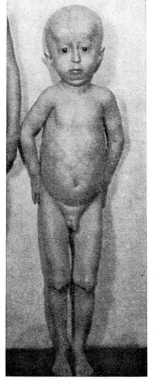

Fig. 2

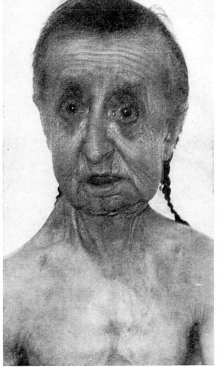

Fig. 3A

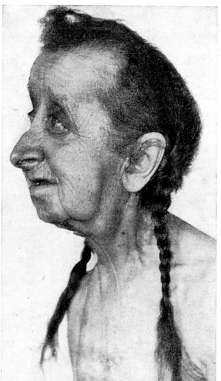

Fig. 3B

BIRD-HEADED DWARFISM

Nanosomia nanocephalica, i.e., bird-headed dwarfism, is a rare form of dwarfism. Its main characteristics are striking shortness of stature, proportionally decreased dimensions of the face and skull and narrow face with protruding and beaked nose, underdeveloped mandible, resembling that of a bird. There is mental deficiency. Sexual development is delayed and deficient; other congenital anomalies may be found. Bone age is delayed in the first decade, but it approaches normal in the second decade. Roentgenograms of the hand and wrist reveal anomalies such as fusion (synostosis) of the semilunate with triangular bones, decreased dimensions of all the bones, or irregular appearance of ossification centers. Skull roentgenograms may reveal underdevelopment of the mandible and zygomatic arches, precocious fusion of the sutures. Other skeletal anomalies are sometimes seen.

Fig. 1A. A 46-year-old patient with bird-headed dwarfism and mandibular ocular facial dyscephaly of Ullrich-Fremerey (Dohn-François) type. Height 124 cm (49 in.). Marked dwarfism, sexual infantilism, pseudogynecomastia, fat deposits on the abdomen are seen.

Fig. 1B. Face of the same patient showing hypotrichosis, prominent frontal bosses, sparse eyebrows and eyelashes, microphthalmos (with blindness) and lack of facial hair growth.

Figs. 1C and 1D. Roentgenograms of the same patient showing triangular shape of the skull (frontal view), elongation of the nasal bone, undeveloped and deformed mandible with enlarged angle, loss of all teeth and recessed chin.

PLATE 3

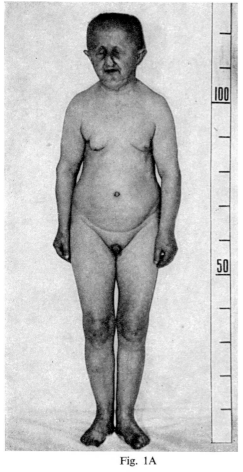

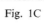

Fig. 1A

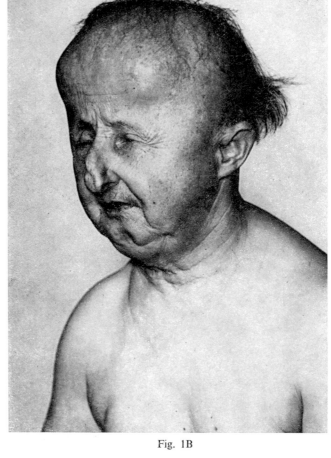

Fig. 1B

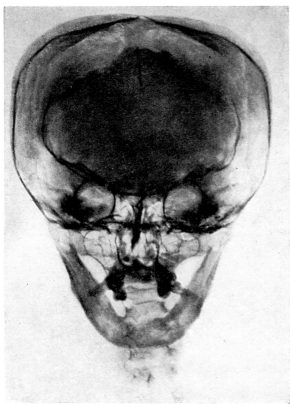

Fig. 1C

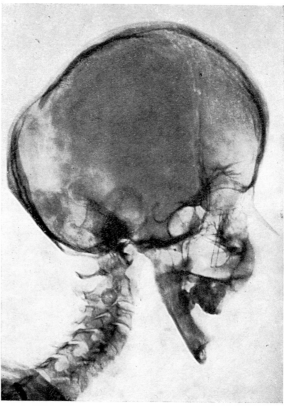

Fig. 1D

D₁ TRISOMY SYNDROME

(TRISOMY 13–15)

The condition presents many developmental anomalies. The basis of the syndrome is autosomal trisomy, that is, the presence of an additional chromosome in the D group. The most frequent clinical findings are cleft palate, cleft lip, microphthalmos or coloboma, malformed and low-set ears, capillary hemangiomas. Simian creases and distal axial triradii are frequently found on the palms. The thumbs are often retroflexible, the distal phalanges narrowed; the nails show longitudinal hyperconvexity.

In roentgen examinations, or in autopsy, additional anomalies are detected, e.g., brain incompletely differentiated due to lack of olfactory tracts and poor frontal lobe development, cardiac anomalies, renal anomalies and others. Cryptorchidism and abnormal scrotal development (in males), and bicornuate uterus (in females) are common. The patients exhibit a lack of mental development, apnea and motor seizures, and usually die in the first months of life, rarely surviving past the first 2 to 3 years.

E₁ TRISOMY SYNDROME

(TRISOMY 17–18)

The syndrome was first described in 1960 by Edwards, *et al.*, and its basis was found to be an additional chromosome, No. 18.

The main features include low birth weight (averaging 5 pounds), retarded physical and mental development, mottled appearance of the skin, persistence of downy body hair and malformation of the auricles which are low set and slanted away from the eyes. The head has a protruding occiput and a small jaw. The sternum is shortened and defectively ossified.

A finding peculiar of E₁ trisomy is the unusual means of clenching of the fingers; the index finger overlaps the third. Sometimes there is elongation of the fifth finger. The dermal ridge pattern is also characteristic; unusually low arches are found on all, or almost all, the fingers. The nails are frequently hypoplastic. There is a limited hip abduction; the big toe is sometimes shortened and in a dorsiflexed position; talipes equinovarus, or rocker-bottom feet, and posterior displacement of the heel are frequent. Cardiac anomalies, especially ventricular septal defects associated with patent ductus arteriosus, and renal anomalies, chiefly horseshoe kidney, or duplication of the pelvis and ureters, are common. Diaphragmatic hernia, eventration or defective development of the musculoskeletal system have also been found. As a rule death occurs in early infancy.

Fig. 1. Head of a patient with trisomy 17–18 showing prominent occiput, low-set ears, recessed chin, and hypermobility of the shoulders due to sternum defect.

Fig. 2. Position of the hand in trisomy 17–18. The second finger is flexed and overlaps the third. The nails are hypoplastic.

Fig. 3. The lower extremities of a patient with trisomy 17–18 showing typical anomalies, i.e., the big toes in retroflexed position and rocker-bottom feet.

Fig. 4. Abnormalities in the external genitalia show strikingly undeveloped, "empty" scrotum and deformed penis in a patient with trisomy 17–18.

Fig. 5. Roentgenogram of the chest of a patient with trisomy 17–18 showing thin and wavy ribs, congenital heart defect and diaphragmatic hernia.

PLATE 4

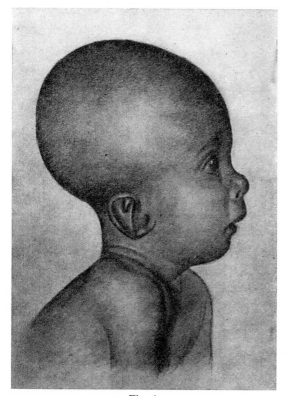

Fig. 1

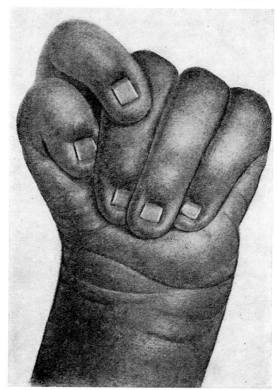

Fig. 2

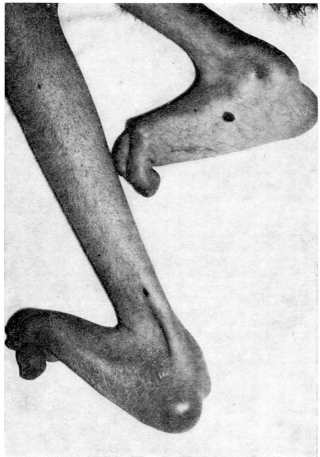

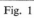

Fig. 3

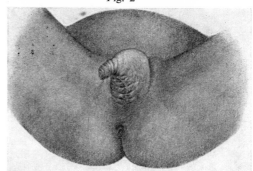

Fig. 4

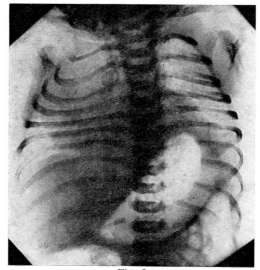

Fig. 5

MONGOLISM

(DOWN'S DISEASE; TRISOMY 21-22)

Mongolism is a frequent congenital disorder associated with chromosomal anomalies, usually trisomy 21-22, or translocations. It is more common among offspring of older mothers. The main manifestations are classic facial features, moderate to severe mental retardation and delayed physical development. There is a marked delay in speech and walking; growth is stunted. Microcephaly, flattening of the occiput, rosy cheeks, small and simply convoluted auricles, shortened palpebral fissures slanting upwards and, on occasion, epicanthal folds are characteristic manifestations. The tongue is usually fissured and, in some cases, protrudes from the mouth; the voice is frequently hoarse.

The fingers are short; additionally, the fifth finger is curved medially. Simian creases on the palm are frequently seen. Dermatoglyphic findings include a high axial triradius in the hypothenar, 10 ulnar loops on fingertips, a third interdigital loop on the palm and tibial arch or small distal loop in the area of the hallux.

Delay in physical and mental development, constipation, abdominal protrusion and umbilical hernia are common to both mongolism and congenital hypothyroidism, however, the typical facial features and hypermobility of the patients enable a diagnosis of mongolism at first glance, and typical changes of the hand confirm it.

Roentgen examinations of the hip joints show bilateral widening and flaring of iliac wings, the acetabular and iliac angles are decreased, and there is a low iliac index. No roentgen manifestations of congenital hypothyroidism such as epiphyseal dysgenesis, deformity of the lumbar vertebra, large skull with underdeveloped sinuses are present in mongolism, only delayed bone age.

Fig. 1. Face of a 5-year-old girl with mongolism (Down's syndrome) shows changes typical of this disease: small palpebral fissures slanting upwards, widely set eyes, undeveloped bridge of the nose, half-open mouth with slightly protruding tongue. Stunted growth, microcephaly and mental retardation are present.

Fig. 2. Hand of a 9-year-old patient with Down's syndrome is short and broad, the fingers shortened (especially the fifth). There is a simian crease, a transverse palm crease running from the radial to the ulnar border of the palm; on the fifth digit only one crease is seen instead of two.

Figs. 3A and 3B. Pelvis, based on roentgenograms of a patient with mongolism and of a control subject, shows the differences in the acetabular angle. In mongolism the iliac bones are flared and widened and the acetabular and iliac angles have decreased.

PLATE 5

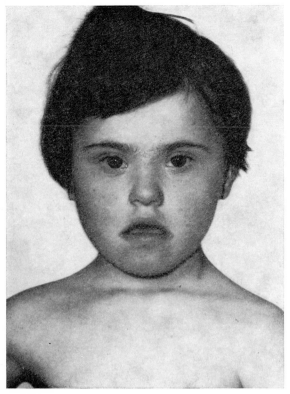

Fig. 1

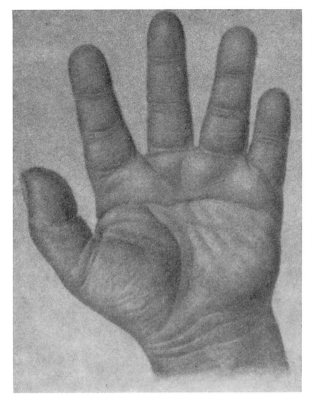

Fig. 2

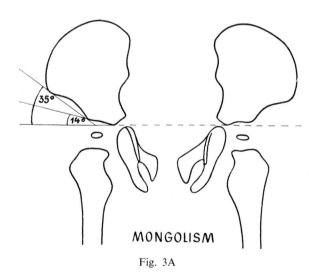

MONGOLISM

Fig. 3A

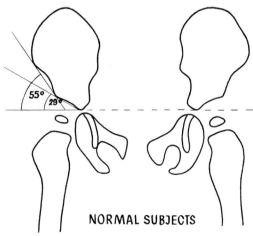

NORMAL SUBJECTS

Fig. 3B

MARFAN'S SYNDROME
(ARACHNODACTYLIA)

The disease is a congenital and familial disorder that affects the musculoskeletal system, the eyes and the cardiovascular system. The incidence of this syndrome is equal in both sexes. The patients are tall with very slender body build, and thin, long extremities. The fingers are very long and thin, giving a spider-like appearance. Frequently there are deformities of the chest and spine, laxity in the joints and poor muscle development. In addition, congenital heart disease, dilatation of the aorta and ocular abnormalities such as ectopia lentis or retinal detachment may be present. Excretion of urinary mucopolysaccharides is increased.

Some patients with homocystinuria present the same clinical manifestations as those with Marfan's syndrome, excessive height, arachnodactylia, pale skin, ectopic lens, skeletal malformations and myopathy. In contrast to Marfan's syndrome, patients with homocystinuria are frequently mentally deficient and already in the first weeks of life show increased urinary excretion of cystine, cysteine, methionine and L-homocystine.

SILVER'S SYNDROME

Silver's syndrome is a rare congenital form of dwarfism associated with hemiatrophy. One of the lower limbs is shorter than the other; in some cases the upper extremity and one side of the face may also be undeveloped. The bone age is normal. There are no hormonal, metabolic or other skeletal abnormalities.

Figs. 1A and 1B. A typical case of Marfan's syndrome in a 20-year-old patient. Note increased height (182 cm, 72 in.), excessively long extremities, poor muscle development and marked kyphoscoliosis.

Fig. 1C. Forearm and hand of the same patient. The fingers are thin and markedly elongated; the muscles are poorly developed.

Fig. 2A. A 7-year-old patient with Silver's syndrome. Note deficient growth (height 108 cm, 43 in.) and asymmetry of the body, the upper and lower extremities on the left side are underdeveloped. The left leg is 3 cm shorter than the right one.

Fig. 2B. Head of the same patient showing protruding frontal bosses.

PLATE 6

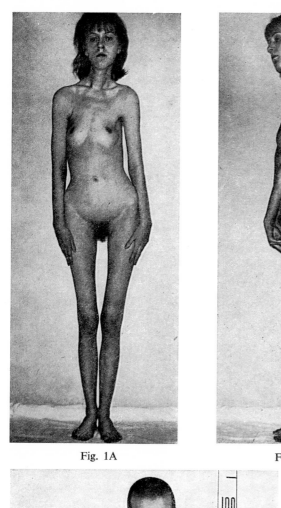

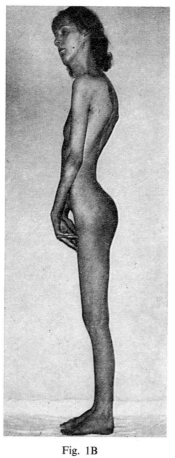

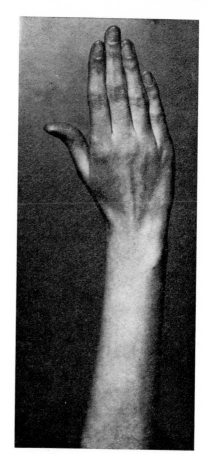

Fig. 1A

Fig. 1B

Fig. 1C

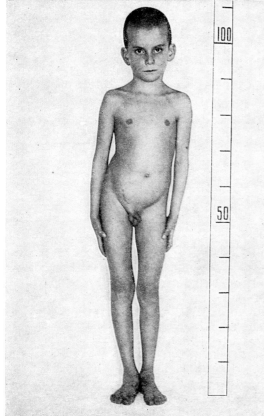

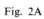

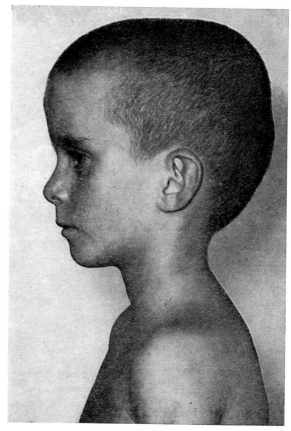

Fig. 2A

Fig. 2B

ACHONDROPLASIA

(ACHONDROPLASTIC DWARFISM; CHONDRODYSTROPHIA FETALIS; MICROMELIA)

This hereditary and congenital disorder is one of the most common types of dwarfism. The main clinical manifestations, already obvious at birth, are short stature, large head and short limbs. The arms and thighs are strikingly short in comparison to the normal-sized trunk. Due to the marked shortness of the limbs, the span is greatly diminished, and the midpoint of stature lies above the umbilicus. The dwarfs usually attain an ultimate height of from 100 to 135 cm (39 to 53 in.).

The head is large with prominent forehead; the base of the nose is depressed. The spine shows increased lumbar lordosis; the buttocks are prominent. The muscles are well developed and the dwarfs are strong. Occasionally, there is genu varum; extension of the elbow joints may be limited. Mental and sexual development is normal. The hands are short and broad with thick, short fingers; the second, third and fourth fingers are nearly equal in length ("trident hand").

Roentgenograms of the hand show that the bone age is normal; the phalanges and metacarpals are short and thick. The ends of the antebrachia are splayed and contain irregular terminal plates; the ulna is shortened is some cases. In the second finger, the epiphyseal plates of the proximal phalanx and metacarpal run obliquely diverging radially instead of being straight. The long bones, especially the femora and the humeri, are of greatly reduced length. Their shafts appear thickened, with exaggerated impressions of the tendons and muscles seen. The ends of the long bones — especially around the knee joints — into which the epiphyses fit closely, are splayed and centrally notched. The epiphyses of long bones are of normal shape and density. The skull is large, while its base is of reduced dimensions, the foramen magnum is often diminished in size and is funnel-shaped. In some patients one of the lumbar vertebral bodies is deformed, i.e., wedge-shaped, causing angular kyphosis. The pelvis is reduced in size. The ilium is abnormal in shape in that the acetabulum is broader than normal. The acetabular angle is reduced and the wing is narrowed.

Laboratory data do not reveal any abnormalities. Diagnosis is based on typical, unmistakable clinical and roentgenographic findings.

Figs. 1A and 1B. A 12-year-old female with achondroplasia. Typical manifestations of the disease are seen: short stature (height 107 cm, 41 in.), large head, short nose with depressed bridge, very short extremities in comparison to the trunk, lumbar lordosis and prominent buttocks. Upper extremities are flexed at the elbows; the arms are extremely shortened.

Fig. 2A. Face of a 10-year-old patient with achondroplasia shows shortened nose with depressed bridge.

Fig. 2B. Hand of the same patient shows broad and stunted fingers of approximately the same length ("trident hand").

Fig. 3. Roentgenogram of the hand and wrist of an 8-year-old patient with achondroplasia. The bone age is normal. The phalanges and metacarpals are broad and short. There is a radial slant to the epiphyseal plate of the second metacarpal and a distal slant to the plate of the adjacent phalanx (arrows). The metaphyses of forearm bones are splayed; epiphyseal plates are irregular.

Fig. 4. Roentgenogram of the knee joint of an 8-year-old achondroplastic dwarf reveals splayed metaphyses of the femur and tibia and irregular epiphyseal plates.

PLATE 7

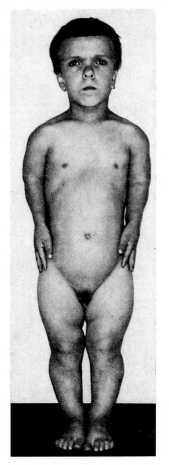
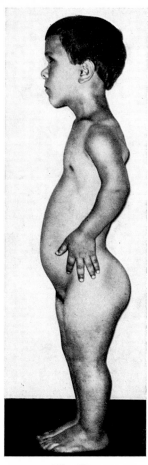
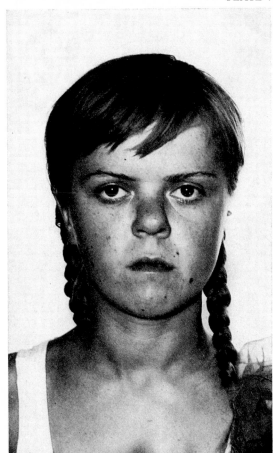

Fig. 1A   Fig. 1B   Fig. 2A

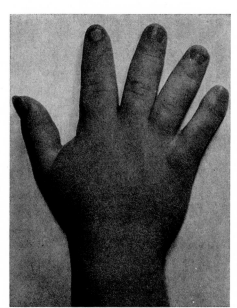
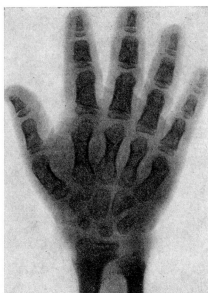
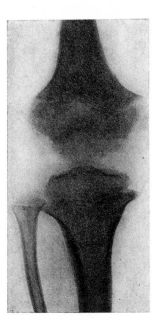

Fig. 2B   Fig. 3   Fig. 4

MULTIPLE EPIPHYSEAL DYSPLASIA

This is a congenital disorder of the skeletal system typified by short stature, shortening of the fingers, limitation of joint movement, and characteristic roentgenographic changes. The disease was formerly often referred to as atypical achondroplasia, dyschondroplasia, Ribbing's disease or epiphyseal dysostosis.

The affected children are normal at birth. The symptoms are noticed usually between the ages of 2 and 5 years, when difficulties in walking are observed. Pains in the knees are common. In the majority of patients, growth is stunted. The shape of the skull is normal. There is usually some flexion in the hip and knee joints. Limitation of movement, especially rotation in the hip joints, is a constant finding; the movements in other joints may also be limited to varying degrees.

Roentgenograms show normal bone age, but there are abnormalities of the epiphyses that are most pronounced in the hips. The femoral heads develop from several irregular ossification centers that later fuse to form an epiphysis flattened and irregular in shape. The femoral neck appears to be shortened and convex in shape, and the acetabula may be irregular and displaced upward. Other epiphyses of long bones, usually the knee joints and metacarpal heads, and the carpal and tarsal bones, are abnormally shaped and develop from irregular ossification centers. Degenerative changes in the hip and in other joints appear in young adults.

Short stature and epiphyseal dysgenesis are common for both multiple epiphyseal dysplasia and congenital hypothyroidism. However, no hormonal abnormalities are found in the former.

METAPHYSEAL DYSOSTOSIS

The common manifestations of this congenital defect of the mataphyses of the long bones are pains in the legs, short stature, genu varum, waddling gait. Roentgen studies demonstrate enlarged and irregular metaphyses, and gross irregularity, widening and occasional fragmentation of the metaphyseal lines. Following epiphyseal fusion, enlargement of the ends of the bones — especially at the ankle and knee — and coarse trabecular structure are seen. No hormonal abnormalities are seen. Clinical and roentgen manifestations resemble vitamin D-refractory rickets; however, in metaphyseal dysostosis the biochemical changes typical of rickets do not occur, nor do the skeletal changes regress upon vitamin D administration.

Fig. 1. A 7-year-old female with hypochondroplasia. Stunted growth (height 104 cm, 41 in.) and shortened extremities, especially the arms and forearms, are evident. Face and hands show no abnormalities.

Fig. 2. Roentgenogram of the hand of a 9-year-old female with multiple epiphyseal dysplasia accompanied by stunted growth and limitation of movements, especially at the hip joints and metacarpal–phalangeal joints. Epiphyses of many long bones of irregular shape and outline. The figure shows short phalanges and metacarpals and grossly abnormal, flattened epiphyses of the metacarpals, radius and ulna.

Figs. 3 and 4. Roentgenograms of the femoral heads in 2 patients with multiple epiphyseal dysplasia resembling epiphyseal dysgenesis in congenital hypothyroidism. The epiphyses are formed of several small, completely irregular ossification centers of uneven density.

Fig. 5. Roentgenogram of the knee joint and lower limb of a 6-year-old female with multiple metaphyseal–epiphyseal dysplasia. The metaphyses are deformed and splayed, with irregular epiphyseal line and grossly disturbed trabecular structure. The epiphyses are of abnormal shape and uneven density.

PLATE 8

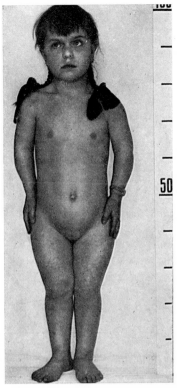

Fig. 1

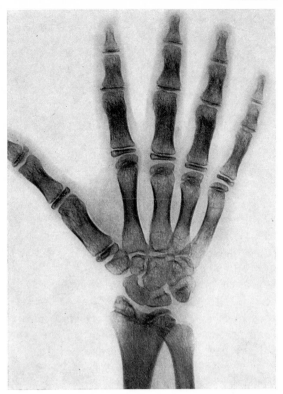

Fig. 2

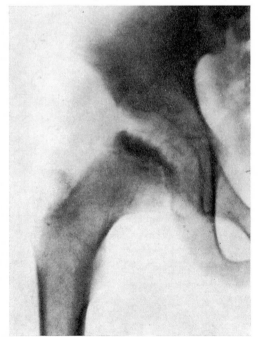

Fig. 3

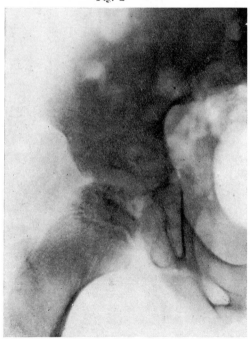

Fig. 4

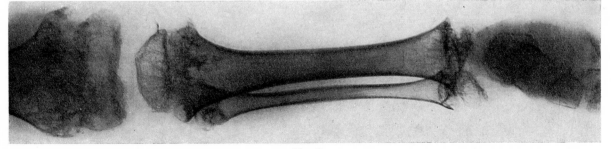

Fig. 5

MUCOPOLYSACCHARIDOSES

Mucopolysaccharidoses are diseases characterized by inborn defects in the metabolism of polysaccharides associated with mental deficiency, short stature, skeletal anomalies, corneal opacities. Five types may be distinguished: Hurler's, Hunter's, Sanfilippo's, Morquio's and Scheie's syndromes.

Type I Mucopolysaccharidosis: Hurler's Syndrome

Hurler's syndrome is a congenital disorder characterized by dwarfism, mental deficiency, skeletal changes, enlargement of the liver and spleen, and corneal opacities. The large head, wide set eyes, underdeveloped bridge of the nose, open mouth and protruding tongue often lead to a mistaken diagnosis of congenital hypothyroidism. The body build is stocky, the neck very short; there is often kyphosis with protruding abdomen and umbilical hernia, flexed knees and hips. The fingers are short and reveal flexion contractures. Urinary mucopolysaccharides, chondroitin sulfate and heparin sulfate, are increased. Reilly-Alder granulations in the lymphocytes may be found.

Typical roentgenographic findings are always present: the skull is large and the pituitary fossa flattened and greatly elongated. The vertebral bodies are not of usual quadratic shape but their upper and lower surfaces are convex. Sometimes a deformity of the first or second lumbar vertebra occurs: the body is small, wedge-shaped or beak-like, displaced backwards and resembling changes found in hypothyroidism. Roentgenograms of the hand show normal bone age, shapeless metacarpals with shafts expanded in the middle, abnormal bone structure with deformed distal ends of the radius and ulna and flexion contractures of the fingers. Coxa valga is common. In young patients the femoral heads may develop from several irregular ossification centers. Enzymatic defects comprise reduced activity of β-galactosidase and increased activity of β-glucuronidase and α-fucosidase.

Type II Mucopolysaccharidosis: Hunter's Syndrome

The manifestations of this syndrome are similar to that of Hurler's syndrome, but of a lesser degree. Mental development may be nearly normal; there are no corneal opacities; deafness is common.

Fig. 1. A 6-year-old patient with type I mucopolysaccharidosis (Hurler's syndrome). Dwarfism (height 92 cm, 36 in.), mental deficiency, large head with prominent frontal bosses and exophthalmos, short neck, protruding abdomen with umbilical hernia, lower extremities flexed at the hips and knees are evident. The liver and spleen are greatly enlarged. Corneal opacities are present.

Fig. 2A. A 4-year-old patient with Hurler's syndrome. Large head rests directly on the shoulders; protruding abdomen with prominent umbilical hernia, flexion contractures at the elbows, hips and knees, imbecility are present.

Fig. 2B. Head of the patient shown in Fig. 2A. Note broad face, widely set eyes, underdeveloped bridge of the nose, open mouth with protruding tongue.

Fig. 2C. Roentgenogram of the pelvis of the same patient reveals coxa valga and flattened, grossly irregular ossification centers of the femoral heads that resemble epiphyseal dysgenesis in congenital hypothyroidism.

Fig. 2D. Roentgenogram of the hand and wrist of the same patient shows shapeless shafts of the metacarpals and phalanges expanded in the middle, flexion contractures of the fingers, deformed radial and ulnar metaphyses and epiphyseal lines slanting medially.

PLATE 9

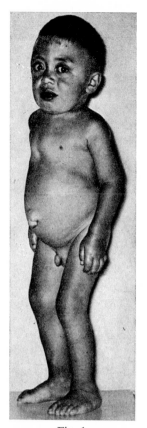

Fig. 1

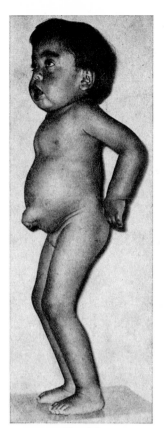

Fig. 2A

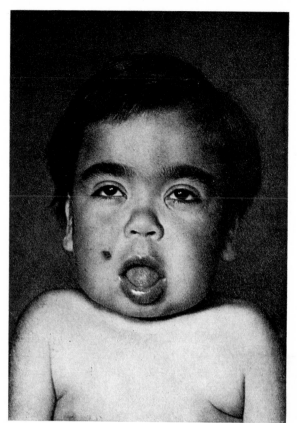

Fig. 2B

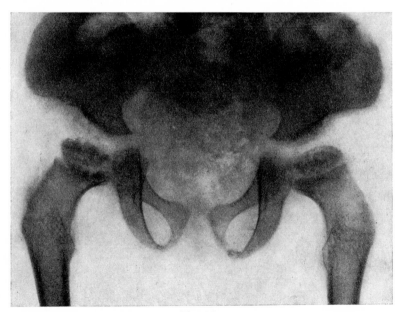

Fig. 2C

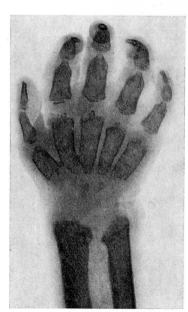

Fig. 2D

Type III Mucopolysaccharidosis: Sanfilippo Syndrome

In this syndrome mental deficiency is greatly pronounced, while somatic manifestations are not very prominent. Mental deficiency is already evident by age 5, then gradually progresses with time to imbecility. Increased amounts of heparin sulfate are found in the urine.

Type IV Mucopolysaccharidosis: Morquio Syndrome

The disease is characterized by dwarfism, marked kyphosis, platyspondylia, genu varum and changes in the hip joints. Mental development is normal. The disorder is usually noted at about age 4, when dwarfism and walking difficulties become conspicuous. Marked kyphosis and shortening of the spine also shorten the trunk. The head is set directly on the hunched shoulders due to shortening of the cervical spine. Owing to flexed knees and hips the patients assume a crouching position. Increased amounts of mucopolysaccharides of the keratine sulfate-type are found in the urine.

Roentgenograms of the spine show osteoporosis and marked flattening of the vertebral bodies, especially in the lower dorsal vertebrae, which may appear as a tonque-like projection anteriorly. One of the vertebral bodies, usually D_{12} or L_1, may be smaller and displaced posteriorly, thus giving rise to angular kyphosis. In roentgenograms of the hip joints the femoral heads are flattened and of irregular shape and outline; the femoral necks are shortened. Coxa vara is common. The acetabula are deformed. Other epiphyses are affected to a lesser degree, while the metaphyses are splayed to accomodate the deformed epiphyses. Roentgenograms of the hand reveal metacarpals and phalanges to be short and stubby with epiphyses tending to point. The carpal bones may be irregular in shape. The metaphyses of the radius and ulna are splayed with the epiphyseal lines tilted toward each other.

Type V Mucopolysaccharidosis: Scheie's Syndrome

The characteristic manifestations are contractures of the fingers of the hands and feet, coarse facial features, pronounced corneal opacities, especially at the periphery, which become progressively worse, and slight mental deficiency.

Fig. 1. An 11-year-old patient with type II mucopolysaccharidosis (Hunter's syndrome) exhibits stunted growth, large head, short neck, contractures of the fingers, flexed knees and hips. Mental development is only slightly retarded.

Fig. 2. An 8-year-old patient with Morquio's syndrome (type IV mucopolysaccharidosis). Walking difficulties noted at age 3 years. Height is greatly stunted (102 cm, 40 in.). Note backward tilt to head, normal facial features, conspicuous shortening of the spine and skeletal deformities, with flexion contractures in several joints. Mental development is completely normal.

Fig. 3A. A 6-year-old patient with type IV mucopolysaccharidosis (Morquio's syndrome). Note crouched position, low-set, tilted head, many skeletal deformities, the extremities severely flexed with restriction of movements. Mental development is normal. No hepatomegaly and no corneal changes are present.

Fig. 3B. Roentgenogram of the pelvis and hip joints of the same patient shows flattened femoral heads of irregular shape and outline and gross deformity of the acetabula.

Fig. 3C. Face of the same patient shows large eyes, intelligent expression and flattened bridge of the nose.

PLATE 10

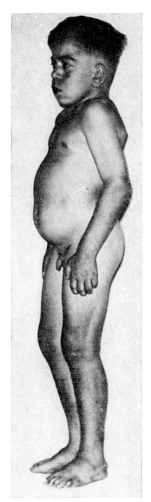

Fig. 1

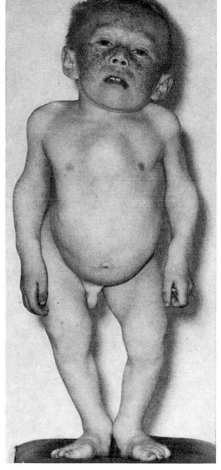

Fig. 2

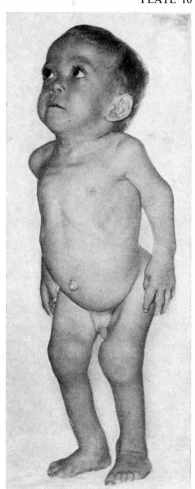

Fig. 3A

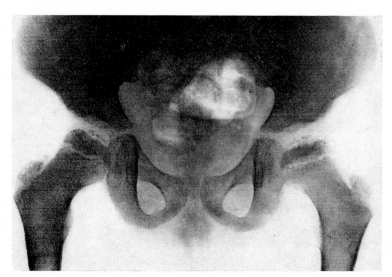

Fig. 3B

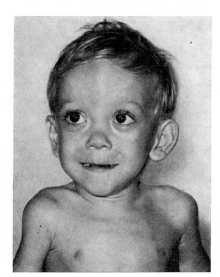

Fig. 3C

RENAL TUBULAR DEFECTS WITH RICKETS

There are 3 main types of renal tubular dysfunction which exhibit similar clinical manifestations but differ in severity and in their biochemical abnormalities. Children affected by the disorder complain of muscular weakness, back pains and pains in the legs. They are of short stature and frequently exhibit genu valgum or other skeletal deformities, enlarged epiphyses, rachitic rosary, transverse Harrison's sulcus and kyphosis. Roentgenograms of the bones show a generalized decrease in bone density, increased intervals between the epiphyses and metaphyses, enlarged and cupped metaphyses with irregular zones of provisional calcification, thinning of the cortex of the long bones and, occasionally, subperiosteal bone resorption as a result of secondary hyperparathyroidism. In some cases, bending of the long bones and deformities of the pelvis, thorax and spine may be seen.

Vitamin D-Resistant Rickets

(Renal Tubular Phosphaturia)

The disease, frequently familial, is one of the milder tubular defects in which laboratory studies reveal hypophosphatemia unresponsive to administration of normal amounts of vitamin D, elevated plasma alkaline phosphatase and hyperphosphaturia.

Fanconi's Syndrome

Fanconi's syndrome is a severe disease characterized by rickets, dwarfism, aminoaciduria, glycosuria without hyperglycemia, hypophosphatemia, hypercalciuria, alkaline hyperphosphatasia, sometimes hypopotassemia and acidosis. The progression of the disease may lead to chronic renal failure resulting in death.

Fig. 1. A 7-year-old patient with vitamin D-resistant rickets. Short stature (109 cm, 43 in.), marked genu varum and protruding abdomen are evident. Serum calcium 4.1 mEq/liter.

Fig. 2. A 10-year-old female with vitamin D-resistant rickets. Marked rachitic changes of the lower extremities are seen. Decreased plasma calcium (3.8 mEq/liter) and phosphorus (1.6 mEq/liter).

Fig. 3. A 16-year-old patient with kidney hypoplasia, renal insufficiency (associated with rickets) and generalized psoriasis. The height is stunted (121 cm, 48 in.). There is enlargement of the ends of the bones at the knee joints and roentgenographic evidence of rickets. Blood urea 120 mg/100 ml, serum phosphorus 4.9 mEq/liter.

Fig. 4A. The hand and wrist of a 7-year-old female with Fanconi's syndrome, glycosuria, aminoaciduria and phosphaturia. There is pronounced bracelet sign, i.e., protrusion of the splayed distal ends of the forearm bones.

Fig. 4B. The lower extremities of the patient show shortening of the femoral bones with lateral bending, genu valgum and conspicuous thickening of the bones at the knees and ankle joints.

Fig. 4C. Roentgenogram of the hand of the same patient with Fanconi's syndrome shows typical rachitic changes: increased width of the zones of provisional calcification — especially of the distal ends of the forearm bones — osteoporosis, delayed bone age and subperiosteal bone resorption.

336

PLATE 11

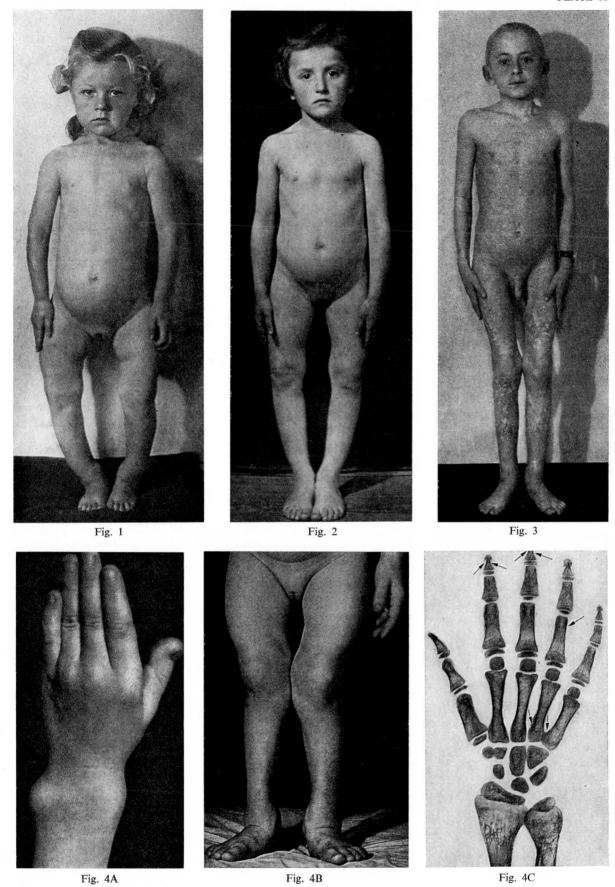

Fig. 1   Fig. 2   Fig. 3

Fig. 4A   Fig. 4B   Fig. 4C

Renal Tubular Acidosis

This form of renal tubular disorder, sometimes familial, is characterized by an inability to excrete urine of normal acidity, hypophosphatemia and severe acidosis with a low plasma bicarbonate, hyperchloremia and increased excretion of calcium and phosphate. The common symptoms are anorexia, loss of weight, pronounced muscular weakness and bone pain. Infections of the urinary tract, renal calculi and nephrocalcinosis are common.

Renal Osteodystrophy

(Renal Rickets)

In some children with chronic renal failure, rickets, osteitis fibrosa and secondary hyperparathyroidism may develop. The disease usually appears in cases of congenital anomalies of the kidneys, and is often complicated by urinary tract infections, renal failure and acidosis. Deficiency in 1,25-dihydrocholecalciferol, a renal metabolite of vitamin D, leads to poor intestinal calcium absorption and subsequent lowering of plasma calcium. This evokes hyperplasia of the parathyroids and their hyperfunction. Clinical manifestations are stunted growth, muscular weakness, waddling gait, bone tenderness and skeletal deformities. Radiologic examination reveals widening of and irregularities in the epiphyseal lines, cupping of the metaphyses, decrease in bone density and sometimes, subperiosteal bone resorption, undistinguishable from that in primary hyperparathyroidism.

Fig. 1A. An 11-year-old patient with renal acidosis and pronounced rickets. Short stature (height 106 cm, 42 in.), emaciation, conspicuous genu valgum and thickening of the epiphyses at the knees, ankles and wrists are seen.

Fig. 1B. Roentgenogram of the same patient showing multiple patchy calcifications in both kidneys (nephrocalcinosis), flattened vertebral bodies, wide intervertebral spaces and increased width in the zones of provisional calcification in the femora. Figs. 1C and 1D. Roentgenograms of the knee in the same patient with renal acidosis before and after treatment with sodium citrate and vitamin D_3. C. Before therapy. A marked widening of the zone of provisional calcification in the tibia and femoral bone, irregular epiphyseal line and decreased bone density are seen. D. After therapy. Considerable improvement is evident; the zone of provisional calcification is of normal width, the epiphyseal line is wavy but well densified.

PLATE 12

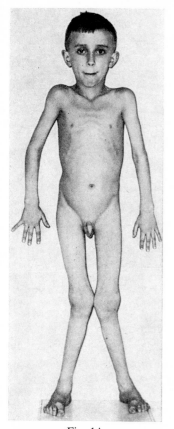

Fig. 1A

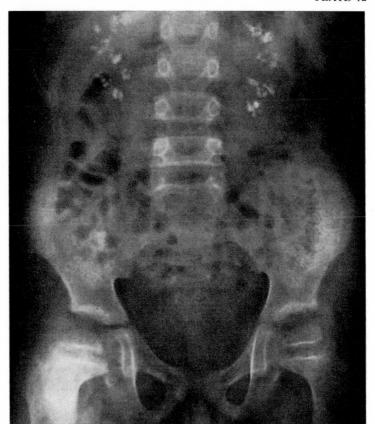

Fig. 1B

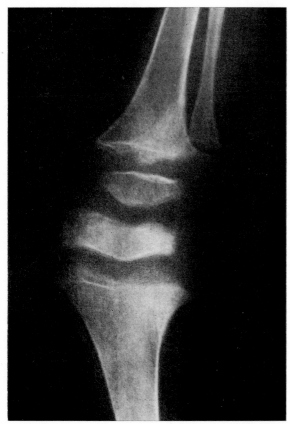

Fig. 1C

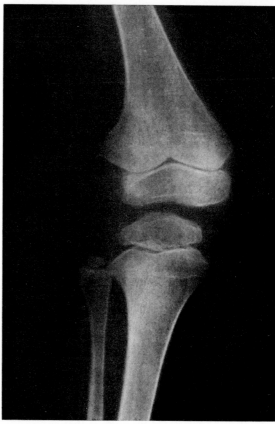

Fig. 1D

PRADER-WILLI SYNDROME

The main manifestations of the Prader-Willi syndrome are stunted growth, obesity, hypogonadism, hypotonia and mental deficiency. The face is frequently rounded with fish-like mouth, almond-shaped eyes, squint, low forehead and micrognathia. The genitalia are underdeveloped consisting of a small penis, cryptorchidism and hypoplastic scrotum. The hands and feet are small, sometimes puffy; syndactylia and clinodactylia may be present. Diabetes mellitus may develop at puberty.

POLYOSTOTIC FIBROUS DYSPLASIA

Fibrous dysplasia of bone has the following characteristics: cystlike lesions localized mainly in the diaphysis and metaphysis, bone deformations and pathologic fractures at the site of the cysts. Due to similar skeletal changes the disease was often confused with primary hyperparathyroidism. However, in contrast to bone lesions in hyperparathyroidism in fibrous dysplasia no osteoporosis is present, plasma calcium and phosphate are normal, and plasma parathyroid hormone concentration is not increased. Fibrous dysplasia of bone, areas of skin pigmentation and precocious puberty in girls indicate Albright's syndrome which is discussed in the Chapter 7.

Cranial localization of fibrous dysplasia known as leontiasis ossea usually involves the mandible, zygoma, the base of the skull and particularly the wings of sphenoid bones. The gross enlargement of the mandible and facial deformity leading to a leonine appearance may suggest acromegaly. However, grossly irregular trabecular structure of the affected facial bones with areas of mottled sclerosis and overgrowth of the cranial base distinguish this disease from acromegaly. In addition serum growth hormone concentration is normal in fibrous dysplasia while it is increased in acromegaly.

Fig. 1A. General appearance of a patient with Prader-Willi syndrome. Obesity and mental retardation are seen.
Fig. 1B. Facial appearance of the same patient with Prader-Willi syndrome includes a rounded face, almond-shaped eyes, strabismus and low forehead (Courtesy SS Gellis and M Feingold: reproduced from the Amer J Dis Child 120, 49, 1970).
Figs. 2A and 2B. Gross facial deformation, massive mandible and displacement of the eyes are seen in a 25-year-old patient with fibrous dysplasia of the facial bones (leontiasis ossea). Serum HGH is 2 ng/ml.

PLATE 13

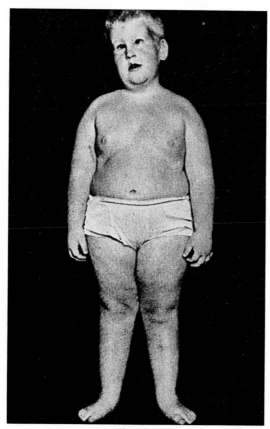

Fig. 1A

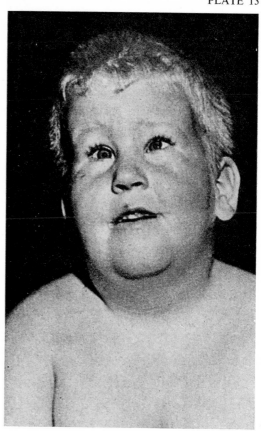

Fig. 1B

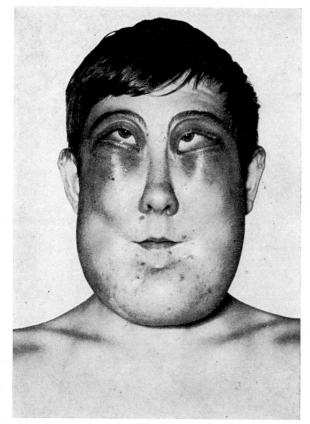

Fig. 2A

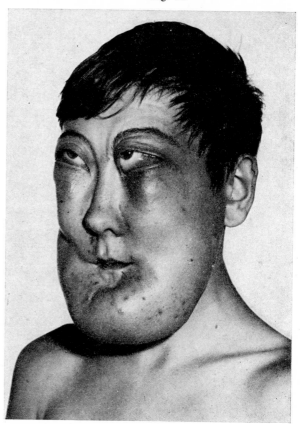

Fig. 2B

REFERENCES

Chapter 1

Amatruda TT, Jr, Mulrow PJ, Gallagher JC, Sawyer WH: Carcinoma of the lung with inappropriate antidiuresis. N Engl. J Med 269:544, 1963

Beardwell CG: Radioimmunoassay of arginine vasopressin in human plasma. J Clin Endocrinol Metab 33:254, 1971

Beck P, Schalch DS, Parker ML, Kipnis DM, Daughaday WH: Correlative studies of growth hormone and insulin plasma concentrations with metabolic abnormalities in acromegaly. J Lab Clin Med 66:366, 1965

Berson SA, Yalow RS: Radioimmunoassay of ACTH in plasma. J Clin Invest 47:2725, 1968

Brasel JA, Wright JC, Wilkins L, Blizzard RM: An evaluation of seventy-five patients with hypopituitarism beginning in childhood. Am J Med 38:484, 1965

Buckman MT, Kaminsky N, Conway M, Peake GT: Utility of L-dopa and water loading in evaluation of hyperprolactinemia. J Clin Endocrinol Metab 36:911, 1973

Burn JH, Truelove LH, Burn I: The antidiuretic action of nicotine and of smoking. Br Med J 1:403, 1945

Butt WR, Lynch S: Radioimmunoassay of gonadotrophins with special reference to follicle-stimulating hormone. Clin Chim Acta 22:79, 1968

Catt KJ: Pituitary function. Lancet 1:827, 1970

Catt KJ: Growth hormone. Lancet 1:933, 1970

Chaussain JL, Garnier PE, Binet E, et al: Effect of synthetic luteinizing hormone-releasing hormone on the release of gonadotropins in hypophyso-gonadal disorders of children and adolescents. III. Hypopituitarism. J Clin Endocrinol Metab 38:58, 1974

Coscia AM, Fleischer N, Besch PK, et al: The effect of synthetic luteinizing hormone-releasing factor on plasma LH levels in pituitary diseases. J Clin Endocrinol Metab 38:83, 1974

Crooke AC, Butt WR: Treatment of infertility and secondary amenorrhea with follicle-stimulating hormone and chorionic gonadotrophin. Lancet 2:636, 1967

Daughaday WH, Parker ML: Sulfation factor measurements as an aid in the recognition of pituitary dwarfism. J Clin Endocrinol Metab 23:638, 1963

Edwards CRW, Kitau MJ, Chard T, Besser GM: Vasopressin analogue DDAVP in diabetes insipidus: Clinical and laboratory studies. Br Med J 3:375, 1973

Fleischer N, Burgus R, Vale W, Dunn T, Guillemin R: Preliminary observations on the effect of synthetic thyrotropin-releasing factor on plasma thyrotropin levels in man. J Clin Endocrinol Metab 31:109, 1970

Foley TP, Owings J, Hayford JT, Blizzard RM: Serum thyrotropin responses to synthetic thyrotropin-releasing hormone in normal children and hypopituitary patients. J Clin Invest 51:431, 1972

Forbes AP, Henneman PH, Griswold GH, Albright F: Syndrome characterized by galactorrhea, amenorrhea and low urinary FSH: Comparison with acromegaly and normal lactation. J Clin Endocrinol Metab 14:265, 1954

Gautvik KM, Weintraub BD, Graeber CT, et al: Serum prolactin and TSH: Effects of nursing and TRH administration in postpartum women. J Clin Endocrinol Metab 36:135, 1973

Glick SM, Roth J, Yalow RS, Berson SA: The regulation of growth hormone secretion. Recent Prog Horm Res 21:241, 1965

Goldberg M: Hyponatremia and the inappropriate secretion of antidiuretic hormone. Am J Med 35:293, 1963

Gual C, Kastin AJ, Midgley AR, Jr, et al: Administration of LH-releasing hormone (LH-RH) as a clinical test of pituitary function. Endocrinology 88:128, 1971

Hartog M, Doyle F, Fraser R, Joplin GF: Partial pituitary ablation with implants of gold-198 and yttrium-90 for acromegaly. Br Med J 2:390, 1965

Hobbs CB, Miller AL: Review of endocrine syndromes associated with tumors of nonendocrine origin. J Clin Pathol 19:119, 1966

Husain MK, Fernando N, Shapiro M, Kagan A, Glick SM: Radioimmunoassay of arginine vasopressin in human plasma. J Clin Endocrinol Metab 37:616, 1973

Jacobs LS, Snyder PJ, Utiger RD, Daughaday WH: Prolactin response to thyrotropin-releasing hormone in normal subjects. J Clin Endocrinol Metab 36:1069, 1973

Jacobs HS, Greenwood FC, Nabarro DN: Changes in plasma growth hormone levels after surgical treatment of acromegaly. Proc R Soc Med 63:223, 1970

James VHT, Landon J: Hypothalamic-pituitary-adrenal function tests. Horsham, Sussex, Ciba Laboratories Ltd, 1971

Kastin AJ, Harate A, Midgley AR, Jr, et al: Ovulation confirmed by pregnancy after infusion of porcine LH-RH. J Clin Endocrinol Metab 33:980, 1971

Kellgren JH, Ball J, Tutton GK: The articular and other limb changes in acromegaly. Q J Med 21:405, 1952

Kleinberg DL, Noel GL, Frantz AG: Chlorpromazine stimulation and L-dopa suppression of plasma prolactin in man. J Clin Endocrinol Metab 33:873, 1971

Kosowicz J, Roguska J: Electrocardiogram in hypopituitarism: Reversibility of changes during treatment. Am Heart J 63:13, 1963

Liddle GW, Estep HL, Kendall JW, Jr, Williams WC, Jr, Townes AW: Clinical application of a new test of pituitary reserve. J Clin Endocrinol Metab 19:875, 1959

Martin LG, Martul P, Connor TB, *et al*: Hypothalamic control of origin of idiopathic hypopituitarism. J Clin Invest 50:64a, 1971

Martin MM, Wilkins L: Pituitary dwarfism: Diagnosis and treatment. J Clin Endocrinol Metab 18:679, 1958

Nabarro JDN: Pituitary tumours and hypopituitarism. Br Med J 1:492, 1972

Nelson DH, Meakin JW, Pealy JG, Jr, Nelson DD, Emerson K, Jr, Thorn GW: ACTH-producing tumor of the pituitary gland. N Engl J Med 259:161, 1959

Newns GG: Hypopituitary dwarfism. Proc R Soc Med 60:665, 1967

Odell WD, Ross GT, Rayford PL: Radioimmunoassay for luteinizing hormone in human plasma or serum: Physiological studies. J Clin Invest 46:248, 1967

Parker ML, Mariz IK, Daughaday WH: Resistance to human growth hormone in pituitary dwarfism: Clinical and immunologic studies. J Clin Endocrinol Metab 24:997, 1964

Randall RV, Clark EC, Bahn RC: Classification of the causes of diabetes insipidus. Proc Mayo Clin 34:299, 1959

Rebar R, Yen SSC, Vandenberg G, *et al*: Gonadotropin responses to synthetic LRF: Dose-response relationship in men. J Clin Endocrinol Metab 36:10, 1973

Roth J, Glick SM, Yalow RS, Berson SA: Hypoglycemia: A potent stimulus to secretion of growth hormone. Science 140:987, 1963

Schalch DS, Gonzales-Barcena D, Kastin AJ, Schally AV, Lee LA: Abnormalities in the release of TSH in response to thyrotropin-releasing hormone in patients with disorders of the pituitary, hypothalamus and basal ganglia. J Clin Endocrinol Metab 35:609, 1972

Schalch DS, Parlow AF, Bonn RC, Reichlin S: Measurement of human luteinizing hormone in plasma by radioimmunoassay. J Clin Invest 47:665, 1968

Schally AV, Kastin AJ, Arimura A: The hypothalamus and reproduction. Am J Obstet Gynecol 114:423, 1972

Schwartz WB, Bennett W, Curelop S, Bartter FC: A syndrome of renal sodium loss and hyponatremia, probably resulting from inappropriate secretion of antidiuretic hormone. Am J Med 23:529, 1957

Sheehan HL, Stanfield JP: The pathogenesis of postpartum necrosis of the anterior lobe of the pituitary gland. Acta Endocrinol 37:479, 1961

Sheehan HL, Summers VK: The syndrome of hypopituitarism. Q J Med 18:319, 1949

Shenkman L: Hypothalamic control of anterior pituitary function. Am J Med Sci 263:433, 1972

Sinha YN, Selby FW, Lewis UJ, Vanderlean WP: A homologous radioimmunoassay for human prolactin. J Clin Endocrinol Metab 36:509, 1973

Steinbach HL, Feldman R, Goldberg MB: Acromegaly. Radiology 73:535, 1959

Thomas WC: Diabetes insipidus (review). J Clin Endocrinol Metab 17:565, 1957

Wright AD, Hartog M, Palter H, Tevaarwerk G, Doyle FD, Arnot R, Joplin GF, Fraser TR: The use of yttrium-90 implantation in the treatment of acromegaly. Proc R Soc Med 63:221, 1970

Young DG, Bahn RC, Randall RV: Pituitary tumors associated with acromegaly. J Clin Endocrinol Metab 25:249, 1965

Chapter 2

Adams DD, Kennedy TH: Evidence to suggest that LATS protector stimulates the human thyroid gland. J Clin Endocrinol Metab 33:47, 1971

Ashkar FS, Bezjian AA: Normalized serum thyroxine (T_4N): The test for thyroid function in pregnancy. Obstet Gynecol 40:575, 1972

Beling U, Einhorn J: Incidence of hypothyroidism and recurrences following I^{131} treatment of hyperthyroidism. Acta Radiol 56:275, 1961

Brauman H, Smets P, and Corvilain J: Comparative study of growth hormone response to hypoglycemia in normal subjects and in patients with primary myxedema or hyperthyroidism before and after treatment. J Clin Endocrinol Metab 36:1162, 1973

Burgess JA, Smith BR, Merimee TJ: Growth hormone in thyrotoxicosis: Effect of insulin-induced hypoglycemia. J Clin Endocrinol Metab 26:1257, 1966

Catt KJ: The thyroid gland. Lancet 1:1183, 1970

Chan V, Landon J: Urinary thyroxine excretion as an index of thyroid function. Lancet 1:4, 1972

Chan V, Landon J, Besser GM, Ekins RP: Urinary triiodothyronine excretion as index of thyroid function. Lancet 2:253, 1972

DeGroot LJ, Hall R, McDermott WV, Jr, Davis AM: Hashimoto's thyroiditis, a genetically conditioned disease. N Engl J Med 267:267, 1962

Doniach D, Hudson RV, Roitt IM: Human auto-immune thyroiditis: Clinical studies. Br Med J 1:365, 1960

Evered D, Hall RH: Hypothyroidism. Br Med J 1:290, 1972

Evered DC, Ormston BJ, Smith PA, Hall RH, Bird T: Grades of hypothyroidism. Br Med J 1:657, 1973

Evered D, Young ET, Ormston BJ, Menzies R, Smith PA, Hall RH: Treatment of hypothyroidism: A reappraisal of thyroxine therapy. Br Med J 3:131, 1973

Grayson RR: Factors which influence the radioactive iodine thyroidal uptake test. Am J Med 28:397, 1960

Green M, Wilson GM: Thyrotoxicosis treated by surgery or iodine-131. With special reference to development of hypothyroidism. Br Med J 1:1005, 1964

Haigler ED, Jr, Pittman JA, Jr, Hershman JM, Baugh CM: Direct evaluation of pituitary thyrotropin reserve utilizing synthetic thyrotropin releasing hormone. J. Clin Endocrinol Metab 33:573, 1971

Hall RH, Besser GM, Ormston BJ, Cryer RJ: The thyrotrophin-releasing hormone test in diseases of the pituitary and hypothalamus. Lancet 2:10, 1971

Hall RH: Immunologic aspects of thyroid function. N Engl J Med 266:1204, 1962

Havard CWH: Which test of thyroid function. Br Med J 1:553, 1974

Havard CWH: Endocrine exophthalmos. Br Med J 1:360, 1972

Hershman JM, Givens JR, Cassidy CE, Astwood EB: Long-term outcome of hyperthyroidism treated with antithyroid drugs. J Clin Endocrinol Metab 26:803, 1966

Hollander CS, Shenkman L: The physiological role of triiodothyronine. Am J Med Sci 264:5, 1972

Ingbar SH: Management of emergencies. IX. Thyrotoxic storm. N Engl J Med 274:1252, 1966

Lancet (editorial): Radioiodine treatment of thyrotoxicosis. Lancet 1:23, 1972

Larsen PR: Triiodothyronine: Review of recent studies of its physiology and pathophysiology in man. Metabolism 21:1073, 1972

Mäenpää J, Hiekkala H, Lamberg BA: Childhood hyperthyroidism: Report on 39 cases. Acta Endocrinol 51:321, 1966

McBrien DJ, Hindle W: Myxoedema and heart-failure. Lancet 1:1066, 1963

Miller JM, Horn RC, Block MA: The evolution of toxic nodular goiter. Arch Intern Med 113:72, 1964

Nauman J, Nauman A, Werner SC: Total and free triiodothyronine in human serum. J Clin Invest 46:1346, 1967

Nofal MM, Beierwaltes WH, Patno ME: Treatment of hyperthyroidism with sodium iodide I^{131}. JAMA 197:605, 1966

Nuttal FQ, Doe R: Achilles reflex in thyroid disease. Ann Intern Med 64:217, 1966

Pitt-Rivers R, Trotter WR (eds): The Thyroid Gland. Washington, Butterworths, 1964

Russel WO, Ibanez ML, Clark RL, White EC: Thyroid carcinoma. Classification, intraglandular dissemination, and clinicopathological study based upon whole organ sections of 80 glands. Cancer 16:1425, 1963

Schally AV, Redding TW, Bowers CY: Thyrotropic hormone releasing factor (TRF). Gunma Symposia Endocrinol 3:15, 1966

Shenkman L, Mitsuma T, Hollander CS: Modulation of pituitary responsiveness to thyrotropin-releasing hormone by triiodothyronine. J Clin Invest 52:205, 1973

Shenkman L, Suphavai A, Mitsuma T, Hollander CS: Triiodothyronine and thyroid-stimulating hormone response to thyrotrophin-releasing hormone. A new test of thyroidal and pituitary reserve. Lancet 1:111, 1972

Sloan IW: Origin, characteristics and behavior of thyroid cancer. J Clin Endocrinol Metab 14:1309, 1954

Snyder PJ, Utiger RD: Response to thyrotropin releasing hormone in normal man. J Clin Endocrinol Metab 34:380, 1972

Solomon DH, Beck JC, Vanderlaan WP, Astwood EB: Prognosis of hyperthyroidism treated by antithyroid drugs. JAMA 152:201, 1953

Stanbury JB, Chapman EM: Congenital goiter with hypothyroidism: Absence of iodide concentrating mechanism. Lancet 1:1162, 1960

Stanbury JB, DeGroot LJ: Problem of hypothyroidism after I^{131} therapy of hyperthyroidism. N Engl J Med 271:195, 1964

Sterling K, Brenner MA: Free thyroxine in human serum: Simplified method with the aid of magnesium precipitation. J Clin Invest 45:153, 1966

Utiger RD: Radioimmunoassay of human plasma thyrotropin. J. Clin Invest 44:1277, 1965

Van Herle AJ, Uller RP, Mathews NL, Brown J: Radioimmunoassay for measurement of thyroglobulin in human serum. J Clin Invest 52:1320, 1973

Volpé R, Johnston MU, Huber N: Thyroid function in subacute thyroiditis. J Clin Endocrinol Metab 18:65, 1958

Werner SC: Response to triiodothyronine as index of persistence of disease in the thyroid remnant of patients in remission from hyperthyroidism. J Clin Invest 35:57, 1956

Wilkins L: Epiphysial dysgenesis associated with hypothyroidism. Am J Dis Child 61:13, 1941

Chapter 3

Addison T: On the constitutional and local effects of disease of suprarenal capsules. London, D. Highley, 1855

Biglieri EG, McIlroy MB: Abnormalities of renal function and circulatory reflexes in primary aldosteronism. Circulation 33:78, 1966

Biglieri EG, Slaton PE, Jr, Kronfield SJ, Schambelan M: Diagnosis of an aldosterone-producing adenoma in primary aldosteronism: An evaluative maneuver. JAMA 201:510, 1967

Biglieri EG, Slaton PE, Jr, Kronfield SJ, Schambelan M: Primary aldosteronism with unusual secretory pattern. J Clin Endocrinol Metab 27:715, 1967

Blizzard RM, Kyle M: Studies of the adrenal antigens and antibodies in Addison's disease. J Clin Invest 42:1653, 1963

Bongiovanni AM: The adrenogenital syndrome with deficiency of 3-β-hydroxysteroid dehydrogenase. J Clin Invest 41:2086, 1962

Bongiovanni AM, Eberlein WR: Clinical and metabolic variations in the adrenogenital syndrome. Pediatrics 16:628, 1955

Bongiovanni AM, Root AW: Adrenogenital syndrome. N Engl J Med 268:1283, 1362, 1391, 1963

Burke CW, Doyle FH, Joplin GF, Arnot RN, Macerlean DP, Fraser TR: Cushing's disease. J Med 42:693, 1973

Carman CT, Brashear RE: Pheochromocytoma as an inherited abnormality. Report of the tenth affected kindred and review of the literature. N Engl J Med 263:419, 1960

Catt KJ: Adrenal cortex. Lancet 1:1275, 1970

Childs B, Grumbach MM, Van Wyk JJ: Virilizing adrenal hyperplasia: A genetic and hormonal study. J Clin Invest 35:213, 1956

Conn JW: Evolution of primary aldosteronism as a highly specific clinical entity. JAMA 172:1650, 1960

Conn JW, Cohen EL, Rovner DR, Nesbit RH: Normokalemic primary aldosteronism: A detectable cause of curable "essential hypertension." JAMA 193:200, 1965

Crandell DL, Myers RT: Pheochromocytoma anesthetic and surgical considerations. JAMA 187:12, 1964

Crout JR, Pisano JJ, Sjöerdsma A: Urinary excretion of catecholamines and their metabolites in pheochromocytoma. Am Heart J 61:375, 1961

Cushing H: The basophil adenomas of the pituitary body and their clinical manifestations (pituitary basophilism). Bull Johns Hopkins Hosp 50:137, 1932

Eberlein, WR, Bongiovanni AM: Plasma and urinary corticosteroids in the hypertensive form of congenital adrenal hyperplasia. J Biol Chem 223:85, 1956

Eberlein WR, Bongiovanni AM: Congenital adrenal hyperplasia with hypertension: Unusual steroid pattern in blood and urine. J Clin Endocrinol Metab 15:1531, 1955

Ekman H, Hakansson B, McCarthy JD, Lehmann J, Sjögren B: Plasma 17-hydroxycorticosteroids in Cushing's syndrome. J Clin Endocrinol Metab 21:684, 1961

Engelman K, Mueller PS, Sjöerdsma A: Elevated plasma free-fatty-acid concentrations in patients with pheochromocytoma. N Engl J Med 270:865, 1964

Evans JA: Difficulties in the diagnosis of pheochromocytoma. Med Clin North Am 44:411, 1960

Farber JE, Gustina FJ, Postoloff AV: Cushing's syndrome in children. Am J Dis Child 65:593, 1943

Forsham PH (ed): The Endocrine System and Selected Metabolic Diseases. Summit NJ Ciba Corp, 1965, p. 90

Fraser TR, Joplin GF, Steiner R, Laws J, Jones E: Partial pituitary ablation by needle implantation of gold-198 seeds for acromegaly and Cushing's disease. Lancet 2:1277, 1961

Gabrilove JL, Sharma DC, Dortman RI: Adrenocortical 11 β-hydroxylase deficiency and virilism first manifest in the adult woman. N Engl J Med 272:1189, 1965

Genest J: Angiotensin, aldosterone and human arterial hypertension. Can Med Assoc J 84:403, 1961

Gifford RW, Jr, Roth GM, Kvale WF: Evaluation of new adrenolytic drug (regitine) as test for pheochromocytoma. JAMA 149:1628, 1962

Gold EM, Kent JR, Forsham PH: Clinical use of a new diagnostic agent methopyrapone (SU-4885) in pituitary and adrenocortical disorders. Ann Intern Med 54:175, 1961

Goldfein A: Treatment of pheochromocytoma. Mod Treat 3:1360, 1966

Green OC, Cleveland WW, Wilkins L: Triamcinolone therapy in the adrenogenital syndrome. Pediatrics 27:292, 1961

Hermann H, Mornex R: Human Tumours Secreting Catecholamines. Oxford, Pergamon Press, 1964

Higgins GA, Brownlee WE, Mantz FA, Jr: Feminizing tumors of the adrenal cortex. Am Surg 22:56, 1956

Insley J, Smallwood WC: Pheochromocytoma in children. Arch Dis Child 37:606, 1962

Irvine WJ, Stewart AG, Scarth L: A clinical and immunological study of adrenocortical insufficiency (Addison's disease). Clin Exp Immunol 2:31, 1967

Jenkins D, Forsham PH, Laidlew JC, Reddy WJ, Thorn GW: Use of ACTH in the diagnosis of adrenal cortical insufficiency. Am J Med 18:3, 1955

Kosowicz J, Pruszewicz A: The taste test in adrenal insufficiency. J Clin Endocrinol Metab 27:214, 1967

Landau RL, Stimmel BF, Humphreys E, Clark DE: Gynecomastia and retarded sexual development resulting from a long-standing estrogen-secreting adrenal tumor. J Clin Endocrinol Metab 14:1097, 1955

Liddle GW: Tests of pituitary-adrenal suppressibility in the diagnosis of Cushing's syndrome. J Clin Endocrinol Metab 20:1539, 1960

Liddle GW, Givens JR, Nicholson WE, Island DP: The ectopic ACTH syndrome. Cancer Res 25:1057, 1965

Liddle GW, Island D, Meador CK: Normal and abnormal regulation of corticotropin secretion in man. Recent Prog Horm Res 18:125, 1962

Meador CK, Liddle GW, Island DP, Nicholson WE, Lucas CP, Nuckton JG, Luetscher JA: Cause of Cushing's syndrome in patients with tumors arising from "non-endocrine" tissue. J Clin Endocrinol Metab 22:693, 1962

Migeon CJ, Green OC, Eckert JP: Study of adrenocortical function in obesity. Metabolism 12:718, 1963

Moses AM, Gabrilove JL, Soffer LJ: Simplified water loading test in hypoadrenocorticism and hypothyroidism. J Clin Endocrinol Metab 18:1413, 1958

Mosier HD, Goodwin WE: Feminizing adrenal adenoma in a seven-year-old boy. Pediatrics 27:1016, 1961

Nelson DH, Meakin JW, Thorn GW: ACTH-producing pituitary tumors following adrenalectomy for Cushing's syndrome. Ann Intern Med 52:560, 1960

Ney RL, Shimizu N, Nicholson WE, Island DP, Liddle GW: Correlation of plasma ACTH concentration with adrenocortical response in normal human subjects, surgical patients and patients with Cushing's disease. J Clin Invest 42:1669, 1963

Nugent CA, Nichols T, Tyler FH: Diagnosis of Cushing's syndrome. Single dose dexamethasone suppression test. Arch Intern Med 116:170, 1965

O'Donnell WM: Changing pathogenesis of Addison's disease. Arch Intern Med 36:266, 1965

Perkoff GT, Eik-Nes K, Nugent CA, Fred HL, Nimer RA, Rush L, Samuels LT, Tyler FH: Studies of the diurnal variation of plasma 17-hydroxycorticosteroids in man. J Clin Endocrinol Metab 19:432, 1959

Peterson RF: Plasma corticosterone and hydrocortisone levels in man. J Clin Endocrinol Metab 17:1150, 1957

Pisano JJ, Crout JR, Abraham D: Determination of 3-methoxy-4-hydroxymandelic acid in urine. Clin Chim Acta 7:285, 1962

Plotz CM, Knowlton AI, Ragan C: The natural history of Cushing's syndrome. Am J Med 13:597, 1952

Salassa RM, Kearns TP, Kernohan JW, Sprague RG, MacCarty CS: Pituitary tumors in patients with Cushing's syndrome. J Clin Endocrinol Metab 19:1523, 1959

Silen W, Biglieri EG, Slaton P, Galante M: Management of primary aldosteronism. Ann Surg 164:600, 1966

Sjöerdsma A, Engelman K, Waldmann TA, Cooperman LH, Hammond WG: Pheochromocytoma: Current concepts of diagnosis and treatment. Ann Intern Med 65:1302, 1966

Soffer LJ, Dorfman RI, Gabrilove IL: The Human Adrenal Gland. Philadelphia, Lea and Febiger, 1961

Steinbach HL, Smith DR: Extraperitoneal pneumography in diagnosis of retroperitoneal tumors. Arch Surg 70:161, 1955

Tucci JR, Jagger PI, Lauler DP, Thorn GW: Rapid dexamethasone suppression test for Cushing's syndrome. JAMA 199:129, 1967

Ulick S, Gauthier E, Vetter K, Markello JR, Lowe CU: An aldosterone biosynthetic defect in a salt-losing disorder. J Clin Endocrinol Metab 24:669, 1964

Wilkins L: Adrenal disorders. Cushing's syndrome and its puzzles. Arch Dis Child 37:1, 1962

Wilkins L: Diagnosis and treatment of congenital virilizing adrenal hyperplasia. Postgrad Med 29:31, 1961

Wurtman RJ: Catecholamines. N Engl J Med 273:637, 693, 746, 1965

Chapter 4

Albert A, Underdahl LO, Greene LF, Lorenz N: Male hypogonadism. IV. The testis in prepubertal or pubertal gonadotropic failure. Proc Mayo Clin 29:131, 1954

Albert A, Underdahl LO, Greene LF, Lorenz N: Male hypogonadism. III. The testis in pituitary dwarfism. Proc. Mayo Clin 28:698, 1953

Anderson H, Andreassen M, Quaade F: Testicular biopsies in cryptorchidism. Acta Endocrinol 18:567, 1955

Avin J: The male Turner syndrome. Am J Dis Child 91:630, 1956

Balleev JW, Mastes WH: Mumps: A cause of infertility: I. Present consideration. Fertil Steril 5:536, 1954

Barr ML: Dysgenesis of the seminiferous tubules. Br J Urol 29:251, 1957

Barr ML, Carr DH: Correlations between sex chromatin and sex chromosomes. Acta Cytol 6:34, 1962

Becker KL, Hoffman DL: Klinefelter's syndrome: Clinical and laboratory findings in 50 patients. Arch Intern Med 118:314, 1966

Bergadá C, Cleveland WW, Jones HW, Jr, Wilkins L: Gonadal histology in patients with male pseudohermaphroditism and atypical gonadal dysgenesis: Relation to theories of sex differentiation. Acta Endocrinol (Kbh) 40:493, 1962

Biben RL, Gordon GS: Familial hypogonadotrophic eunuchoidism. J Clin Endocrinol Metab 15:931, 1966

Bradbury JT, Bunge RG, Boccabella RA: Chromatin test in Klinefelter's syndrome. J Clin Endocrinol Metab 16:689, 1956

Carr DH, Barr ML: An XXXY sex chromosome complex in Klinefelter subjects with duplicated sex chromatin. J Clin Endocrinol Metab 21:491, 1961

Charney CW, Wolgin W: Cryptorchidism. New York, Hoeber, 1957

de la Balze FA, Mancini RA, Arrilaga F, Andrada JA, Vilar O, Gurtman AJ, Davidson OW: Histologic study of the undescended human testis during puberty. J Clin Endocrinol Metab 20:286, 1960

del Castillo EB, Traubucco A, de la Balze FA: Syndrome produced by absence of the germinal epithelium without impairment of the Sertoli or Leydig cells. J Clin Endocrinol Metab 7:493, 1947

Deming C: The evaluation of hormonal therapy in cryptorchidism. J Urol 68:354, 1952

Dey DL: Management of maldescended testes. Med J Aust 2:214, 1961

Dorfman RI, Forchielli E, Gut M: Androgen biosynthesis and related studies. Recent Prog Horm Res 19:251, 1963

Dorfman RI, Ungar F: Metabolism of Steroid Hormones. New York, Academic Press, 1965

Drucker WD, Blanc WA, Rowland LP, Grumbach MM, Christy NP: The testis in myotonic muscular dystrophy: A clinical and pathologic study with a comparison with the Klinefelter syndrome. J Clin Endocrinol Metab 28:59, 1963

Ferguson-Smith MA: The prepubertal testicular lesion in chromatin-positive Klinefelter's syndrome (primary micro-orchidism) as seen in mentally handicapped children. Lancet 1:219, 1959

Ferguson-Smith MA, Johnston AW, Handmaker SD: Primary amentia and micro-orchidism associated with an XXXY sex chromosome constitution. Lancet 2:184, 1960

Ferguson-Smith MA, Lennox B, Mack WS, Stewart JSS: Klinefelter's syndrome: Frequency and testicular morphology in relation to nuclear sex. Lancet 2:167, 1957

Ferguson-Smith MA, Lennox B, Stewart JSS, Mack WS: Klinefelter's syndrome. Mem Soc Endocrinol 1:173, 1960

Fraccaro M, Ekkos D, Lindsten J, Luft R, Tillinger KB: Testicular germinal dysgenesis (male Turner's syndrome). Acta Endocrinol (Kbh) 36:98, 1961

Fraser JH, Boyd E, Lennox B, Dennison WM: A case of XXXXY Klinefelter's syndrome. Lancet 2:1064, 1961

Gemzell C, Kjessler B: Treatment of infertility after partial hypophysectomy with human pituitary gonadotrophins. Lancet I:644, 1964

Gross RE, Jewett TC: Surgical experience from 1222 operations for undescended testis. JAMA 160:634, 1956

Grumbach MM, Morishima A: Sex chromatin and the sex chromosomes: On the origin of sex chromatin from a single X chromosome. Acta Cytol 6:46, 1962

Grumbach MM, Van Wyk JJ, Wilkins L: Chromosomal sex in gonadal dysgenesis (ovarian agenesis): Relationship to male pseudohermaphroditism and theories of sex differentiation. J Clin Endocrinol Metab 15:1161, 1955

Hand JR: Undescended testes: Report of 153 cases with evaluation of clinical findings, treatment, and results on followup up to thirty-three years. Trans Am Assoc Genitourin Surg 47:9, 1955

Heller CG, Nelson WO: Classification of male hypogonadism and a discussion of pathologic physiology, diagnosis and treatment. J Clin Endocrinol Metab 8:345, 1948

Hortling H, de la Chapelle A, Johansson GJ, Niemi H, Sulamaa: An endocrinologic follow-up study of operated cases of cryptorchidism. J Clin Endocrinol Metab 27:120, 1967

Jacobs PA, Brunton M, Melville MM, Brittain RP, McClemont WF: Aggressive behavior, mental sub-normality and the XYY male. Nature 208:1351, 1965

Johnsen SG: A study of human testicular function by the use of human menopausal gonadotrophin and of human chorionic gonadotrophin in male hypogonadotrophic eunuchoidism and infantilism. Acta Endocrinol (Kbh) 53:315, 1966

Johnsen SG: Studies on the testicular-hypophyseal feedback mechanism in man. Acta Endocrinol [Suppl] 90:99, 1964

Jull JW, Bonser GM, Dossett JA: Hormone excretion studies of males with gynaecomastia. Br Med J 2:797, 1964

Kirshner MA, Lipsett MB, Collins DR: Plasma ketosteroids and testosterone in man: A study of the pituitary, testicular axis. J. Clin Invest 44:657, 1965

Klinefelter HF, Jr, Reifenstein EC, Jr, Albright F: Syndrome characterized by gynecomastia, aspermatogenesis without a-Leydigism and increased excretion of follicle-stimulating hormone. J Clin Endocrinol Metab 2:615, 1942

Lipsett MB, Davis TE, Wilson H, Craig JC: Testosterone production in chromatin-positive Klinefelter's syndrome. J Clin Endocrinol Metab 25:1027, 1965

Lipsett MB, Korenman SG: Androgen metabolism. JAMA 190:757, 1964

MacLeod J, Pazianos A, Ray BS: Restoration of human spermatogenesis by menopausal gonadotrophins. Lancet 1:1196, 1964

Maddock WW, Nelson WO: The effects of chorionic gonadotropin in adult men: Increased estrogen and 17-ketosteroid excretion, gynecomastia, Leydig cell stimulation and seminiferous tubule damage. J Clin Endocrinol Metab 12:985, 1952

Mellinger RC, Thompson RJ: The effect of clomiphene citrate in male infertility. Fertil Steril 17:94, 1966

Mroueh A, Lytton B, Kore N: Effects of human chorionic gonadotropin and human menopausal gonadotropin (Pergonal) in males with oligospermia. J Clin Endocrinol Metab 27:53, 1967

Nielsen J: Klinefelter's syndrome and behaviour. Lancet 2:587, 1964

Nydick M, Bustos J, Dale JH, Jr, Rawson RW: Gynecomastia in adolescent boys. JAMA 178:449, 1961

Odell WD, Ross GT, Rayford PL: Radioimmunoassay for luteinizing hormone in human plasma or serum: Physiological studies. J Clin Invest 46:248, 1967

Pritchard M: Klinefelter's syndrome and behaviour. Lancet 2:762, 1964

Raboch J, Sipova I: The mental level in 47 cases of true Klinefelter's syndrome. Acta Endocrinol (Kbh) 36:404, 1961

Robinson JN, Engle ET: Cryptorchidism: Pathology and treatment. Pediat Clin North Am 2:729, 1955

Sniffen RC: Histology of the normal and abnormal testis at puberty. Ann NY Acad Sci 55:609, 1952

Sohval AR: "Mixed" gonadal dysgenesis: A variety of hermaphroditism. Am J Hum Genet 15:155, 1963

Sohval AR: Histopathology of cryptorchidism: Study based upon comparative histology of retained and scrotal testes from birth to maturity. Am J Med 16:347, 1954

Stewart JSS: Gonadal dysgenesis: The genetic significance of unusual variants. Acta Endocrinol (Kbh) 33:89, 1960

Tanner JM, Prader A, Habich H, Ferguson-Smith MA: Genes on the Y chromosome influencing rate of maturation in man: Skeletal-age studies in children with Klinefelter's (XXY) and Turner's (XO) syndromes. Lancet 2:141, 1959

Thannhauser SJ: Werner's syndrome (progeria of the adult) and Rothmund's syndrome. Two types of closely related hereditofamilial atrophic dermatoses with juvenile cataracts and endocrine features: A critical study with five new cases. Ann Intern Med 23:599, 1945

Werner SC: Spermatogenesis and apparent fertility in eunuchoid male in eleventh year of androgen therapy. J Clin Endocrinol Metab 11:612, 1951

Werner SC: Clinical syndrome associated with gonadal failure in men. Am J Med 3:52, 1947

Chapter 5

Acheson RM, Zampa GA: Skeletal maturation in ovarian dysgenesis and Turner's syndrome. Lancet 1:917, 1961

Archibald RM, Finby N, De Vito F: Endocrine significance of short metacarpals. J Clin Endocrinol Metab 19:1312, 1959

Astley R: Chromosomal abnormalities in childhood, with particular reference to Turner's syndrome and mongolism Br J Radiol 36:2, 1963

Baikie AG, Garson OM, Weste SM, Ferguson J: Numerical abnormalities of the X chromosome. Frequency among inpatients of a general hospital and in a general population. Lancet 1:398, 1966

Barr ML, Carr DH: Correlations between sex chromatin and sex chromosomes. Acta Cytol 6:34, 1962

Boczkowski K, Teter J: Clinical, histological, and cytogenic observations in pure gonadal dysgenesis. Acta Endocrinol (Kbh) 51:497, 1966

Carr DH, Barr ML, Plunkett ER: An XXXX sex chromosome complex in two mentally deficient females. Can Med Assoc J 84:131, 1961

Carr DH, Barr ML, Plunkett ER, Grumbach MM, Morishima A, Chu EHY: An XXXY sex chromosome complex in Klinefelter subjects with duplicated sex chromatin. J Clin Endocrinol Metab 21:491, 1961

Carr DH, Morishima A, Barr ML, Grumbach MM, Lüers T, Boschann HW: An XO/XX/XXX mosaicism in relationship to gonadal dysgenesis in females. J Clin Endocrinol Metab 22:671, 1962

Catt KJ: Reproductive Endocrinology. Lancet 1:1097, 1970

Engel E, Forbes AP: Cytogenetic and clinical findings in 48 patients with congenitally defective or absent ovaries. Medicine 44:135, 1965

Finby N, Archibald RM: Skeletal abnormalities associated with gonadal dysgenesis. Am J Roentgenol Radium Ther Nucl Med 89:1222, 1963

Forbes AP, Jacobson JG, Carroll EL, Pechet MM: Studies of growth arrest in gonadal dysgenesis. Metabolism 11:56, 1962

Ford CE, et al: A sex-chromosomal anomaly in a case of gonadal dysgenesis (Turner's syndrome). Lancet 2:711, 1959

Goldzieher JW, Green JA: The polycystic ovary. I. Clinical and histological features. J Clin Endocrinol Metab 22:325, 1962

Grady HG, Smith DE (eds): The Ovary. Baltimore, Williams Wilkins, 1963

Greenblatt RB: The Hirsute Female. Springfield, Charles C. Thomas, 1963

Grumbach MM, Barr ML: Cytologic tests of chromosomal sex in relation to sexual anomalies in man. Recent Prog Horm Res 14:335, 1958

Grumbach MM, Van Wyk JJ, Wilkins L: Chromosomal sex in gonadal dysgenesis (ovarian agenesis): Relationship to male pseudohermaphroditism and theories of human sex differentiation. J Clin Endocrinol Metab 15:1161, 1955

Haddad HM, Wilkins L: Congenital anomalies associated with gonadal aplasia. Pediatrics 23:885, 1959

Job JC, Garnier PE, Chaussain JIL, Milhaud G: Elevation of serum gonadotropins (LH and FSH) after releasing-hormone (LH-RH) injection in normal children and in patients with disorders of puberty. J Clin Endocrinol Metab 35:473, 1972

Kastin AJ, Zarate A, Midgley AR, Canales ES, Schally AV: Ovulation confirmed by pregnancy after infusion of porcine LH-RH. J Clin Endocrinol Metab 33:980, 1971

Kosowicz J: The roentgen appearance of the hand and wrist in gonadal dysgenesis. Am J Roentgenol Radium Ther Nucl Med 93:354, 1965

Kosowicz J: The carpal sign in gonadal dysgenesis. J Clin Endocrinol Metab 22:949, 1962

Kosowicz J: The deformity of the medial tibial condyle in nineteen cases of gonadal dysgenesis. J Bone Joint Surg 42A:600, 1960

Kosowicz J, Bialecki M, Wojtowicz M, Sobieszczyk S: Unilateral gonadal dysgenesis. Am J Obstet Gynecol 105:116, 1969

Lindsten J: The nature and origin of X chromosome aberrations in Turner's syndrome: A cytogenetical and clinical study of 57 patients. Stockholm, Almqvist and Wiksell, 1963

Lipsett MB: Decreased adrenal androgen biosynthesis in patients with gonadal dysgenesis. J Clin Endocrinol Metab 22:119, 1962

Lloyd CW, Lobotsky J, Segre EJ, Kobayashi T, Taymor ML, Batt RE: Plasma testosterone and urinary 17-ketosteroids in women with hirsutism and polycystic ovaries. J Clin Endocrinol Metab 26:314, 1966

Lloyd CW, Moses AM, Lobotsky J, Klaiber EL, Marshall LD, Jacobs RD: Studies of adrenocortical function of women with idiopathic hirsutism: Response to 25 units of ACTH. J Clin Endocrinol Metab 23:413, 1963

Lyon MF: Sex chromatin and gene action in the mammalian X-chromosome. Am J Hum Genet 14:135, 1962

Mahesh VB, Greenblatt RB, Aydar CK, Roy S, Puebla RA, Ellegood JO: Urinary steroid excretion patterns in hirsutism. I. Use of adrenal and ovarian suppression tests in the study of hirsutism. J Clin Endocrinol Metab 24:1283, 1964

Melicow MM, Uson AC: Dysgenetic gonadomas and other gonadal neoplasms in intersexes: Report of 5 cases and review of the literature. Cancer 12:552, 1959

Mellman WJ, Bongiovanni AM, Hope JW: The diagnostic usefulness of skeletal maturation in an endocrine clinic. Pediatrics 23:530, 1959

Mellman WJ, Klevit HD, Yakovac WC, Moorhead PS, Saksela E: XO/XY chromosome mosaicism. J Clin Endocrinol Metab 23:1090, 1963

Midgley AR, Jr: Radioimmunoassay: A method for human chorionic gonadotropin and human luteinizing hormone. Endocrinology 79:10, 1966

Midgley AR, Jr, Jaffe RB: Regulation of human gonadotropins. X. Episodic fluctuations of LH during the menstrual cycle. J Clin Endocrinol Metab 33:962, 1971

Miller OJ: The sex chromosome anomalies. Am J Obstet Gynecol 90:1078, 1964

Mittwoch U: Sex chromatin (review). J Med Genet 1:50, 1964

Noall MW, Kaufman RH: Estrogen synthesis by ovarian cortex and medulla from Stein-Leventhal patients. Fertil Steril 17:83, 1966

Polani PE: Turner's syndrome and allied conditions. Clinical features and chromosome abnormalities. Br Med Bull 17:200, 1961

Segre EJ, Klaiber EL, Lobotsky J, Lloyd OW: Hirsutism and virilizing syndromes. Annu Rev Med 15:315, 1964

Simmer H, Pion RJ, Dignam WJ: Testicular Feminization. Springfield, Charles C Thomas, 1965

Sohval AR: The syndrome of pure gonadal dysgenesis. Am J Med 38:615, 1965

Stein IF, Leventhal ML: Amenorrhoea associated with bilateral polycystic ovaries. Am J Obstet Gynecol 29:181, 1955

Teter J, Philip J, Wecewicz G, Potocki J: A masculinizing mixed germ cell tumour (gonocytoma III). Acta Endocrinol (Kbh) 46:1, 1964

Teter J, Tadowski R: Tumors of the gonads in cases of gonadal dysgenesis and male pseudohermaphroditism. Am J Obstet Gynecol 79:321, 1960

Turner HH: A syndrome of infantilism, congenital webbed neck and cubitus valgus. Endocrinology 23:566, 1938

Vague J, Nicolino J, Anselmi E: La déformation en enclume de l'extrémité supérieure du tibia l'agénésie gonadale. Ann Endocrinol (Paris) 22:40, 1961

Wilkins L, Fleischmann W: Ovarian agenesis: Pathology, associated clinical symptoms and the bearing on the theories of sex differentiation. J Clin Endocrinol Metab 4:357, 1944

Chapter 6

Bergada C, Cleveland WW, Jones HW, Wilkins L: Gonadal histology in patients with male pseudohermaphroditism and atypical gonadal dysgenesis: Relation to theories of sex differentiation. Acta Endocrinol (Kbh) 40:493, 1962

Boczkowski K, Teter J: Familial male pseudohermaphroditism. Acta Endocrinol (Kbh) 49:497, 1965

Bowen P, Lee CS, Migeon CJ, Kaplan NM, Whalley PJ, McKusick VA, Reifenstein EC: Hereditary male pseudohermaphroditism with hypogonadism, hypospadias and gynecomastia: Reifenstein's syndrome. Ann Intern Med 62:252, 1965

Chu EHY, Grumbach MM, Morishima A: Karyotypic analysis of a male pseudohermaphrodite with the syndrome of feminizing testes. J Clin Endocrinol Metab 20:1608, 1960

Goldberg MB, Maxwell AF: Male pseudohermaphroditism proved by surgical exploration and microscopic examination: A case report with speculations concerning pathogenesis. J Clin Endocrinol Metab 8:367, 1948

Goldberg MB, Scully AL: Gonadal malignancy in gonadal dysgenesis: Papillary pseudomucinous cystadenocarcinoma in a patient with Turner's syndrome. J Clin Endocrinol Metab 27:341, 1967

Grumbach MM, Ducharme JR: The effects of androgens on fetal sexual development: Androgen-induced female pseudohermaphroditism. Fertil Steril 11:157, 1960

Ferguson-Smith MA, Johnston AW, Weinberg AN: The chromosome complement in true hermaphroditism. Lancet 2:126, 1960

French FS, Baggett B, Van Wyk JJ, Talbert LM, Hubbard WR, Weaver RP, Forchielli E, Rao GS, Sarda IR: Testicular feminization: Clinical morphological and biochemical studies. J Clin Endocrinol Metab 25:661, 1965

Harnden DG, Armstrong CN: The chromosomes of a true hermaphrodite. Br Med J 2:1287, 1959

Hauser GA, Keller M, Koller T, Wenner R, Gloor F: "Testikulare Feminisierung" bei Erwachsenen. Schweiz Med Wochenschr 87:1573, 1957

Hayles AB, Nolan RB: Female pseudohermaphroditism: Report of a case in an infant born of a mother receiving methyltestosterone during pregnancy. Proc Staff Meeting Mayo Clin 32:41, 1957

Herrmann WL, Buckner F, Baskin A: Interstitial-cell tumor of the testis with gynecomastia. J Clin Endocrinol Metab 18:834, 1958

Jacobs PA, Baikie AG, Court-Brown WM, Forrest H, Roy JR, Stewart JSS, Lennox B: Chromosomal sex in the syndrome of testicular feminisation. Lancet 2:591, 1959

Johnson JE: Virilizing congenital adrenal hyperplasia: Twenty-five years later. Ann Intern Med 54:924, 1960

Jones HW, Scott WW: Hermaphroditism: Genital anomalies and related endocrine disorders. Baltimore, Williams and Wilkins, 1958

Lubs HA, Jr, Vilar O, Bergenstal DM: Familial male pseudohermaphroditism with labial testes and partial feminization: Endocrine studies and genetic aspects. J Clin Endocrinol Metab 19:1110, 1959

Melicow MM, Uson AC: Dysgenetic gonadomas and other gonadal neoplasms in intersexes: Report of 5 cases and review of the literature. Cancer 12:552, 1959

Money J, Hampson JG, Hampson JL: Hermaphroditism: Recommendations concerning assignment of sex, change of sex and psychologic management. Bull Johns Hopkins Hosp 97:284, 1955

Moore KL, Barr ML: Smear from the oral mucosa in detection of chromosomal sex. Lancet 2:57, 1955

Morris JM: The syndrome of testicular feminization in male pseudohermaphrodites. Am J Obstet Gynecol 65:1192, 1953

Morris JM, Mahesh VB: Further observations on the syndrome, "testicular feminization." Am J Obstet Gynecol 87:731, 1963

Overzier C (ed): Intersexuality. New York, Academic Press, 1963

Philip J, Trolle D: Familial male hermaphroditism with delayed and partial masculinization. Am J Obstet Gynecol 93:1076, 1965

Rosenberg HS, Clayton GW, Hsu TC: Familial true hermaphroditism. J Clin Endocrinol Metab 23:203, 1963

Simmer H, Pion RJ, Digman WJ: Testicular feminization. Springfield, Ill, Charles C. Thomas, 1965

Southren A, Ross H, Sharma DC, Gordon G, Weingold AB, Dorfman RI: Plasma concentration and biosynthesis of testosterone in the syndrome of feminizing testes. J Clin Endocrinol Metab 25:518, 1965

Teter J, Boczkowski K: Errors in management and assignment of sex in patients with abnormal sex differentiation. Am J Obstet Gynecol 93:1084, 1965

Wilkins L: Masculinization of the female fetus due to the use of orally given progestins. JAMA 172:1028, 1960

Wilkins L, Jones HW, Jr, Holman GH, Stempfel RS, Jr: Masculinization of the female fetus associated with administration of oral and intramuscular progestins during gestation: Non-adrenal female pseudohermaphroditism. J Clin Endocrinol Metab 18:559, 1958

Chapter 7

Albright F, Butler AM, Hampton AO, Smith P: Syndrome characterized by osteitis fibrosa disseminata, areas of pigmentation and endocrine dysfunction, with precocious puberty in females: Report of five cases. N Engl J Med 216:727, 1937

Benedict PH: Endocrine features in Albright's syndrome (fibrous dysplasia of bone). Metabolism 11:30, 1962

Bruk I, Dancaster CP, Jackson WPU: Granulosa-cell tumors causing precocious puberty: Oestrogen fractionations in two patients. Br Med J 2:26, 1960

Camin AJ, Dorfman RI, McDonald JH, Rosenthal IM: Interstitial cell tumor of the testis in a seven-year-old child. Am J Dis Child 100:389, 1960

Cook CD, Gross RE, Landing BH, Zygmuntowicz AS: Interstitial-cell tumor of the testis: Study of a 5-year-old boy with pseudo-precocious puberty. J Clin Endocrinol Metab 12:725, 1952

Eberlein WR, Bongiovanni AM, Jones IT, Yakovac WC: Ovarian tumors and cysts associated with sexual precocity. J Pediat 57:484, 1960

Hain AM: An unusual case of precocious puberty associated with ovarian dysgerminoma. J Clin Endocrinol Metab 9:1349, 1949

Hampson JG, Money J: Idiopathic sexual precocity in the female. Psychosom Med 17:16, 1955

Hoge RH: Precocious puberty in girls. Am J Obstet Gynecol 57:388, 1949

Jacobsen AW, Macklin MT: Hereditary sexual precocity: Report of a family with twenty-seven affected members. Pediatrics 9:682, 1952

Jolly H: Sexual precocity. Springfield, Ill, Charles C. Thomas, 1955

Jungck EC, Thrash AM, Ohlmacher AP, Knight AM, Jr, Dyrenforth LY: Sexual precocity due to interstitial-cell tumor of testis: Report of 2 cases. J Clin Endocrinol Metab 17:291, 1957

Kupperman HS, Epstein JA: Medroxyprogesterone acetate in the treatment of constitutional sexual precocity. J Clin Endocrinol Metab 22:456, 1962

Mason LW: Precocious puberty. J Pediat 34:730, 1949

McCullagh EP, Rosenberg HS, Norman N: Tumor of the tuber cinereum with precocious puberty: Case report with hormone assays. J Clin Endocrinol Metab 20:1286, 1960

McCune DJ, Bruch H: Osteodystrophia fibrosa: Report of a case in which the condition was combined with precocious puberty, pathologic pigmentation of the skin and hyperthyroidism, with a review of the literature. Am J Dis Child 54:806, 1937

Money J, Hampson JG: Idiopathic sexual precocity in the male. Psychosom Med 17:1, 1955

Morley TP: Hypothalamic tumor and precocious puberty. J Clin Endocrinol Metab 14:1, 1954

Novak E: The constitutional type of female precocious puberty: With a report of 9 cases. Am J Obstet Gynecol 47:20, 1944

Piotti A: Pubertas Praecox bei Tumor der Regio Hypothalamica und Neurofibromatose Recklinghausen. Acta Endocrinol [Suppl. 9] 10:66, 1952

Pomer FA, Stiles RE, Graham JH: Interstitial-cell tumors of testis in children: Report of a case and review of the literature. N Engl J Med 250:233, 1954

Reeves RL, Tesluk H, Harrison CE: Precocious puberty associated with hepatoma. J Clin Endocrinol Metab 19:1651, 1959

Reuben MS, Manning GR: Precocious puberty. Arch Pediatr 39:769, 1922; and 40:27, 1923

Richter RB: True hamartoma of the hypothalamus associated with pubertas praecox. J Neuropathol Exp Neurol 10:368, 1951

Seckel HPG: Precocious sexual development in children. Med Clin North Am 30:183, 1946

Seckel HPG, Scott WW, Benditt EP: Six examples of precocious sexual development. I. Studies in diagnosis and pathogenesis. Am J Dis Child 78:484, 1949

Sobel EH, Sniffen RC, Talbot N: The testis. V. Use of testicular biopsies in the differential diagnosis of precocious puberty. Pediatrics 8:701, 1951

Thamdrup E: Precocious sexual development: A clinical study of 100 children. Springield, Charles C Thomas, 1961

Walker SH: Constitutional true sexual precocity. J Pediatr 41:251, 1952

Weinberger LM, Grant FC: Precocious puberty and tumors of the hypothalamus: Report of a case and review of the literature with a pathophysiologic explanation of the precocious sexual syndrome. Arch Intern Med 67:762, 1941

Chapter 8

Albright F: A page out of the history of hyperparathyroidism. J Clin Endocrinol Metab 8:637, 1948

Albright F, Burnett CH, Smith PH, Parson W: Pseudohypoparathyroidism: Example of "Sebright-Bantam Syndrome"; Report of 3 cases. Endocrinology 30:922, 1942

Albright F, Reifenstein EC, Jr: The parathyroid glands and metabolic bone disease. Baltimore, Williams and Wilkins, 1948

Aurbach GD, Potts JT, Jr: Radioimmunoassay of parathyroid hormone. Arch Intern Med 124:413, 1969

Avioli LV: The diagnosis of primary hyperparathyroidism. Med Clin North Am 52:451, 1968

Becker KL, Purnell DC, Jones JD: Tubular reabsorption of phosphate in primary hyperparathyroidism — before and after administration of parathyroid hormone. J Clin Endocrinol Metab 24:347, 1964

Chase LR, Melson GL, Aurbach GD: Pseudohypoparathyroidism: Defective excretion of 3′, 5′-AMP in response to parathyroid hormone. J Clin Invest 48:1832, 1969

Conner TB, Hopkins TR, Thomas WC, Jr, Carey RA, Howard JE: The use of cortisone and ACTH in hypercalcemic states. J Clin Endocrinol Metab 16:949, 1956

Davis RH, Fourman P, Smith JWG: Prevalence of parathyroid insufficiency after thyroidectomy. Lancet 2:1432, 1961

Dent CE: Some problems of hyperparathyroidism. Br Med J 2:1419, 1962

Dent CE: Cortisone test for hyperparathyroidism. Br Med J 1:230, 1956

Dent CE: Rickets and osteomalacia from renal tubule defects. J Bone Joint Surg 34B:266, 1952

Fonseca OA, Calverley JR: Neurological manifestations of hypoparathyroidism. Arch Intern Med 120:202, 1967

Gaillard PJ, Talmage RV, Budy AM (eds): The Parathyroid Glands. Chicago, University of Chicago Press, 1965

Goldsmith RS: Hyperparathyroidism. N Engl J Med 281:67, 1969

Greep RO, Talmage RV (eds): The Parathyroids. Springfield, Ill, Charles C Thomas, 1961

Hawker CD, Glass J, Rasmussen H: Further studies on the isolation and characterization of parathyroid polypeptides. Biochemistry 5:344, 1966

Hodges M, Waterhouse C: Hypercalcemia of hyperparathyroidism responsive to prednisone. Arch Intern Med 120:75, 1967

Leifer E, Hollander W: Idiopathic hypoparathyroidism and chronic adrenal insufficiency. J Clin Endocrinol Metab 13:1264, 1953

Lloyd HM, Rose GA: Ionized, protein-bound, and complexed calcium in the plasma in primary hyperparathyroidism. Lancet 2:1258, 1958

Massey JG, Coburn JW, Popovtzer MM, Shinaberger JH, Maxwell MH, Kleeman CR: Secondary hyperparathyroidism in chronic renal failure. Arch Intern Med 124:431, 1969

Miles J, Elrick H: Pseudo-pseudohypoparathyroidism. J Clin Endocrinol Metab 15:576, 1955

Potts JT, Jr, Aurbach GD, Sherwood LM: Parathyroid hormone: Chemical properties and structural requirements for biological and immunological activity. Recent Prog Horm Res 22:101, 1966

Potts JT, Jr, Aurbach GD, Sherwood LM, Sandoval A: Structural basis of biological and immunological activity of parathyroid hormone. Proc Nat Acad Sci 54:743, 1965

Pugh DG: Subperiosteal resorption of bone: A roentgenologic manifestation of primary hyperparathyroidism and renal osteodystrophy. Am J Roentgenol 66:577, 1951

Raddick FA: Primary hyperparathyroidism. Med Clin North Am 51:871, 1967

Rasmussen H, De Luca A, Arnaud C, Hawker D, von Stedingk M: The relationship between witamin D and parathyroid hormone. J Clin Invest 42:1940, 1963

Reiss E: Primary hyperparathyroidism: A simple approach to diagnosis. Med Clin North Am 54:183, 1970

Reiss E, Canterbury JM: Primary hyperparathyroidism: Application of radioimmunoassay to differentiation of adenoma and hyperplasia and to preoperative localization of hyperfunctioning parathyroid glands. N Engl J Med 280:1381, 1969

Stanbury SW, Lumb GA: Parathyroid function in chronic renal failure. Q J Med 35:1, 1966

Sutphin A, Albright F, McCune DJ: Five cases (3 in siblings) of idiopathic hypoparathyroidism associated with moniliasis. J Clin Endocrinol Metab 3:625, 1943

Walsh FB, Howard JE: Conjunctival and corneal lesions in hypercalcemia. J Clin Endocrinol Metab 7:644, 1947

Chapter 9

Boley SJ, Lin J, Schiffmann A: Functioning pancreatic adenomas in infants and children. Surgery 48:592, 1960

Boshell BR, Kirschenfeld JJ, Soteres PS: Extrapancreatic insulin-secreting tumor. N Engl J Med 270:338, 1964

Fajans SS, Schneider, JM, Schteingart DE, Conn JW: The diagnostic value of sodium tolbutamine in hypoglycemic states. J Clin Endocrinol Metab 21:371, 1961

Floyd JC, Jr, Fajans SS, Knopf RF, Conn JW: Plasma insulin in organic hyperinsulinism: Comparative effects of tolbutamide, leucine and glucose. J Clin Endocrinol Metab 24:747, 1964

Howard JM, Moss NH, Rhoads JE: Hyperinsulinism and islet-cell tumors of the pancreas: With 398 recorded tumors. Int Surg [Abst] 90:417, 1950

Marshall FS: Islet-cell tumors of the pancreas producing hypoglycemia. Surg Clin North Am 38:775, 1958

McGavran MH, Unger RH, Recant L, Polk HC, Kilo CH, Levin ME: Glucagonoma: The identification of a glucagon-secreting-α-cell carcinoma of the pancreas. N Engl J Med 274:1408, 1966

McQuarrie I: Idiopathic spontaneously occurring hypoglycemia in infants. Am J Dis Child 87:399, 1954

Underdahl LC, Woolner LB, Black BM: Multiple endocrine adenomas: Report of eight cases in which the parathyroids, pituitary and pancreatic islets were involved. J Clin Endocrinol Metab 13:30, 1953

Chapter 10

Albright F, Butler AM, Bloomberg E: Rickets resistant to vitamin D therapy. Am J Dis Child 54:529, 1937

Benda CE: Mongolism and Cretinism. New York, Grune and Stratton, 1946

Brante G: Gargoylism — a mucopolysaccharidosis. Scand J Clin Lab Invest 4:43, 1952

Carter CO, Hamerton JL, Polani PE, Gunlap A, Weller SDV: Chromosome translocation as a cause of familial mongolism. Lancet 2:678, 1960

Cremin BJ, Beighton P: Dwarfism in the newborn: The nomenclature, radiological features and genetic significance. Br J Radio 47:77, 1974

Dent CE: Rickets and osteomalacia from renal tubular defects. J Bone Joint Surg 34B:266, 1952

De Toni G: Renal rickets with phospho-gluco-amino renal diabetes (De Toni-Debré Fanconi syndrome). Ann. Paediatr 187:42, 1956

Fanconi G: Tubular insufficiency and renal dwarfism. Arch Dis Child 29:1, 1954

Flosi AZ, Assis LM, Coelho-Neto AS, Bloise W, Ulhôa-Cintra AB, Barros RP: Hormonal treatment of Hand-Schüller-Christian disease: Report on a case with disappearance of the bone lesions. J Clin Endocrinol Metab 19:239, 1959

Follis RH, Jr: Renal rickets and osteitis fibrosa in children and adolescents. Bull Johns Hopkins Hosp 87:593, 1950

Jenkinson EL, Kinzer RE: Achondroplasia foetalis (chondrodystrophia foetalis). Radiology 37:581, 1941

Kozlowski K, Zychowicz C: Hypochondroplasie. Fortschr Geb Roentgenstr Nuklearmed 100:529, 1964

LeJeune J: The 21-trisomy — current state of chromosomal research. Steinberg AG, Beam A (eds). Vol 3. Prog Med Genet, 1963

LeJeune J: Le mongolisme, trisomie degressive. Ann Genet (Paris) 2:1, 1960

Lindsay S, Reilly WA, Gotham TJ, Skahen R: Gargoylism. II. Study of pathologic lesions and clinical review of twelve cases. Am J Dis Child 76:239, 1948

McKusick VA: Hereditable disorders of connective tissue. III. The Marfan syndrome. J Chronic Dis 2:609, 1955

McKusick VA: Hereditable Disorders of Connective Tissue, 2nd Ed. St Louis, CV Mosby, 1960

McKusick VA et al.: The genetic mucopolysaccharidoses. Medicine 44:45, 1965

Rados A: Marfan's syndrome (arachnodactyly coupled with dislocation of lens). Arch Ophthalmol 27:477, 1942

Reilly WA, Lindsay S: Gargoylism (lipochondrodystrophy). I. A review of clinical observations in eighteen cases. Am J Dis Child 75:595, 1948

Rosenbloom AL, Smith DW: Natural history of metaphyseal dysostosis. J Pediatr 66:857, 1965

GENERAL REFERENCES

Jones HW, Jr, Scott WW: Hermaphroditism: Genital Anomalies and Related Endocrine Disorders. Baltimore, Williams and Wilkins, 1958

Lisser H, Escamilla RF: Atlas of Clinical Endocrinology. St. Louis, Mosby, 1962

Wilkins L, Blizzard RM, Migeon CJ: The Diagnosis and Treatment of Endocrine Disorders in Childhood and Adolescence. 3rd Ed. Springfield, Ill, Charles C Thomas, 1965

Williams RH (ed): Textbook of Endocrinology. 5th Ed. Philadelphia, WB Saunders, 1974

Jerzy Kosowicz, M.D., obtained his degree in medicine from the University of Poznań and started clinical work at the Department of Internal Diseases. His main interest has always been in endocrine disorders and all associated diagnostic procedures. His early studies and publications were on electrocardiograms in hypopituitarism (Am Heart J 65:17, 1963), taste hypersensitivity in primary and secondary adrenal insufficiency (J Clin Endocrinol Metab 27:214, 1967) and observations on variants of gonadal dysgenesis (Am J Obstet Gynecol 105:1116, 1969). He obtained his M.D. degree for a thesis on *Pituitary dwarfism: Diagnosis and therapy*. Later, his interest focused on roentgen manifestations of endocrine diseases, and he published several original papers, the best known of which are the descriptions of deformity of the medial condyle of the tibia in Turner's syndrome (J Bone Joint Surg 42A:600, 1960), the carpal sign in gonadal dysgenesis (J Clin Endocrinol Metab 22:949, 1962), abnormal basal angle (Acta Radiol 17:669, 1976) and skull abnormalities in sex chromosome aberrations (Clin Radiol 26:371, 379, 1975). Some of these roentgenographic findings, first described by Dr. Kosowicz, were reproduced in several books on radiology, endocrinology and bone surgery.

He spent some time in research in the Department of Pathology, Liverpool University, under Professor H.L. Sheehan; in the Institute of Child Health in Birmingham; and later was engaged in radioimmunoassay in the Endocrine Unit of Hammersmith Hospital, London, under Professor T. Russell Fraser. On his return to Poland he has been involved in the development and application of radioimmunoassay for protein, steroid and thyroid hormones. He opened the radioimmunoassay laboratory in the Department of Endocrinology, School of Medicine in Poznań, where he introduced the radioimmunoassay of numerous hormones and trained the staff of the Department, as well as visiting scientists from various Polish universities in these procedures. He has organized radioimmunoassay courses on a national scale and was a member and chief lecturer at the Interregional Training Course of the International Atomic Energy Agency, held in the Department of Endocrinology, Poznań, in June 1975. In 1976 Dr. Kosowicz, as an expert of the International Atomic Energy Agency, was sent on a mission to Ecuador to expand the radioimmunoassay laboratories in Quito. Dr. Kosowicz is a member of the Royal Society of Medicine (London), chairman of the Clinical Section, Polish Society of Endocrinology, member of the Committee for Endocrinology of the Polish Academy of Sciences, and other scientific committees, and chairman of the working group in endocrinology of the Poznań School of Medicine.

Dr. Kosowicz was appointed Associate Professor in Endocrinology in 1970 and is at present Head of the Radioimmunoassay Laboratory in the Department of Endocrinology, School of Medicine in Poznań.